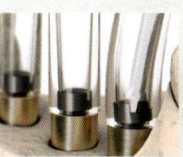
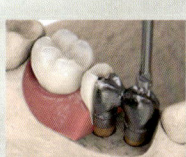
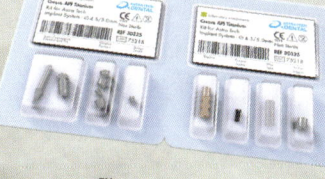
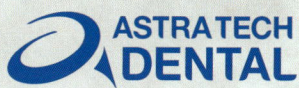
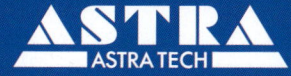
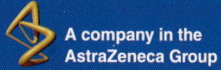

EDITORIAL

THIS IS WHO WE ARE

Writing an editorial commemorating an anniversary is a tough task. By the time the list of acknowledgments and accolades, self-serving words and patting on the back, meaningless and boring reflections, and an agonizing grocery list of landmarks in time are completed, the reader is likely to be dozing off or moving on to less formal and more entertaining activities. It is the ceremonial and somewhat pompous nature of such editorials that make them such a turn-off.

So how can one discuss such an important event from a slightly different angle? Well, first try to understand the major reason for the QDT's longevity. After all, it is a busy market filled with multiple excellent scientific publications and numerous free pseudoscientific advertisement-based publications. The main reason for the QDT's long-lasting success is our readers, to be sure. Without a readership that has a profound interest and passion for true clinical and technical excellence, the QDT would not survive.

Pure scientific data are of paramount importance, but the profession needs a venue that emphasizes clinical and technical excellence, demonstrating how to execute clinical and technical procedures in depth, and in an uncompromised manner. While scientific publications provide the core around which the profession is forged, clinical reports also play a unique role. Those who tend to look down at clinical and technical publications are usually those who could not prepare a tooth or fabricate a restoration if their life were dependent on it. While clinical publications do not constitute science, they do constitute a state of mind that strives for and appreciates true excellence. On this forefront of clinical and technical excellence, QDT really shines.

Although we have received many compliments over the years, I have also heard that it is not right to focus only on the very high end, presenting outcomes that are literally unattainable in daily practice. One year I read a review of the book that was very positive in nature but also stated that such beautiful photos must have been manipulated by computer imaging. This is far from being the case; raising the bar gives everyone a goal to which they can aspire, a motivating target that keeps them pushing forward and improving. Eventually, this standard of excellence raises the clinical standard of care.

So what's next? As always, the previous generation expresses sincere concern when their time has come to pass the torch to the younger generation. You always hear that the younger generation does not show the same level of commitment and dedication that their predecessors have demonstrated. This notion, faulty across the boundaries of all professions, can easily be proven wrong by the QDT. The addition of young readers and authors is what is keeping QDT young and fresh, and it is a sure sign that the torch will continue to pass with ease.

At 30 it's just getting started.

Avishai Sadan, DMD
Editor-in-Chief
Avishai.Sadan@Case.edu

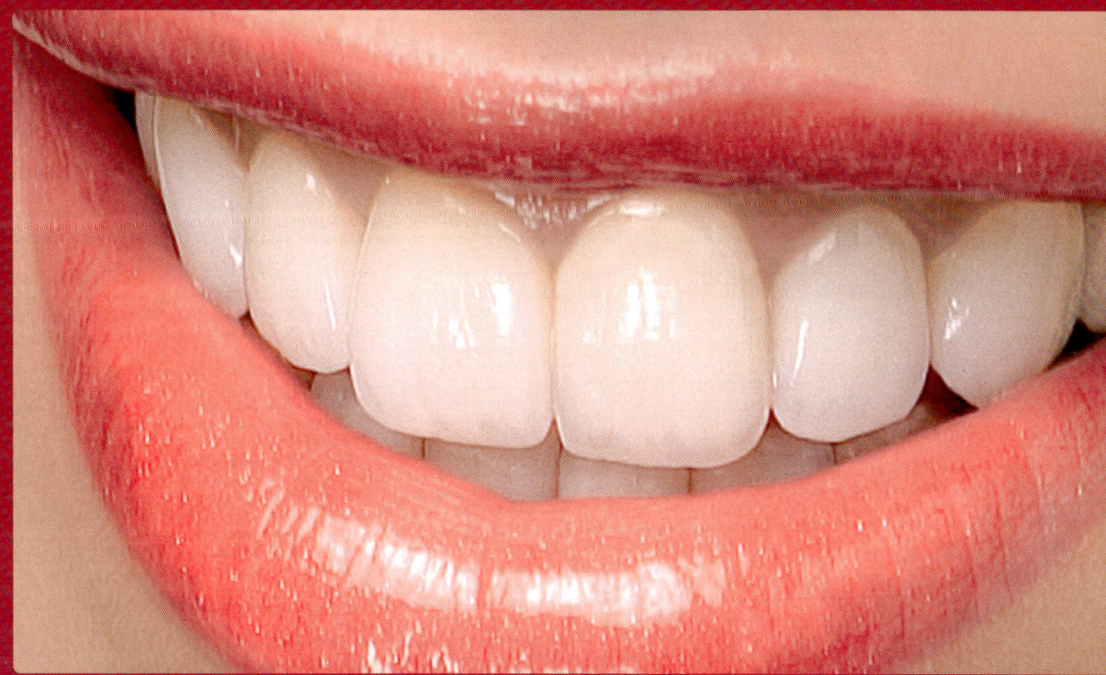
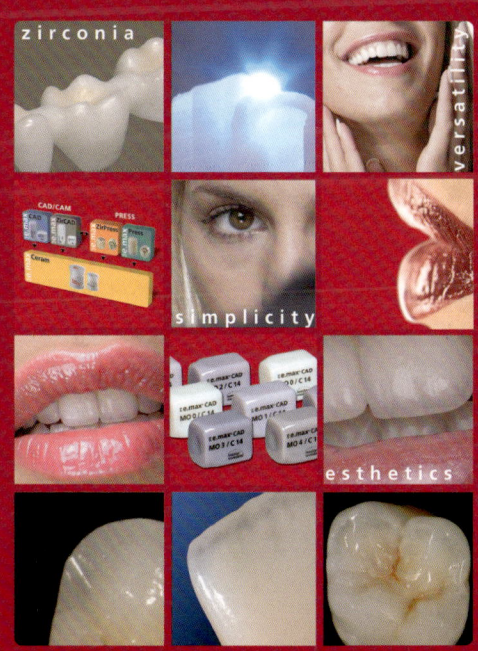
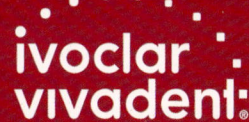

QDT 2007

QUINTESSENCE OF DENTAL TECHNOLOGY

Cover photograph by Naoki Aiba.
For additional information, see page 118.

PUBLISHER
H.W. Haase

ASSOCIATE PUBLISHER
Tomoko Tsuchiya

JOURNAL DIRECTOR
Lori A. Bateman

MANUSCRIPT EDITOR
Jacob Wolff

PRODUCTION EDITOR
Patrick Penney

PRODUCTION MANAGER
Susan Robinson

ADVERTISING SALES
William G. Hartman

**ADVERTISING/EDITORIAL/
SUBSCRIPTION OFFICE**
Quintessence Publishing Co, Inc
4350 Chandler Drive
Hanover Park, Illinois 60133
Phone: (630) 736-3600
Toll-free: (800) 621-0387
Fax: (630) 736-3633
E-mail: service@quintbook.com
Website: http://www.quintpub.com

QDT is published once a year by
Quintessence Publishing Co, Inc,
4350 Chandler Drive, Hanover Park,
Illinois, 60133. Price per copy: $80.

MANUSCRIPT SUBMISSION
QDT publishes original articles covering
dental laboratory techniques and methods.
See Guidelines for Authors at www.quint-
pub.com for submission information.

Printed in Canada
ISSN 0896-6532 / ISBN 978-0-86715-472-6

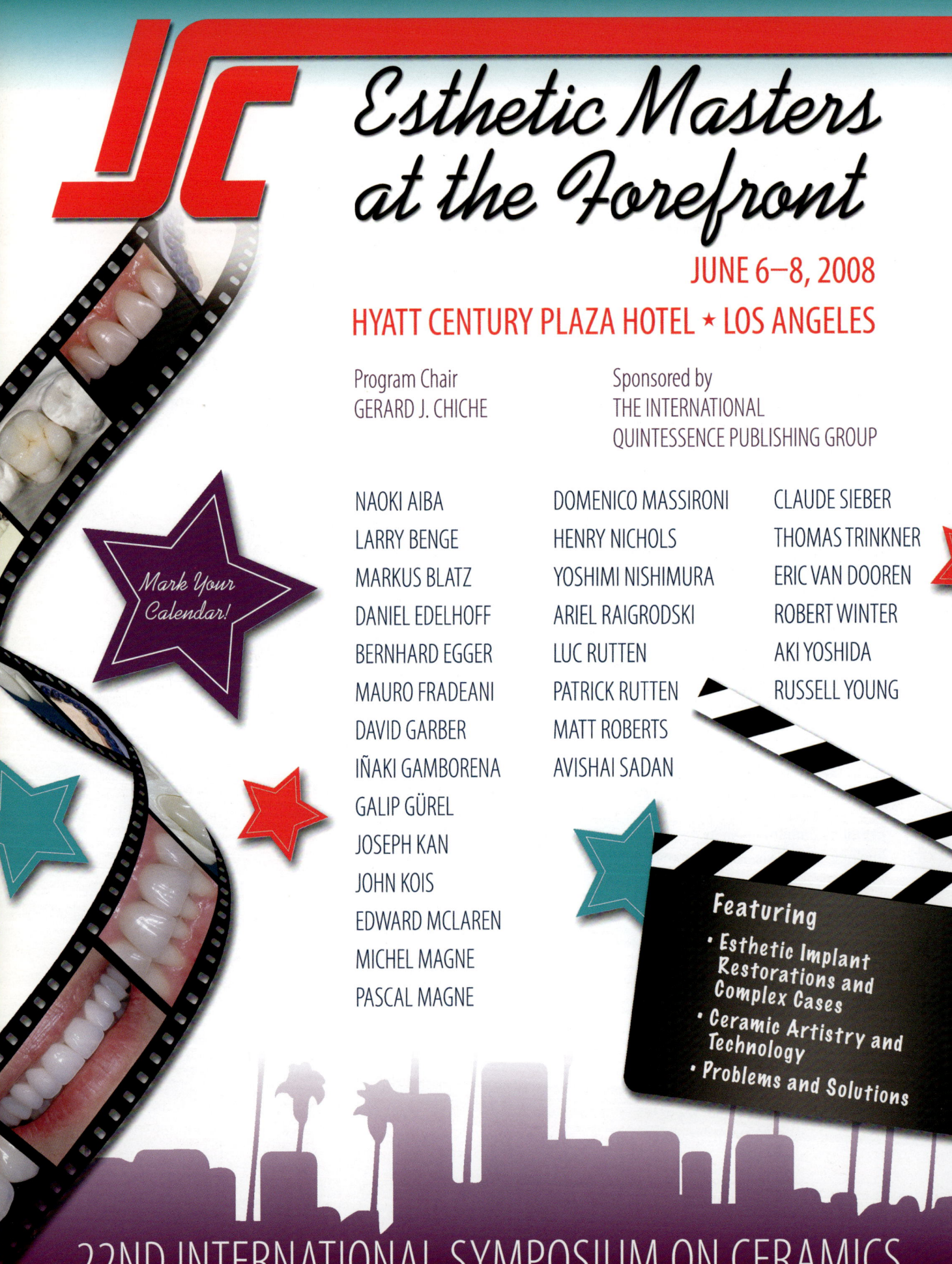

OPALESCENCE:
THE KEY TO NATURAL ESTHETICS

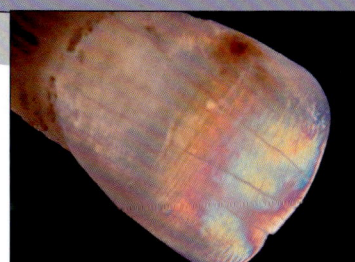

Sillas Duarte, Jr, DDS, MS, PhD[1]

Enamel and dentin have sophisticated optical characteristics.[1,2] Creating esthetic restorations for a missing part of the tooth is an exciting challenge, because the restorative material used must interact with the rest of the mouth. Since restorative materials are monochromatic, a combination of materials with different translucencies and optical properties is fundamental to achieve a natural appearance for the restoration. The characteristics of translucency, opacity, opalescence, and fluorescence must be taken into consideration to exactly reproduce the contiguous tissues.[3–6] In particular, opalescence is vital for repairing fractured incisal edges. Recent studies revealed that some resin composites and ceramics are able to replicate this interesting optical behavior.[7–9] To better comprehend this phenomenon, a comparison of enamel and resin composite structures will be discussed.

[1]Associate Professor, Department of Comprehensive Care, Case Western Reserve University School of Dental Medicine, Cleveland, Ohio, USA.

Correspondence to: Dr Sillas Duarte, Jr, Department of Comprehensive Care, Case Western Reserve University School of Dental Medicine, 10900 Euclid Avenue, Cleveland, OH 44106-4905, USA. E-mail: Sillas.Duarte@case.edu

ENAMEL BIOMINERALIZATION

Enamel is a tissue consisting of mineral and organic phases.[10] During enamel biomineralization, extracellular matrix proteins control the formation of the inorganic component of hard tissues.[11] The structural proteins of the enamel matrix, such as amelogenin, ameloblastin, enamelin, and amelotin, have specific protein-protein interactions to produce a matrix capable of directing the highly ordered structure of the enamel crystallites.[12] Among the proteins, amelogenin regulates the form and size of the hydroxyapatite crystallites.[12] The amelogenin nanospheres allow the crystallite to grow in the preferred orientations; however, ameloblastin may inhibit crystallite growth.[13] Further, lateral branches may grow out of the crystals, and crystal fusing often occurs, thus causing the crystallites to assume pyramidal shapes with their wide bases pointing toward the dentinoenamel junction (DEJ).[14]

Individual crystallites, approximately 100 nm in diameter, agglomerate in bundles that constitute the enamel rods.[14,15] The crystallite organization within the rods is evident.[13] The hydroxyapatite crystallites that are not part of a prism are named interprismatic or interrod. The interrod crystallites surround the prisms at an angle of approximately 60 degrees to their long axis, producing a "honeycomb" appearance.[13]

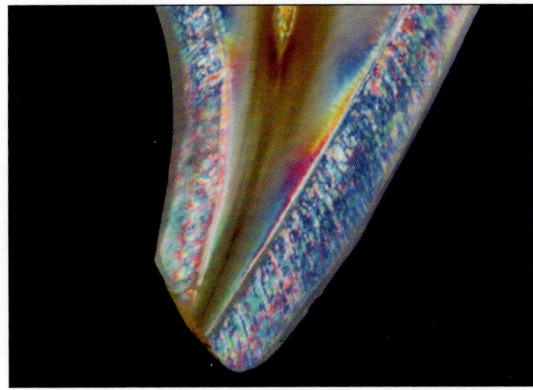

Fig 1 The complex optical behavior of human enamel under polarized light. Note the light contrast in different areas of the tooth.

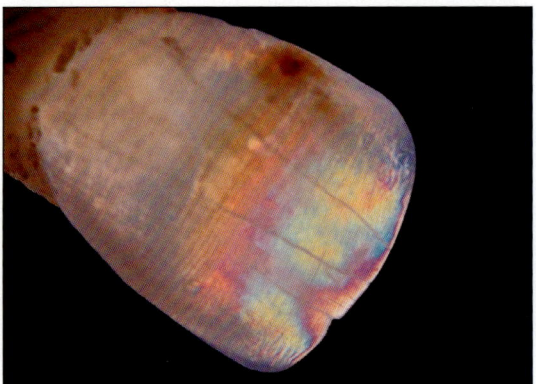

Fig 2 Iridescence of human enamel.

The rods decussate in layers, also called bands. Although each set of layers bifurcates in only one direction, transitional zones may occur between the bands.[16] The spatial arrangement of the layers is related to the DEJ and can be described in two parameters using a tangential view[16]: inclination and orientation. A set of 10 or more layers of enamel rods composes the Hunter-Schreger bands.[10,13]

The highly mineralized prisms function similarly to fiber optics. The light entering the prism is reflected from the surrounding prism sheath and remains within the prism.[16] The set of enamel rods in the Hunter-Schreger bands that intersect at different angles may clinically display light and dark bands on the enamel surface in reflected light.[17] However, the light and dark bands switch under transmitted light.

OPTICAL CHARACTERISTICS OF ENAMEL

Human enamel is translucent, and its translucency is determined by the total transmittance of wavelengths, which ranges from 400 to 700 nm.[18] When a white light reaches the enamel, different wavelengths of light may be absorbed, reflected, or transmitted through its structures.[9] The higher the wavelength, the more translucent the enamel.[18] Because enamel covers dentin in varying thicknesses, different optical behavior must be expected in different regions of the tooth (Fig 1). In particular, the greatest thickness of enamel in the human tooth is found at the incisal third. Transmitted light is clearly observed in this region. The path of incident light is altered by the difference in the speed of light between air and the enamel. The extent of this difference depends on the thickness and refractive index of the enamel, the angle at which the light strikes the enamel surface, and the wavelength of the light.[19] Furthermore, enamel is three-dimensionally organized in layers of prisms,[20] so multilayer interference also occurs.[21] The transmitted light travels through the prism until it meets the prism substructure surface, where again some light is reflected. This light reflected from the prism's substructure surface travels back and rejoins the light reflected from the top surface. The hydroxyapatite crystallites not only contribute significantly to scattering, but are also responsible for the backscattering.[22] For this reason, enamel may also display some iridescence (Fig 2).[23] *Iridescence* is defined as the change in color or luminosity with angle of observation or illumination.[24] This phenomenon is a manifestation of *coherent scattering*, which is the differential scattering of light wavelengths from multiple objects.[24,25] Coherent scattering is determined by phase interactions among scattered light waves.[25]

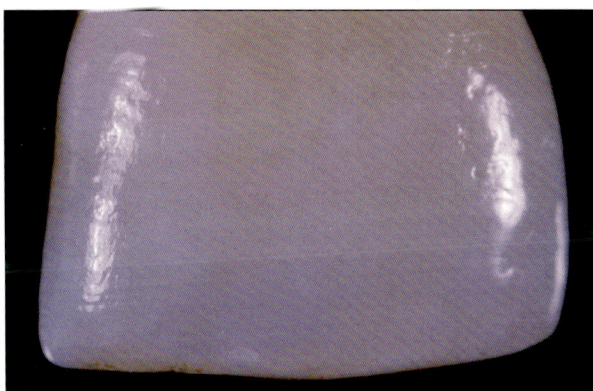

Fig 3a Under reflected light, the tooth displays a bluish appearance.

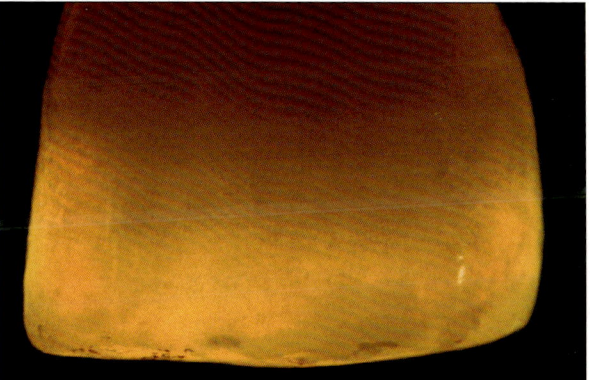

Fig 3b Under transmitted light, the tooth shows opalescence.

OPALESCENCE

Incoherent scattering is produced by particles the size of visible light or smaller.[24] As individual crystallites are 100 nm in diameter,[13] short wavelength hues, such as blue or violet, are produced. Thus, under reflected light, the area between the dentin and the incisal border assumes a bluish appearance (Fig 3a). However, the same area under transmitted light displays an orange-reddish hue (Fig 3b), because the white light transmitted through the enamel disperses the shortest wavelengths.[9,26] Thus, the orange-reddish hue results from the passage of longer wavelengths through the enamel.[6] This occurrence is called *opalescence*.

Opalescence is an optical property.[7] The name is derived from opal, which is renowned for its colors. It has been demonstrated using scanning electron microscopy (SEM) that opalescence is caused by diffraction from a regular three-dimensional structure arising from regular and uniform spherical particles of silica separated by uniform tetrahedral or octahedral voids.[27] Since enamel has a highly organized three-dimensional structure, with different refractive indices of proteinaceous matrix and crystallites, opalescence should be expected.

Restorative materials must have properties of light reflection similar to the natural tooth (Fig 4a). Resin composites are composed of a resin matrix and inorganic fillers, which have different refractive indices.[7] However, opalescence is influenced by the resin composite and shade.[4,7] The organic matrix should serve as an empty space to facilitate the transmission of light scattered by the fillers.[28] The fillers affect the light scattering depending on their size, shape, and number.[29] However, to optimize the light scattering, the particle size should be larger than the wavelength of the incident light.[9] For instance, to maximize opalescence, some fillers with blue-range wavelengths must be dispersed into the material. To improve opalescence, a given material must have: *(1)* one or more internal phases, *(2)* small internal phases of 380 to 500 nm dispersed in the material, *(3)* a large difference in refractive index between the matrix and internal phase, and *(4)* a high dispersion of one or all of the internal phases.[9] Recently developed resin composites have filler sizes ranging from 20 to 800 nm. These fillers, when agglomerated in clusters, may contribute to opalescence (Fig 4b).[7] The amount of pigments and opacifying agents influences the translucency and opalescence of a resin composite.[7,30] Within a single resin composite brand, opalescence may drastically vary from one translucent shade to another. Highly translucent resin composites tend to have more opalescence than shaded resin composites.[7]

It is possible to recreate the bluish appearance of the incisal translucent layer by using tints. A shade guide (Creative Color System, Ducera, Rosbach, Germany) facilitates the identification of tooth characteristics.[31] Interestingly, this shade guide has four different saturations for an incisal blue hue. To ensure

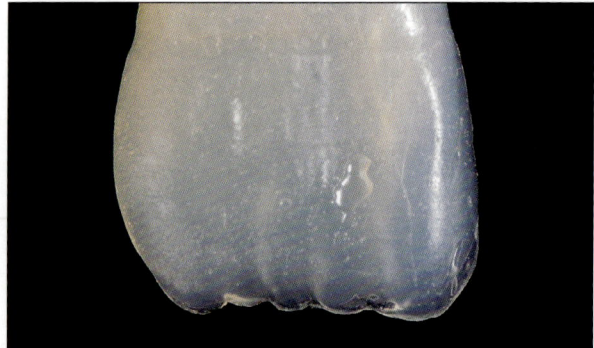

Fig 4a Under reflected light and with a black background, a highly translucent resin composite shows similar behavior to the natural tooth.

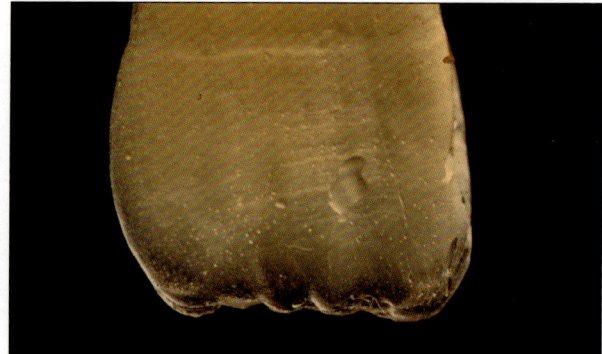

Fig 4b Under transmitted light, a highly translucent resin composite is comparable to the natural tooth.

the correct bluish hue, it is recommended to use a combination of blue, gray, and untinted tints.[28] The percentage of these tints may vary according to the incisal translucency, and the blending effect should be tested prior to fabrication of the restoration. Nevertheless, if intensive colorants were used as a substitute for highly translucent resin composites to reproduce incisal translucency, opalescence should not be expected once the tints have some degree of opacity. Therefore, tints must be used carefully in conjunction with opalescent resin composites to restore the correct hue of an unusual incisal translucency.

INCISAL OPALESCENT LAYER PATTERNS

It is possible to recognize patterns in the opalescent layers in natural teeth.[26,32] Opalescent layer distribution varies not only from individual to individual, but from tooth to tooth. To better understand this concept, a scientific investigation was carried out to recognize and classify patterns of opalescence in human teeth. Junior graduate students (≥ 20 years of age) at the Araraquara School of Dentistry, São Paulo State University, São Paulo, Brazil, volunteered and were selected for this study. The patients' maxillary central (n = 50) and lateral (n = 50) incisors were selected based on the following criteria: (1) healthy marginal tissue, with no evidence of gingival alteration; (2) presence of all anterior teeth; (3) no history of periodontal surgery or orthodontics; (4) no notice-

able incisal wear (80% width/length ratio); and (5) no anterior restorations. Standardized closeup slide photographs (2:1 magnification) were taken of the selected incisors in occlusion and against a black background. The incisal opalescent layer of each incisor was clinically inspected under fiber-optic transillumination and recorded in a drawing.

Additionally, the incisal opalescent/translucent layers of extracted central and lateral incisors were examined (n = 20). The teeth were sectioned through the center with a water-cooled low-speed diamond disk (Isomet 1000, Buehler, Lake Bluff, IL, USA) to a 1.0-mm-wide slab. The specimens were analyzed under a stereomicroscope equipped with a transmitted light base (TLSM) (Carl Zeiss, Oberkochen, Germany).

The obtained data were used to classify the incisal opalescence according to the incidence of the opalescent layers in four categories: type I, mamelons; type II, straight; type III, diffused; and type IV, mixed (Table 1).

Type I featured an incisal translucent and opalescent layer that penetrated the mamelons (Fig 5a). Most patients displayed this category of opalescent layer (53%). It was found that the opalescent layer was either continuous or intermittent, but either way had an intimate relationship with the mamelons. The mamelons' contour was found to be well defined under microscopic evaluation and transillumination (Fig 5b). However, in reflected light, the crest of the mamelons occasionally appeared to feather with the opalescent layer or incisal halo (Fig 5a).

Table 1 Frequency of Different Incisal Opalescent Layer Patterns in Maxillary Incisors

Type	Frequency	Percent	Valid Percent	Cumulative Percent
I	53	53.0	53.5	53.3
II	17	17.2	17.2	70.7
III	4	4.0	4.0	74.7
IV	25	25.3	25.3	100.0
Total	99	99.0	100.0	
Missing	1	1.0		
Total	100	100.0		

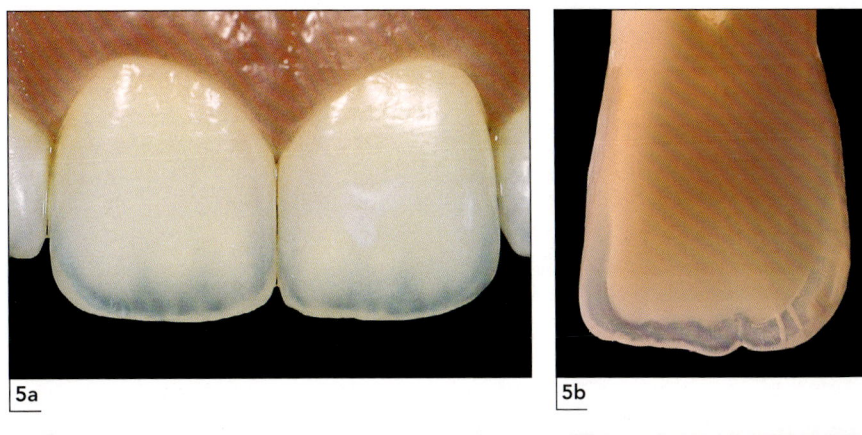

Figs 5a and 5b Type I opalescent layers infiltrate the mamelons.

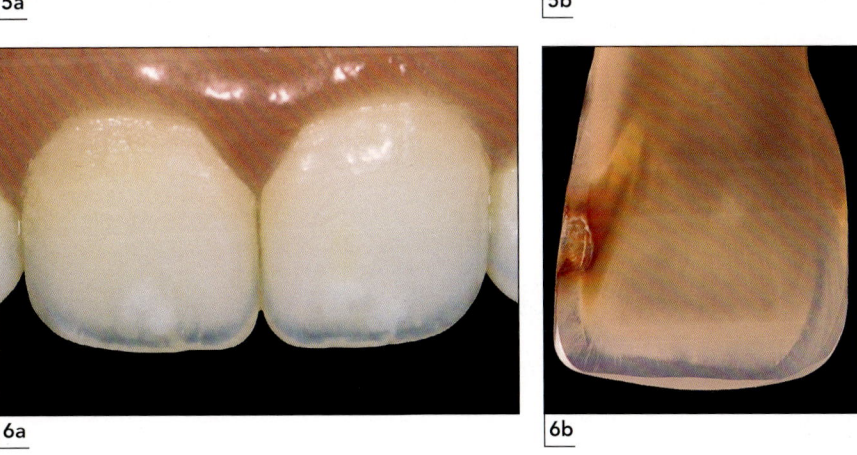

Figs 6a and 6b Type II opalescent layers do not penetrate the mamelons; rather, they maintain a straight line parallel to the incisal border.

On the other hand, some patients (17%) exhibited an opalescent layer that did not penetrate the mamelons, instead maintaining a straight line parallel to the incisal border (Fig 6a). This group of incisal opalescent layers was named type II. In type II patterns, the mamelons appeared to fade away, especially when observed under TLSM (Fig 6b).

Identifying the precise location of the incisal opalescent layer was quite complex for the next group. The opalescent layer was randomly distributed at the entire incisal third (Fig 7a). This small group of patients (4%) with a diffused opalescent layer was classified as type III. SEM observations revealed small but distinct translucent/opalescent regions at the incisal proximal area (Fig 7b), which could also be clinically observed.

Type IV was a mixed opalescent layer plus pigmentation (Fig 8a), and was observed in a large group of patients (25%). The patterns of incisal opalescence varied according to the types de-

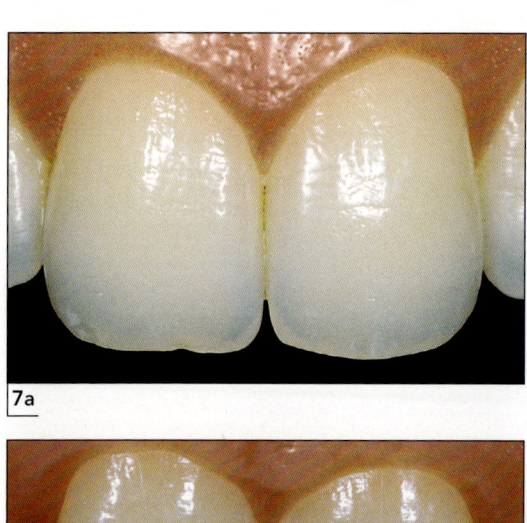

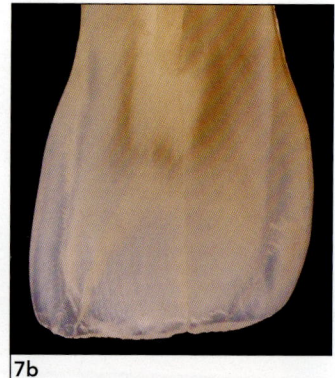

Figs 7a and 7b Type III opalescent layers are randomly distributed at the entire incisal third. However, a more distinct area may be seen at the proximal-incisal angles.

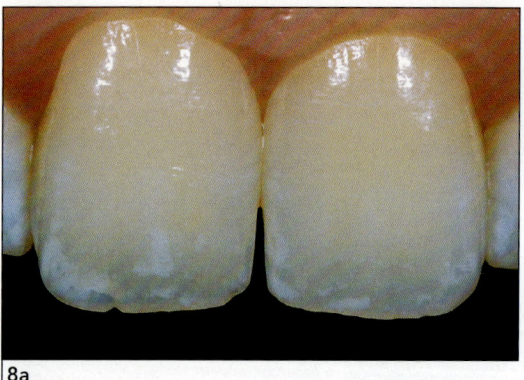

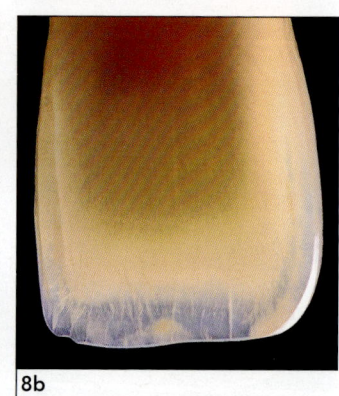

Figs 8a and 8b Type IV opalescent layers are mixed, with some degree of white or amber pigmentation.

scribed earlier; however, type IV was always associated with some degree of pigmentation. White spots, white cloudy pigmentation, or amber staining were recorded both clinically and under microscopy (Fig 8b).

COUNTER-OPALESCENCE

When analyzing photographs of the selected teeth in occlusion (Fig 9a), the incisal translucent layer was barely visible compared to the photographs set against a black background (Fig 9b). The bluish appearance was nearly gone, except for at the mesioincisal and distoincisal line angles.

It has been established that the background affects the opalescence of a given object.[1,3,4,7,9,26,33] Highly opalescent structures help mask the background color, and this appears to be related to the translucency parameter.[7] The incident light reflects onto a white background and again is transmitted through the enamel.[34] Because the antagonist tooth has the same optical properties of the studied tooth,

a complex light distribution should be expected (Fig 10). The more translucent the opalescent layer, the greater the diffuse reflection. In reflective backgrounds, a translucent object may assume a yellowish and reddish hue. It has been speculated that some residual long-wavelength beams are transmitted back throughout the translucent incisal layer, resulting in a form of counter-opalescence.[35]

A similar behavior should also be seen in highly translucent resin composite. Opalescent resin composites must display high translucency in front of nonreflective backgrounds and some yellowish hue under reflective backgrounds (Fig 11). In fact, some resin composites are able to produce an intricate light distribution (Figs 12a and 12b).[7] However, some resin composites, designed to serve as the opalescent layer in the anterior, may not show an ideal performance because of the incorporated pigments. In these cases, the incident light, which is not completely reflected or scattered, is absorbed by intense stains[3] and mostly turns into heat.[36] This absorption attenuates the light beam,[3] thus modifying the appearance of the resin composite in different backgrounds.

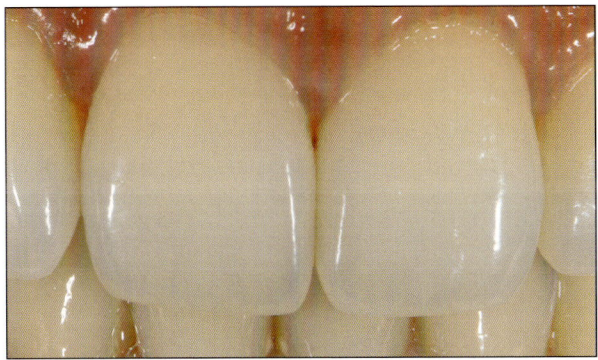

Fig 9a Central incisors in occlusion. Note that the opalescent layer is hardly visible; instead, an orange hue is apparent at the mamelons. This optical phenomenon is called counter-opalescence.

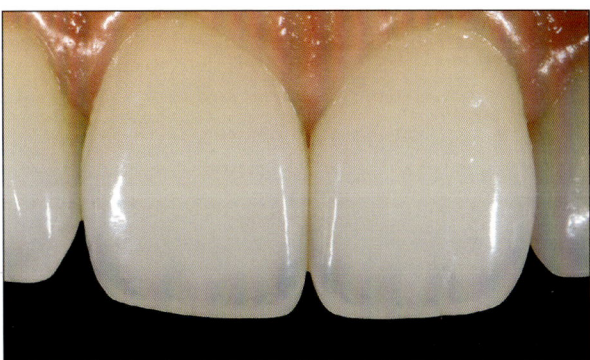

Fig 9b Central incisors against a nonreflective background. The opalescent layer displays a bluish hue.

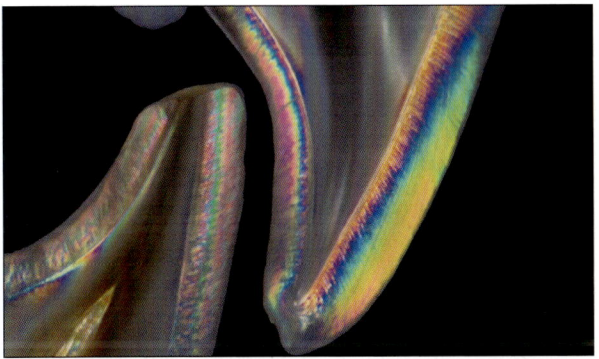

Fig 10 Complex light scattering is visible during occlusion.

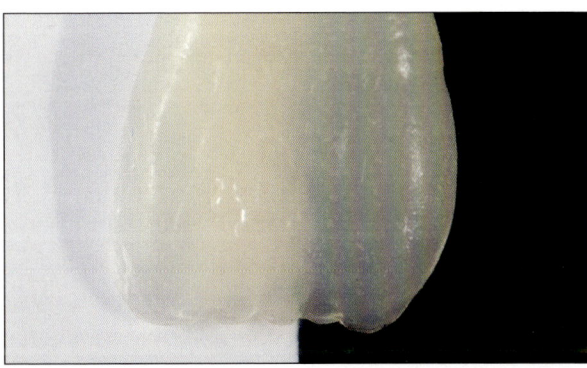

Fig 11 Highly translucent and opalescent resin composite shows an intricate light distribution under reflective and nonreflective backgrounds.

Figs 12a and 12b Highly translucent and opalescent resin composites against a nonreflective **(a)** and reflective **(b)** background. Observe the difference in hue produced by different resin composites. *(left to right)* YT (Filtek Supreme, 3M ESPE); GT (Filtek Supreme, 3M ESPE); Blue (4 Seasons, Ivoclar Vivadent); Clear (4 Seasons, Ivoclar Vivadent).

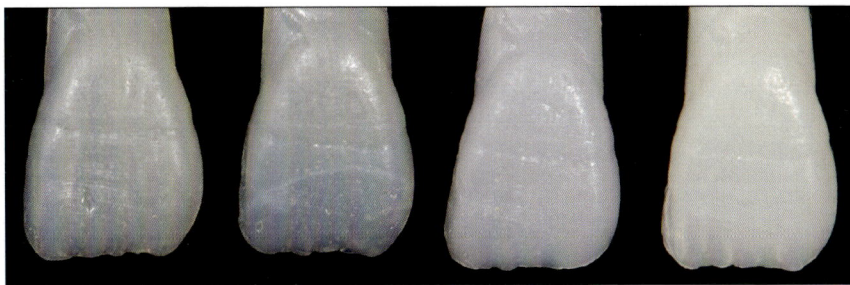

12a

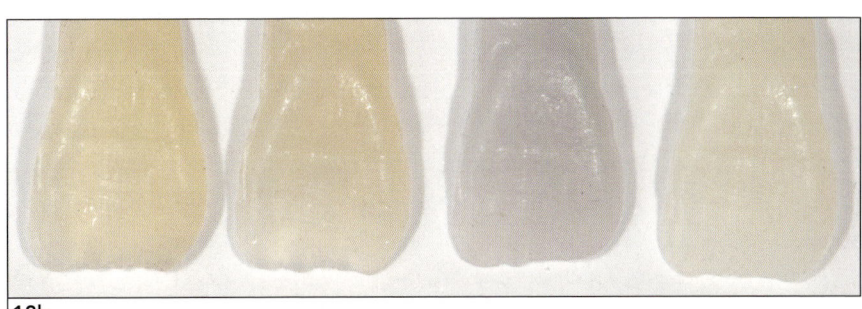

12b

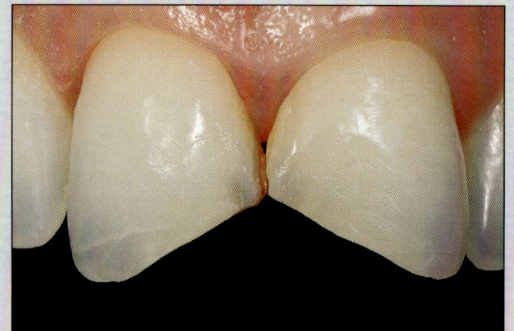

Fig 13 Preoperative view showing the fractured incisal edge of the maxillary central incisors.

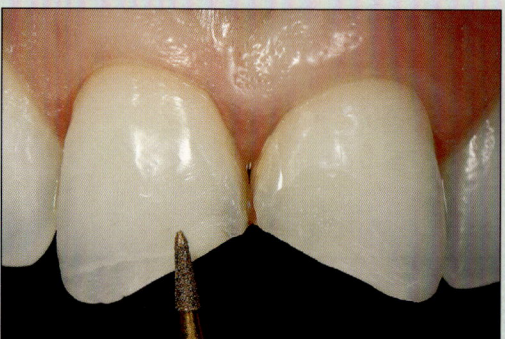

Fig 14 A 1.0-mm bevel was produced at the fracture margins with a tapered flame-head fine diamond bur using a high-speed handpiece under water cooling.

CASE PRESENTATION

An 18-year-old female patient presented with incisal edge fracture on the maxillary central incisors (Fig 13). A direct resin composite restoration was recommended to recreate the anterior esthetics. An irreversible hydrocolloid impression was made, an additive waxup was performed, and a silicone matrix was fabricated.

The shade was selected using a classic ceramic shade guide (VITA Lumin Classic, VITA Zahnfabrik, Bad Säckingen, Germay) and the teeth characteristics were evaluated with a specific shade guide (Creative Color System). The restorative resin composites were selected according to the layering technique in seven different restorative phases: (1) artificial lingual enamel, (2) artificial dentin core, (3) artificial dentin, (4) incisal opalescent layer, (5) incisal halo, (6) characterization, and (7) artificial facial enamel. A mockup was performed prior to fabrication of the restoration to select the ideal thickness of each layer regarding an accurate light transmission. The procedure was carried out with no field isolation to prevent the tooth from dehydrating. All details were recorded in a drawing to serve as reference for the final restoration.

At the restorative appointment, the teeth were cleaned with pumice and water with a soft brush under a low-speed handpiece. A 1.0-mm bevel (Fig 14) was produced at the fracture line with a 46-µm fine diamond bur (1190F, KG Sorensen, Barueri, São Paulo, Brazil) using a water-cooled high-speed handpiece. The diamond bur was positioned parallel to the long axis of the tooth because of its tapered flame head (Fig 15a). However, after the bevel was created, a sharp angle was produced at the cavosurface margins. This sharp angle has been known to make the fracture line visible after the restoration is complete. Therefore, a coarse aluminum oxide disk (Sof-Lex Pop-On, 3M ESPE, St Paul, MN, USA) was used to round and smooth the cavosurface margins (Fig 15b). This way, because the line angles were rounded, the incident light was scattered, thus preventing the fracture line from appearing.

The operative tooth was isolated and the adjacent teeth protected with Teflon tape (DuPont, Wilmington, DE, USA). The enamel was etched with 35% phosphoric acid gel for 15 seconds (Fig 16), washed, and air dried. An ethanol- and water-based adhesive system (Single Bond Plus, 3M ESPE; Excite, Ivoclar Vivadent, Schann, Liechtenstein) was applied (Fig 17) according to the manufacturer's instructions, and light cured for 20 seconds. The Teflon tape was then removed.

Fig 15a A diamond bur was positioned parallel to the long axis of the tooth.

Fig 15b A coarse aluminum oxide disk was used to round the angles and produce diffuse light scattering at the fracture/bevel margins.

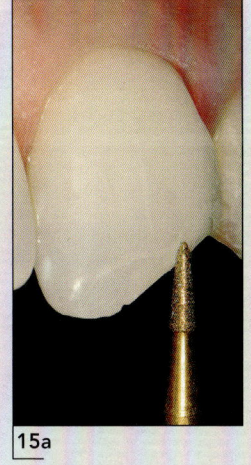
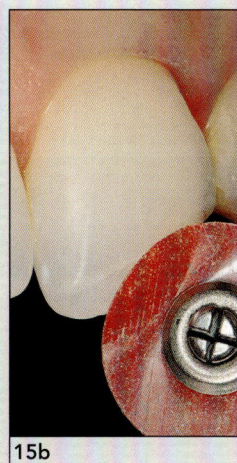

15a

15b

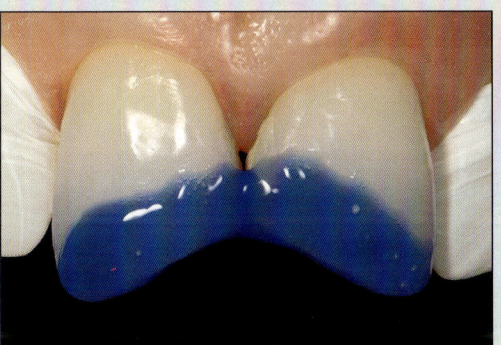

Fig 16 The enamel was etched with 35% phosphoric acid for 15 seconds.

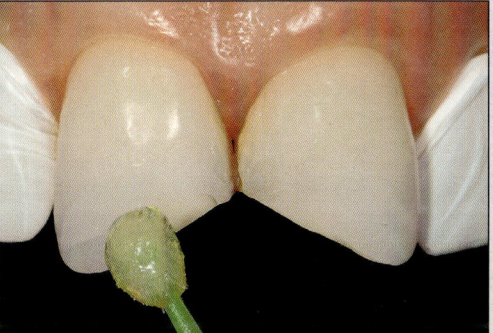

Fig 17 An ethanol- and water-based adhesive was applied per the manufacturer's instructions and light cured for 20 seconds.

Artificial Lingual Enamel

Fabricating the restoration from the lingual aspect to the facial aspect produces a more predicable restoration, since it is possible to determine and control the thickness of each increment.

To reproduce the lingual enamel, a highly translucent resin composite (eg, Translucent, Filtek Supreme, 3M ESPE; Clear, 4 Seasons, Ivoclar Vivadent) was used. The resin composite was inserted to a thickness of 0.5 mm directly into the silicone matrix, and carefully shaped to its final contour with a Gold Microfill Instrument (Almore International, Portland, OR, USA) and a fine

artist brush (no. 1, Cosmedent, Chicago, IL, USA). A solvent-free bonding resin (Scotchbond Multi-Purpose Adhesive, 3M ESPE) was used as a lubricant.[37] Subsequently, the silicone matrix was adapted to the lingual surface of the fractured central incisors (Fig 18). The incisal and proximal outlines of the artificial lingual enamel were confirmed, and the resin composite was light cured for 40 seconds. The silicone matrix was removed and the final contours were evaluated from facial and incisal views (Figs 19 and 20). The incisal view revealed important information concerning the thickness of the resin composite layers.

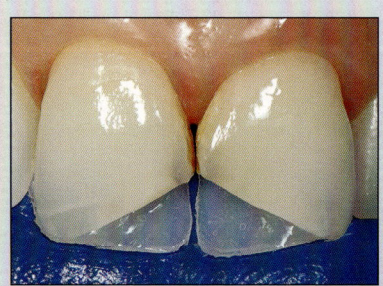

Fig 18 The silicone matrix with a highly translucent resin composite was adapted to the lingual surface of the maxillary central incisors and light cured for 40 seconds.

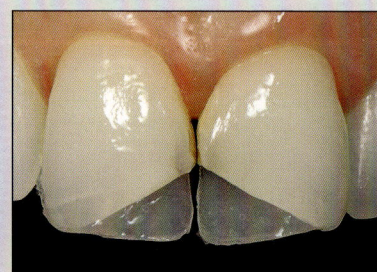

Fig 19 Facial view of the artificial lingual enamel contours.

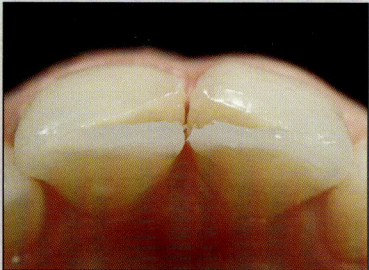

Fig 20 An incisal view of the artificial lingual enamel shows important information regarding the thickness for the coming layers.

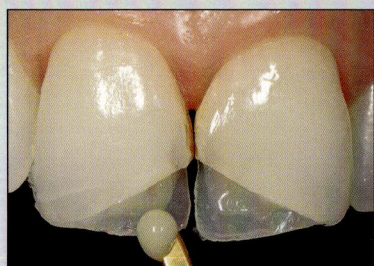

Fig 21 The dentin core was created with a more saturated and less translucent resin composite to reproduce the inner aspect of the dentin.

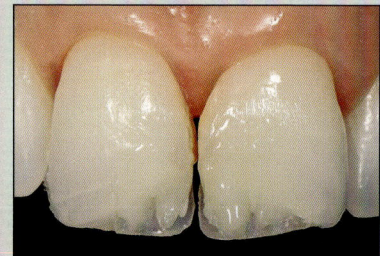

Fig 22 The artificial dentin was sculpted with a less saturated resin composite to generate a chroma progression from inside to outside the restoration.

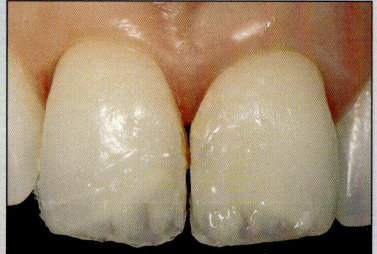

Fig 23 A highly opalescent resin composite was used to reproduce a type I opalescent layer.

Dentin Core

The light must cross a complex tubular structure of dentin. Dentin has 45,000 tubules/mm² near the pulp, but only 20,000 tubules/mm² near the DEJ.[38] Therefore, dentin becomes less translucent and more saturated as it approaches the pulp.[28] The dentin core, which represents the inner dentin, is usually two chroma more saturated than that of the selected shade. For instance, if the selected shade is A1, the dentin core will be A3.

A small amount of a less translucent and fluorescent resin composite (eg, A3D, Filtek Supreme; A3 Dentin, 4 Seasons) was applied directly to the artificial lingual enamel (Fig 21) and light cured for 40 seconds.

Artificial Dentin

The dentin is more opaque than enamel; however, it is also translucent.[39] For this reason, a resin composite that is less translucent than enamel-shaded resin composites should be used for the artificial dentin. The thickness of the dentin layer is fundamental to creating a lifelike result. To restore the gradual change in chroma from the inner to the outer part of the restoration, a less saturated shade than the dentin core should be used. Therefore, if the main shade is A1, the dentin core will be A3, and the artificial dentin will be A2. At this point, the selected incisal opalescent layer pattern must be reevaluated, because the final result depends on the dentin morphology.

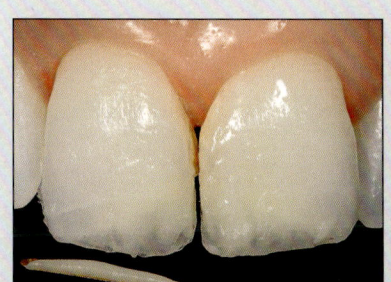

Fig 24 The incisal halo was produced at the incisal edge using a thin layer of dentin shade composite.

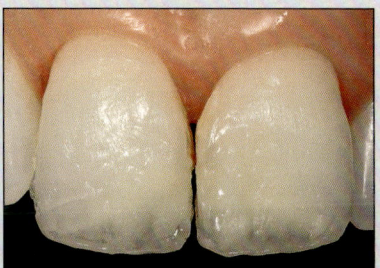

Fig 25 Facial aspect of the layering technique showing the mamelons, incisal opalescent layer, and incisal halo.

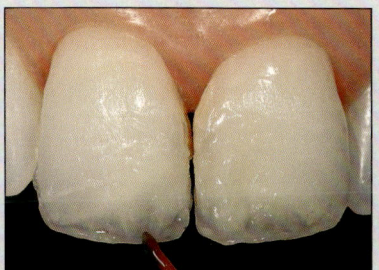

Fig 26 Intense colorants were used to correct the bluish incisal hue and increase the saturation at the mamelons.

A less saturated and less translucent resin composite (eg, A2D, Filtek Supreme; A2 Dentin, 4 Seasons) was used to restore the dentin morphology. The resin composite was inserted, covering the dentin core but keeping 1.0 to 0.5 mm away from the incisal edge. Three developmental lobes (mesial, central, and small distal) were shaped to create a type I opalescent layer (Fig 22). The morphology of the mamelons was sculpted with an explorer and light cured for 40 seconds.

Incisal Opalescent Layer

To produce a natural, convincing restoration, the incisal opalescent layer must be carefully evaluated. An incisal, highly translucent, opalescent resin composite must be applied according to the selected incisal opalescent pattern.

A highly translucent and opalescent resin composite (eg, YT, Filtek Supreme; Super Clear, 4 Seasons) was inserted at the incisal third of the restoration. This layer was cautiously applied among the mamelons toward the incisal edge, without exceeding the incisal border, and then light cured for 20 seconds (Fig 23).

Incisal Halo

When the light reaches the incisal edge, all visible wavelengths are scattered and deflected from their original path because of the divergence of the enamel prisms. This intricate light dispersion makes the incisal border cloudy and opaque in reflected light. An opaque resin composite should be used to reestablish this phenomenon.

The same shade of resin composite used for the artificial dentin was selected to build the incisal halo. A small amount of resin composite was rolled over a paper pad to a "spaghetti-like" shape of 0.2 to 0.3 mm thickness. With the use of an interproximal carver composite instrument (IPC, Cosmedent), the delicate resin composite layer was collected from the paper pad (Fig 24), inserted on top of the restoration's incisal edge, and light cured for 40 seconds (Fig 25).

Characterization

The correct incisal bluish hue was analyzed with a specific shade guide (Creative Color System). To obtain the correct hue of the opalescent layer under reflected light, a mix of blue, gray, and untinted colorants was tested on the adjacent teeth prior to placement of the restoration. A mix of 40% blue tint, 40% gray tint, and 20% untinted resin composite (Vita-l-escence Colors, Ultradent, South Jordan, Utah, USA) was prepared and applied over the incisal opalescent layer, without covering the mamelons (Fig 26).

Additionally, yellow and orange tints diluted with untinted resin composite were mixed and

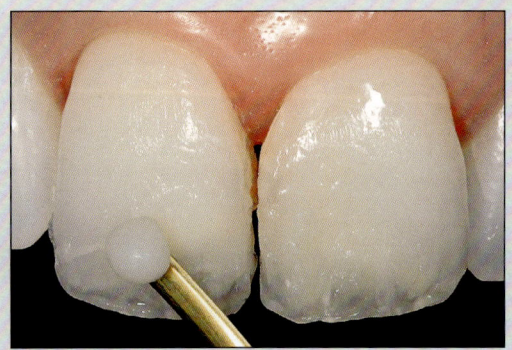

Fig 27 The artificial facial enamel was reestablished using enamel-shaded translucent resin composite.

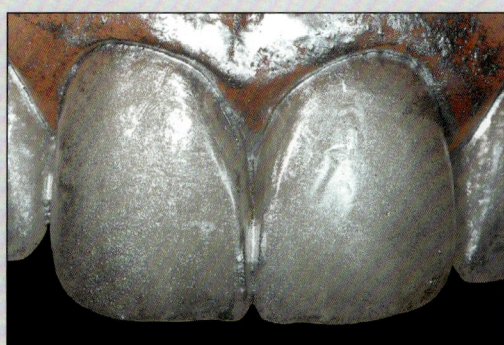

Fig 28 Nontoxic silver powder was used to reveal the overhangs at the restoration margins.

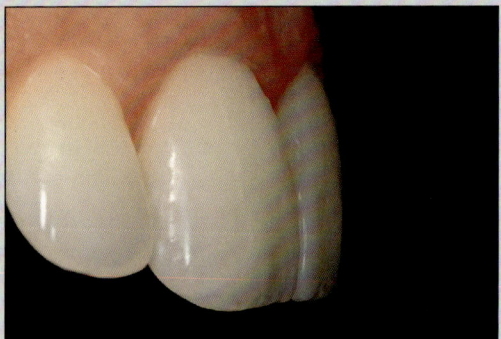

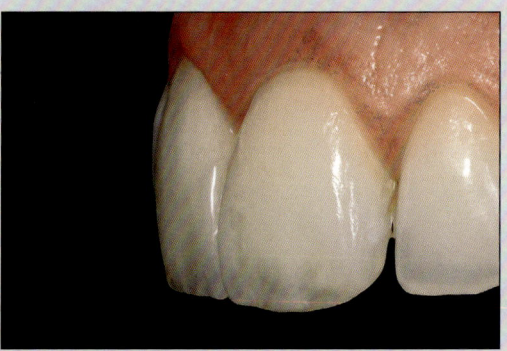

Figs 29a and 29b Postoperative side views of the anterior restorations. Note the esthetic integration with the adjacent teeth.

carefully applied at the lateral side of each mamelon to increase the saturation and reproduce the maverick colors.

Artificial Facial Enamel

Enamel has a highly translucent and colorless structure. Some authors advocate the use of neutral translucent resin composites to restore lost enamel.[32,40] However, most translucent resin composites currently on the market employ some degree of pigmentation. Enamel-shaded resin composites facilitate shade identification and the layering technique.

A translucent and opalescent enamel-shaded resin composite (eg, A1E, Filtek Supreme; A1, 4 Seasons) was used as the artificial enamel (Fig 27). The resin composite was applied, shaped to the desired form with a resin composite instrument followed by an artist brush, and light cured for 40 seconds.

A nontoxic silver powder was applied over the entire surface of the restorations to identify the presence of overhangs at the margins (Fig 28). Initial finishing was performed with medium-grit aluminum oxide disks (Sof-Lex Pop-On). The occlusion was checked and the patient was dismissed.

In a second appointment, nontoxic silver powder was again applied over the entire surface of

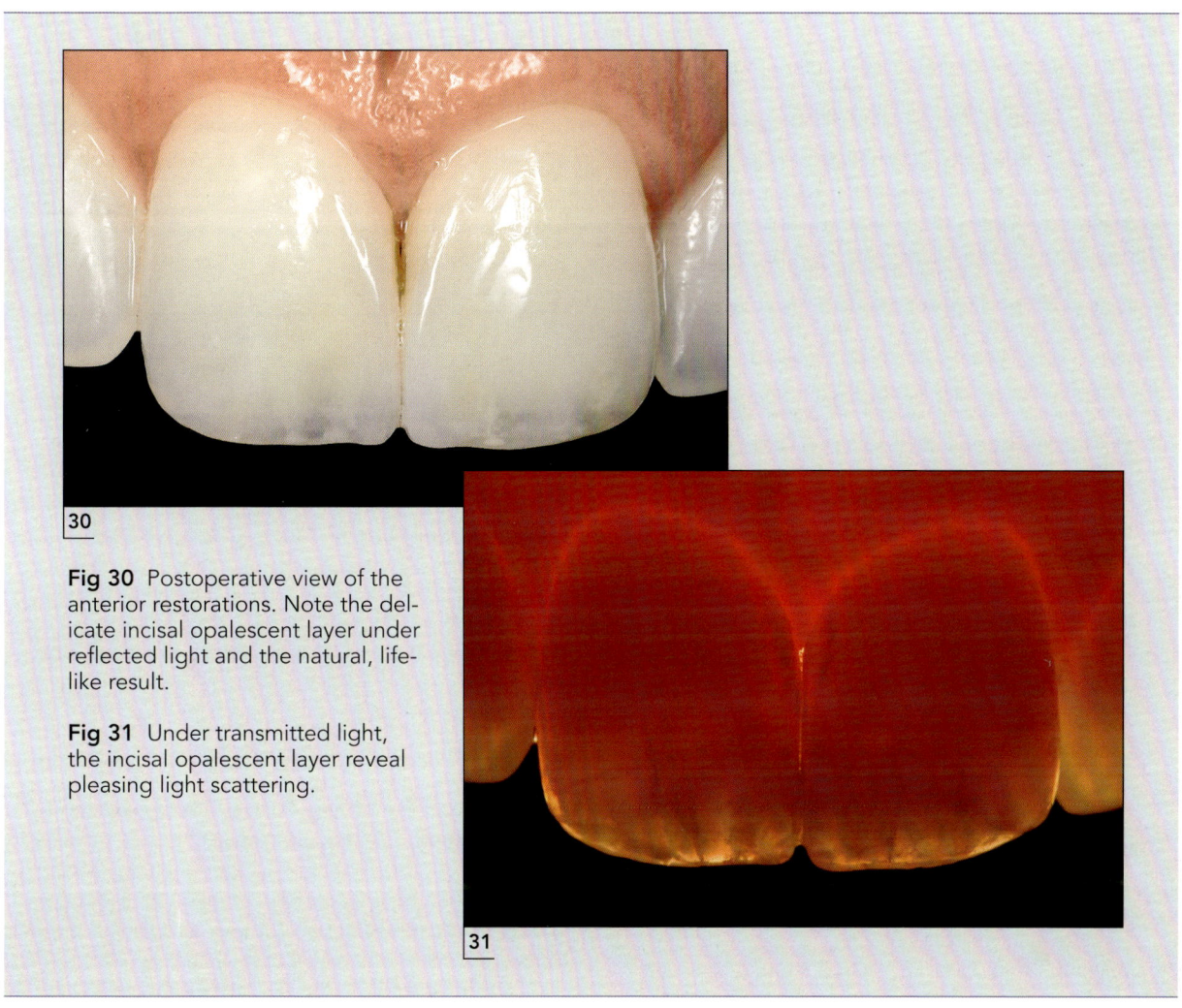

Fig 30 Postoperative view of the anterior restorations. Note the delicate incisal opalescent layer under reflected light and the natural, lifelike result.

Fig 31 Under transmitted light, the incisal opalescent layer reveal pleasing light scattering.

the restoration to emphasize the morphology and texture of the teeth. Morphology and texture were defined with fine diamond burs at a high speed. The restoration was then polished with extra-thin aluminum oxide disks (Sof-Lex Pop-On). A buffing wheel (FlexiBuff, Cosmedent) in conjunction with aluminum polishing paste (Enamelize, Cosmedent) was used to impart a high gloss to the restoration.[41]

Figures 29a and 29b show the final restoration from the proximal sides. The restoration demonstrated a high degree of esthetic integration with the surrounding tissues (Fig 30). Furthermore, a harmonious opalescent effect was observed under transillumination (Fig 31).

CONCLUSION

To achieve full esthetic integration, the optical properties of resin composite must be understood, analyzed, and tested prior to placement of the final restoration.

REFERENCES

1. Cook WD, McAree DC. Optical properties of esthetic restorative materials and natural dentition. J Biomed Mater Res 1985;19:469–488.

2. Sieber C. In light of nature [in German]. Quintessenz Zahntech 1991;17:1301–1314.

3. Grajower R, Wozniak WT, Lindsay JM. Optical properties of composite resins. J Oral Rehabil 1982;9:389–399.

4. Lee YK, Lu H, Powers JM. Optical properties of four esthetic restorative materials after accelerated aging. Am J Dent 2006;19:155–158.

5. Ikeda T, Sidhu SK, Omata Y, Fujita M, Sano H. Colour and translucency of opaque-shades and body-shades of resin composites. Eur J Oral Sci 2005;113:170–173.

6. Winter R. Visualizing the natural dentition. J Esthet Dent 1993;5:102–117.

7. Lee YK, Lu H, Powers JM. Measurement of opalescence of resin composites. Dent Mater 2005;21:1068–1074.

8. Lee YK, Lim BS, Rhee SH, Yang HC, Powers JM. Changes of optical properties of dental nano-filled resin composites after curing and thermocycling. J Biomed Mater Res B Appl Biomater 2004;71:16–21.

9. Primus CM, Chu CC, Shelby JE, Buldrini E, Heckle CE. Opalescence of dental porcelain enamels. Quintessence Int 2002;33:439–449.

10. Boyde A. Microstructure of enamel. Ciba Found Symp 1997;205:18–27.

11. Bartlett JD, Ganss B, Goldberg M, et al. Protein-protein interactions of the developing enamel matrix. Curr Top Dev Biol 2006;74:57–115.

12. Fincham AG, Bessem CC, Lau EC, et al. Human developing enamel proteins exhibit a sex-linked dimorphism. Calcif Tissue Int 1991;48:288–290.

13. White SN, Luo W, Paine ML, Fong H, Sarikaya M, Snead ML. Biological organization of hydroxyapatite crystallites into a fibrous continuum toughens and controls anisotropy in human enamel. J Dent Res 2001;80:321–36.

14. Daculsi G, Menanteau J, Kerebel LM, Mitre D. Length and shape of enamel crystals. Calcif Tissue Int 1984;36:550–555.

15. Boyde A. A 3-D model of enamel development at the scale of one inch to the micron. Adv Dent Res 1987;1:135–140.

16. Koenigswald WV, Sander PM. Tooth Enamel Microstructure. Balkema, Rotterdam: Swets, 1997.

17. Koenigswald WV, Clemens WA. Levels of complexity in the microstructure of mammalian enamel and their application in studies of systematics. Scanning Microsc 1992;6:195–217.

18. Brodbelt RH, O'Brien WJ, Fan PL, Frazer-Dib JG, Yu R. Translucency of human dental enamel. J Dent Res 1981;60:1749–1753.

19. Vukusic P, Sambles JR. Photonic structures in biology. Nature 2003;424:852–855.

20. Kodaka T, Kuroiwa M, Higashi S, Miake K. Three-dimensional observations of the relation between the natural enamel surface and the outermost layer in human permanent tooth. Bull Tokyo Dent Coll 1990;31:105–115.

21. Kinoshita S, Yoshioka S. Structural colors in nature: The role of regularity and irregularity in the structure. Chemphyschem 2005;6:1442–1459.

22. Vaarkamp J, ten Bosch JJ, Verdonschot EH. Propagation of light through human dental enamel and dentine. Caries Res 1995;29:8–13.

23. Terry DA, Geller W, Tric O, Anderson MJ, Tourville M, Kobashigawa A. Anatomical form defines color: Function, form, and aesthetics. Pract Proced Aesthet Dent 2002;14:59–67.

24. Prum RO, Quinn T, Torres RH. Anatomically diverse butterfly scales all produce structural colours by coherent scattering. J Exp Biol 2006;209(Pt 4):748–765.

25. Prum RO, Torres RH. A Fourier tool for the analysis of coherent light scattering by bio-optical nanostructures. Integr Comp Biol 2003;43:59–602.

26. Yamamoto M. Metal Ceramics. Principles and Methods of Makoto Yamamoto. Chicago: Quintessence, 1985.

27. Saunders JV. Color of precious opal. Nature 1964;204:1151–1153.

28. Duarte S Jr, Perdigao J, Lopes M. Composite resin restorations—Natural aesthetic and dynamics of light. Pract Proced Aesthet Dent 2003;15:657–664.

29. Kingery WD, Bowen HK, Uhlmann DR. Introduction to Ceramics, ed 2. New York: Wiley & Sons, 1976.

30. Kim JH, Lee YK, Powers JM. Influence of a series of organic and chemical substances on the translucency of resin composites. J Biomed Mater Res B Appl Biomater 2006;77:21–27.

31. Hegenbarth EA. Creative Ceramic Color: A Practical System. Chicago: Quintessence, 1989.

32. Vanini L. Light and color in anterior composite restorations. Pract Periodontics Aesthet Dent 1996;8:673–682.

33. Lee YK, Lu H, Powers JM. Changes in opalescence and fluorescence properties of resin composites after accelerated aging. Dent Mater 2006;22:653–660.

34. Lee YK, Lim BS, Kim CW. Difference in the colour and colour change of dental resin composites by the background. J Oral Rehabil 2005;32:227–233.

35. Baratieri LN, Araujo EM, Monteiro JS. Composite Restorations in Anterior Teeth: Fundamentals and Possibilities. Chicago: Quintessence Publishing, 2005.

36. Longair M. Light and colour. In: Lamb T, Bourriau J (eds). Colour: Art and Science. Cambridge: Cambridge University Press, 1995:65–102.

37. Perdigao J, Gomes G. Effect of instrument lubricant on the cohesive strength of a hybrid resin composite. Quintessence Int 2006;37:621–625.

38. Perdigao J. Dentin bonding as a function of dentin structure. Dent Clin North Am 2002;46:277–301.

39. Thomas GJ, Whittaker DK, Embery G. A comparative study of translucent apical dentine in vital and non-vital human teeth. Arch Oral Biol 1994;39:29–34.

40. Dietschi D, Ardu S, Krejci I. A new shading concept based on natural tooth color applied to direct composite restorations. Quintessence Int 2006;37:91–102.

41. Turssi CP, Saad JR, Duarte SL Jr, Rodrigues AL Jr. Composite surfaces after finishing and polishing techniques. Am J Dent 2000;13:136–138.

COMPREHENSIVE ESTHETIC AND FUNCTIONAL REHABILITATION WITH A CAD/CAM ALL-CERAMIC SYSTEM

Iñaki Gamborena, DMD, MSD, FID[1]
Markus B. Blatz, DMD, PhD[2]

CAD/CAM technology and all-ceramic systems have become integral parts of modern dentistry and laboratory technology. The Procera system[1] (Nobel Biocare, Göteborg, Sweden) was introduced over a decade ago and offers various components, materials, and techniques within one concept (C&B&I: crown & bridge & implant, Nobel Biocare). The CAD/CAM system allows fabrication of single- and multiple-unit frameworks as well as implant components (Procera Crown, Procera Bridge, Procera Abutment). Each of these restorative components can be fabricated from titanium alloy, densely sintered aluminum oxide ceramic (Alumina), or densely sintered zirconium oxide ceramic (Zirconia).

The advantages, properties, and clinical applications of the all-ceramic components and materials used with the Procera system, based on scientific evidence, are discussed in this article. The featured case presentation, a comprehensive full-mouth rehabilitation, demonstrates the versatility and esthetic capabilities of the Procera system.

ALUMINUM OXIDE CERAMICS

High-strength ceramic materials (eg, aluminum oxide and zirconium oxide) are typically used as coping materials for full-coverage restorations and

[1]Affiliate Associate Professor, University of Washington School of Dentistry, Seattle, Washington, USA; private practice, San Sebastian, Spain.

[2]Professor of Restorative Dentistry and Chairman, Department of Preventive and Restorative Sciences, University of Pennsylvania School of Dental Medicine, Philadelphia, Pennsylvania, USA.

Correspondence to: Dr Iñaki Gamborena, Resureccion Mª De Azkue, 6, 20018 San Sebastian, Spain.
E-mail: gambmila@arrakis.es

fixed partial denture frameworks.[2–5] CAD/CAM technology compensates for the significant shrinkage of metal oxide high-strength ceramic materials during sintering. An industrialized production process bears multiple advantages in respect to the unique sintering temperatures and conditions of high-strength ceramics and outsourcing of a critical laboratory procedure. Procera uses densely sintered, high-purity aluminum oxide (>99.9%) ceramics, which offer a flexural strength of 610 MPa.[6] Procera Alumina has a higher degree of translucency compared to Procera Zirconia and may, therefore, be preferred in anterior, low-pressure-bearing areas of esthetic significance.[4,5] Alumina is used for single crowns, implant abutments, and laminate veneers.[2] The clinical long-term success of Procera Alumina crowns has been validated in many clinical studies.[7–9] Most recently, Galindo et al[10] reported on the follow-up of 39 patients with 135 Procera Alumina crowns. The cumulative survival rate was 99% after 5 and 7 years.

ZIRCONIUM OXIDE CERAMICS

Zirconium oxide ceramics provide superior physical properties (high flexural strength), biocompatibility, and excellent esthetics.[4,5] The inherent strength of zirconia makes it useful in a variety of clinical applications including full-coverage crowns, resin-bonded fixed and conventional fixed partial dentures, implant abutments, and even long-span implant bars.[11,12] Lifetime predictions reveal favorable success rates for zirconium oxide ceramic restorations.[13] In dentistry, zirconium oxide (ZrO_2) ceramic is mostly used in a tetragonal crystalline phase, partially stabilized with yttrium oxide. Polycrystalline zirconium oxide ceramics provide a flexural strength greater than 1,000 MPa and feature a unique material property: active crack resistance. External forces transfer the partially stabilized tetragonal particle into a monoclinic form. The newly acquired monoclinic form has an increased volume, which gives the material the ability to close a crack (transformation toughening).[4,5]

VENEERING CERAMICS FOR HIGH-STRENGTH CERAMIC COPINGS

High-strength ceramic copings are veneered with feldspathic (or silica-based) ceramics, which have a low flexural strength but offer superior esthetics and high translucency.[2,3] Feldspathic veneering ceramics for metal-alloy copings typically fail to provide long-term bonds and adequate physical properties when fired to high-strength ceramics due to a mismatch in the thermal coefficient of expansion, weak ceramic-ceramic bonds, and low fracture strength. Aboushelib et al[14] summarized in an in vitro study that cone cracking of the veneering ceramic is the dominant mode of failure of layered all-ceramic restorations. They conclude that higher strength veneering ceramics are needed to exploit the high strength of zirconia. Newer veneering ceramics and bonding methods modified for alumina and zirconia copings provide higher strengths and improved bonding mechanisms that seem to prevent delamination and fractures. Shear bond strengths of three recently developed veneering ceramics to zirconium oxide ceramic were investigated by Blatz et al.[15] Interestingly, all ceramic-ceramic combinations were different from each other but significantly stronger than the metal-ceramic control.

CEMENTATION

Cementation materials and methods play a critical role in the clinical survival of ceramic restorations.[16–18] Oppes et al[19] conducted an in vitro study on the marginal seal and fracture strength of Procera Alumina crowns after exposure in an artificial chewing simulator. They concluded that the type of luting agent has a significant effect on the fracture strength and microleakage of all-ceramic crowns. Bonding with a composite resin luting agent containing adhesive phosphate monomers significantly increased the fracture strength and improved the marginal seal of alumina crowns. However, all luting agents used in this investigation provided fracture strengths well above the average physiologic chewing forces. Okutan et al[20] investigated the fracture load and marginal fit of shrinkage-free ($ZrSiO_4$) all-ceramic crowns after chewing simulation. In this study, using adhesive composite resin cement resulted in higher mean fracture loads, which were, however, not statistically different from glass-ionomer cement. Even with a reduced coping thickness of 0.4 mm, zirconium oxide ceramic seems to provide adequate strength for nonadhesive cementation.[21]

CERAMIC IMPLANT ABUTMENTS

Conventional metal abutments may cause gray discoloration of the surrounding gingiva. Aluminum oxide or zirconium oxide ceramic implant abutments prevent this phenomenon.[22] Clinical studies demonstrate that zirconium oxide ceramic abutments had a cumulative survival rate of 100% after 4 and 6 years follow-up.[23,24] While zirconium oxide ceramic offers almost twice the strength, aluminum oxide ceramic abutments feature some esthetic advantages.[25] Att et al[26,27] investigated the strength of Procera zirconia and alumina crowns in combination with titanium, zirconia, and alumina abutments after exposure in an artificial chewing simulator. All material combinations exceeded physiologic chewing forces in the anterior jaw. Fracture strengths of zirconia crowns were significantly different when used with either one of the abutment materials.[26] The combination of zirconia crowns and alumina abutments resulted in the lowest fracture strengths. On the other hand, alumina crowns yield similar strength when used with either zirconia or alumina abutments and were comparable to the zirconia-zirconia combination.[27] Therefore, alumina abutments should preferably be used with alumina crowns while zirconia abutments can be used with either crown material.

ALL-CERAMIC FIXED PARTIAL DENTURES

Distinctive multidirectional forces and biomechanic requirements in the connector/pontic areas make zirconia the preferred framework material for all-ceramic multiple-unit fixed partial dentures. Studart et al[28] concluded from a recent study that "in spite of the susceptibility to subcritical crack growth, calculations based on the fatigue parameters and on the stress applied on the prosthesis indicate that posterior bridges with zirconia frameworks can exhibit lifetimes longer than 20 years if the diameter of the bridge connector is properly designed." While short-term clinical studies reveal promising success rates, long-term data are still needed to confirm the reliability of zirconia fixed partial dentures.[29]

CASE PRESENTATION

A 70-year-old man presented with failing restorations (Figs 1 and 2). The existing full-mouth rehabilitation was less than 2 years old and he complained of difficulty with chewing and function. The initial clinical and radiographic examination revealed heavy horizontal bruxism. The occlusal scheme was locked in position by the existing restorations without anterior or lateral freedom (overjet and immediate anterior disclusion). Reduced opening of the vertical dimension of occlusion contributed to an excessive load to the anterior teeth, which caused the restorations to fracture. The crowns were loose and the abutments were decayed to the gingival margin (Figs 3 and 4). Existing implants (3i Implant Innovations, Palm Beach, FL, USA) in the areas of the maxillary right first premolar to first molar and left first and second molars were well integrated and could be preserved for future restorations. Some mandibular restorations revealed recurrent caries. The periodontal diagnosis included advanced generalized gingivitis with localized periodontitis.

The comprehensive restorative treatment plan included implant-supported restorations in the maxilla and tooth-supported restorations in the mandible.

CASE PRESENTATION

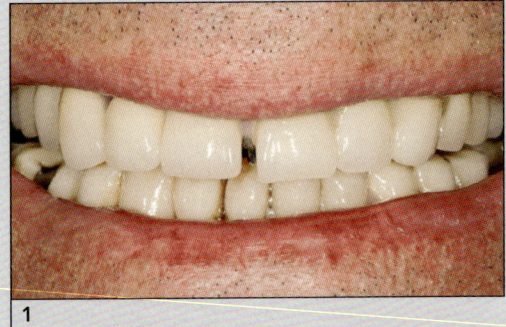

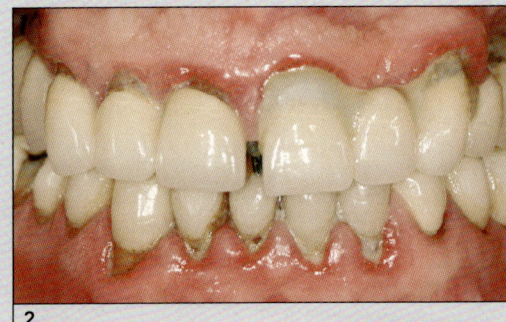

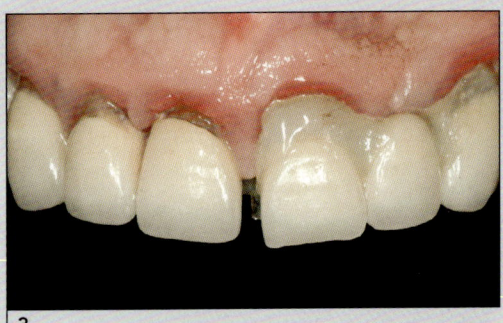

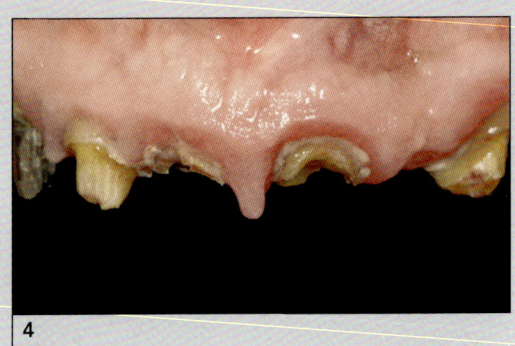

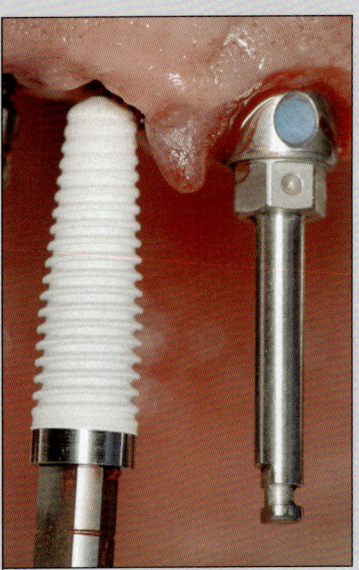

Figs 1 and 2 Failing full-mouth restoration in a 70-year-old patient. Initial clinical situation.

Figs 3 and 4 Preoperative intraoral frontal view of failing restorations.

Figs 5 and 6 Dental implants were placed with a flapless surgical procedure immediately after extraction of the destroyed teeth.

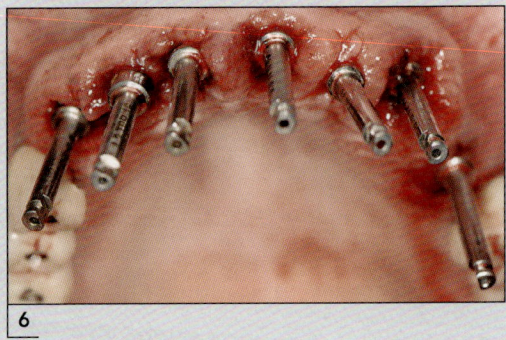

Remaining roots in the maxilla were extracted and immediately replaced with seven implants (Replace Select HA, Nobel Biocare) in a flapless procedure (Figs 5 and 6). Different implant diameters were used to maximize implant-to-bone contact: 5 mm for the central incisors, canines, and left second molar; 4.3 mm for the right lateral incisor; and 3.5 mm for the left lateral incisor. All implants were planned to be immediately loaded with provisional abutments and fixed full-arch provisional restorations, which were fabricated from the diagnostic waxup. After placement of all implants, temporary

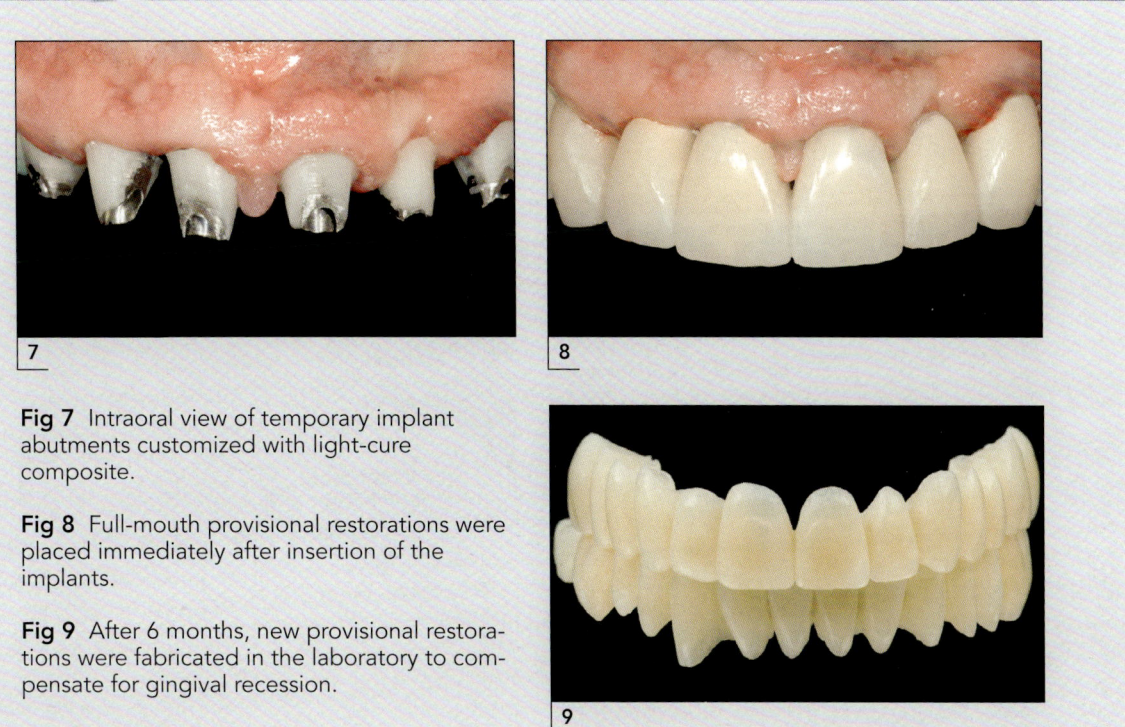

Fig 7 Intraoral view of temporary implant abutments customized with light-cure composite.

Fig 8 Full-mouth provisional restorations were placed immediately after insertion of the implants.

Fig 9 After 6 months, new provisional restorations were fabricated in the laboratory to compensate for gingival recession.

abutments (titanium temporary direct abutments, Nobel Biocare) were screwed onto the implants and used as impression copings to transfer the three-dimensional position of the implants to a stone cast. At this stage, the titanium abutments were prepared and the cast was trimmed around each implant to create an emergence profile that matched the contour of the teeth in the diagnostic waxup. Each individual emergence profile was created by applying a light-cure composite resin (Tetric Ceram HB, Ivoclar Vivadent, Schaan, Liechtenstein) into the carved stone and 360 degrees around the implant abutment to create a customized abutment. The composite resin was cured in the laboratory (Triad 2000, Visible Light Cure System, Dentsply/Trubyte, York, PA, USA) and prepared with diamond burs to its ideal abutment form.

The customized provisional abutments (titanium temporary abutments and composite profile) were connected to the implants, and the full-arch shell provisional restoration was relined directly in the patient's mouth. The screw access holes of all abutments were carefully filled with a light-cure temporary material (Fermit, Ivoclar Vivadent). The abut-

ments were isolated with petroleum jelly before relining the provisional restoration with a self-cure acrylic material (Temporary Bridge Resin, Caulk/Dentsply). The provisional restoration was removed after polymerization. Each abutment was unscrewed and the margins were finalized in the laboratory for optimal fit. The abutments were retightened (Fig 7) and the provisional restoration seated to be adjusted to the mandible. In the meantime, the existing mandibular crowns were removed and the abutment teeth were prepared. The mandibular full-arch provisional shell was relined and occlusion adjusted against the maxilla during the same visit. The provisional restorations were cemented with temporary cement (Temp-Bond NE, Kerr, Orange, CA, USA) after final adjustments, recontouring, and polishing (Fig 8).

Gingival recession of 1 to 2 mm was observed 6 months after tooth extraction and immediate implant placement. The provisional abutments were recontoured and new provisional restorations were fabricated in the laboratory (Fig 9) to compensate for the missing soft tissue. During that period, additional implants were placed to re-

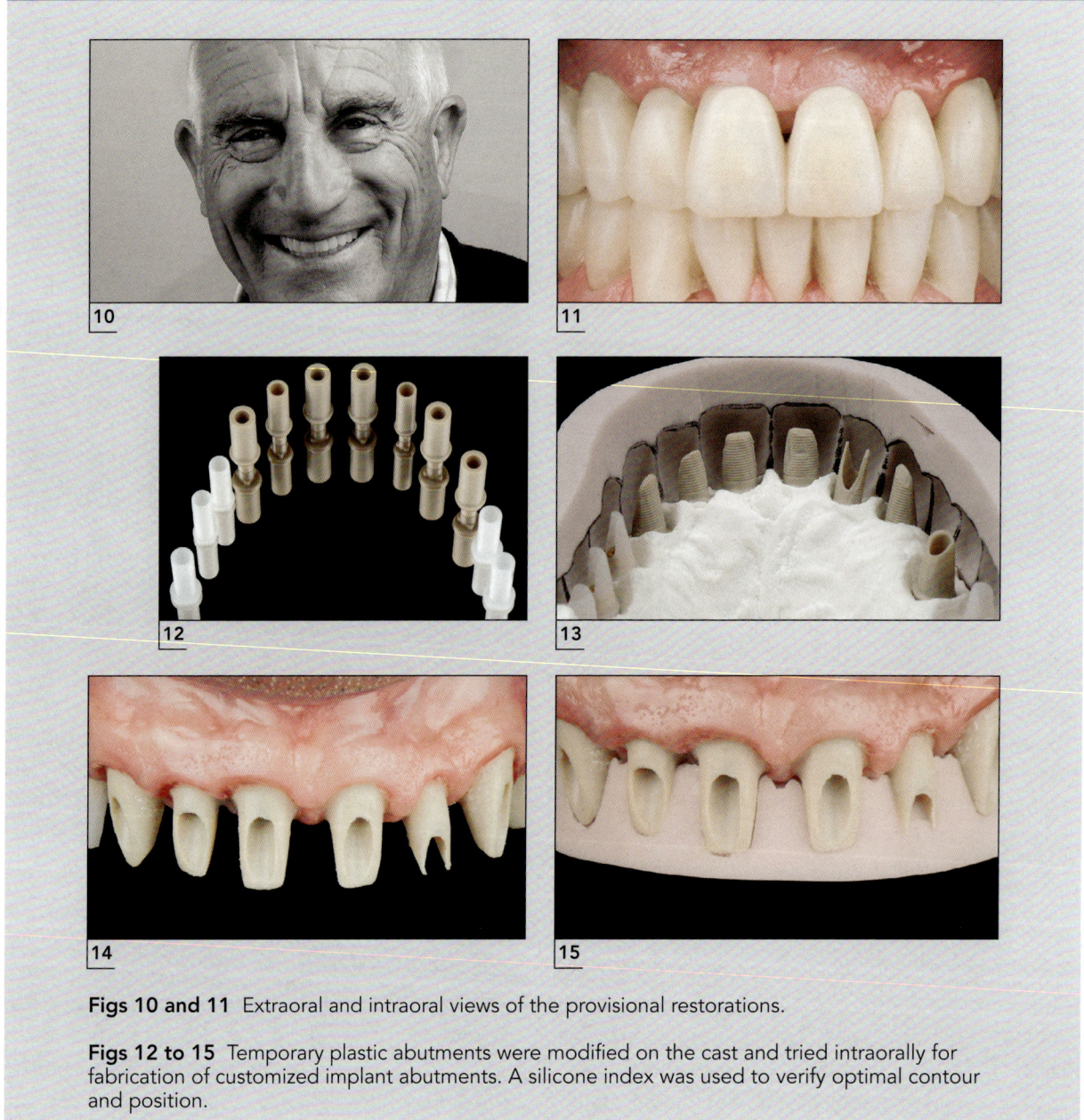

Figs 10 and 11 Extraoral and intraoral views of the provisional restorations.

Figs 12 to 15 Temporary plastic abutments were modified on the cast and tried intraorally for fabrication of customized implant abutments. A silicone index was used to verify optimal contour and position.

store both mandibular first molars (5 × 13-mm Straight Replace Select HA, Nobel Biocare). Periodic follow-up visits did not reveal any loosening of the provisional restorations, which demonstrated an adequate occlusal scheme. Optimal functional and esthetic parameters were established during the provisional phase (Figs 10 and 11), which could then be transferred to the final restorations.

Final impressions of the mandible were taken with the double-cord technique (#000 and #0 Ultrapak, Ultradent, South Jordan, UT, USA) and the double-mix impression technique (Virtual VPS putty base regular set and extra-light-body fast set, Ivoclar Vivadent). A pickup impression of the maxillary full-arch provisional restoration was taken with the double-mix technique (Virtual VPS putty base regular set and extra-light-body fast

Fig 16 Definitive implant abutments were fabricated from zirconia (anterior) and gold (posterior).

Figs 17 and 18 Optimal contour and adequate tissue support of the implant abutments is verified on the master cast and confirmed intraorally.

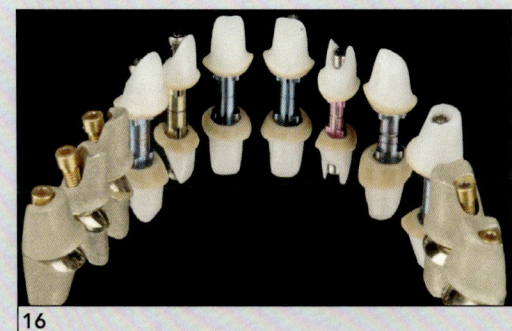

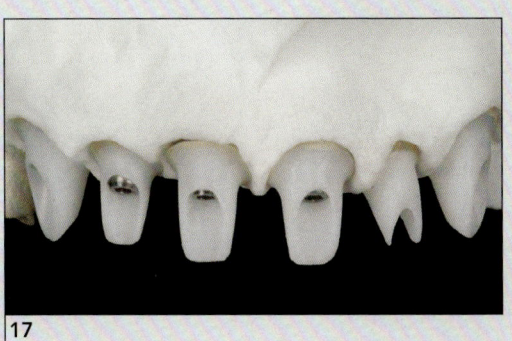

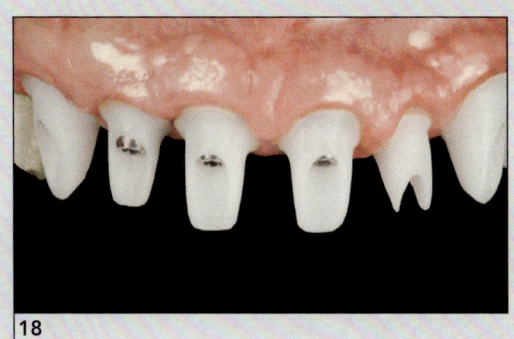

set). The provisional restoration was embedded and locked into the impression material upon removal. The abutments were unscrewed and removed from the mouth, and laboratory implant analogues were connected to the corresponding provisional abutments. The provisional cement was left in place for precise fit and transfer of the tissue topography and implant position to the master cast (GC Fuji-Rock EP Pearl White color, GC, Alsip, IL, USA). Cross-mounted casts were selected to facilitate and transfer the provisional information to the fabrication of the final prosthesis. Acrylic jigs (GC Pattern Resin) were used in addition to interocclusal wax registrations (bite registration wax sheets, Almore International) to maintain the same vertical dimension as established in the provisional restorations.

Materials for the final restorations were selected at this stage. It was decided to apply all components of the Procera product line, single crowns, implant abutments, and fixed partial dentures, and to take advantage of the unique material properties of zirconia (implant abutments, posterior restorations, and fixed partial dentures) and

alumina restorations (anterior crowns). Customized gold abutments were planned for the existing implants in the posterior maxilla.

Two master casts were fabricated from each impression. One was sectioned into individual dies to facilitate scanning of each abutment and pontic site. The second cast was solid and duplicated the provisional restoration for a stable reference of the soft tissue contour and fabrication of zirconia abutments. A silicone index was made from this cast (Zetalabor laboratory high-precision condensation silicone, Zhermack, Badia Polesine, Italy).

The fabrication of a customized zirconia abutment begins with a temporary plastic direct abutment (Nobel Biocare) (Fig 12) that is modified with composite to its ideal contour and form according to the silicone index made from the provisional restoration (Fig 13). The customized plastic abutments should be tried in the mouth and verified with the silicone index (Figs 14 and 15) before final scanning and fabrication of the definitive implant abutments (Figs 16 to 18). The Procera Forte scanner (Nobel Biocare) was used to scan the multiple-unit restorations, the temporary plastic abutments,

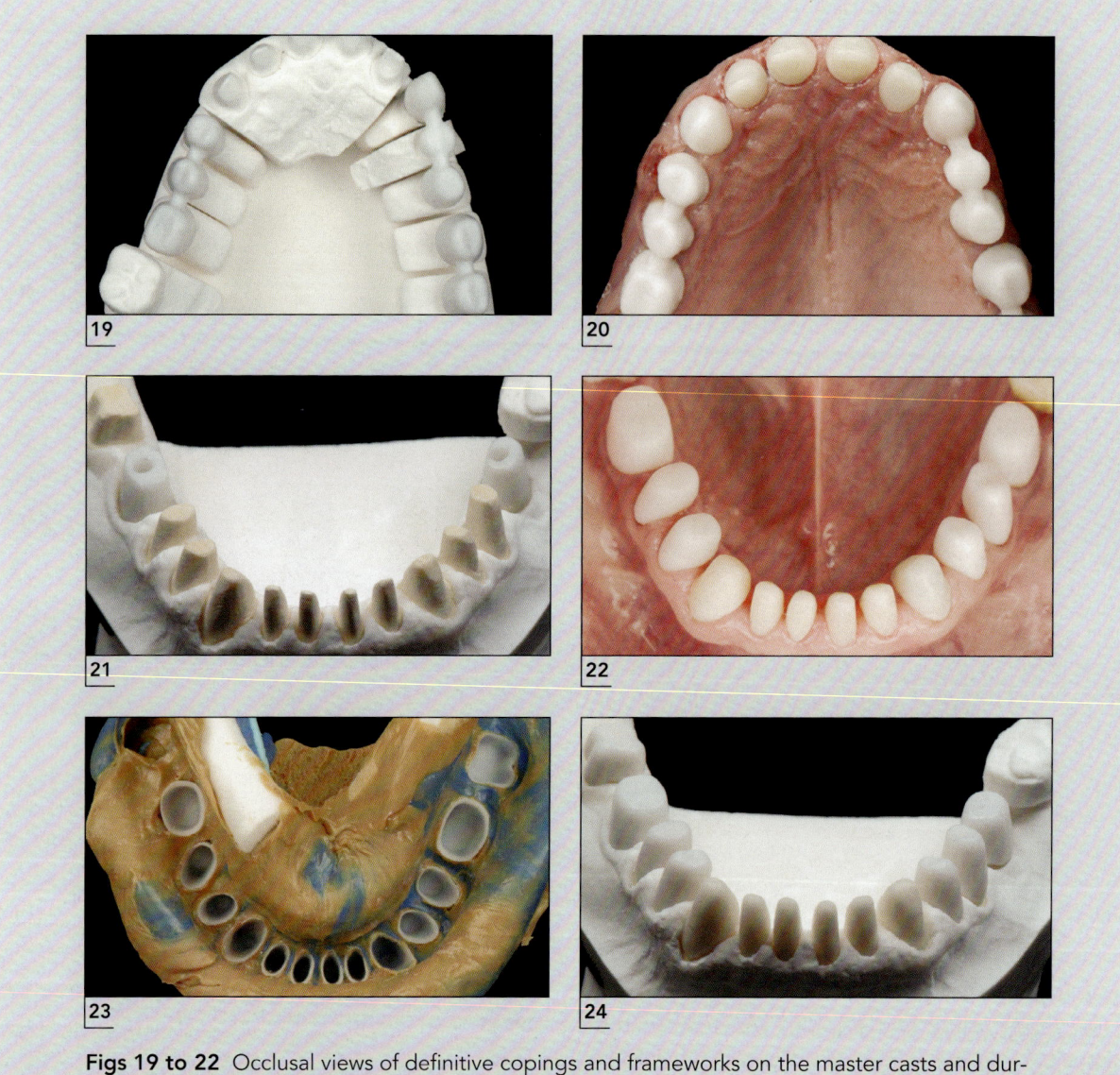

Figs 19 to 22 Occlusal views of definitive copings and frameworks on the master casts and during clinical try-in on the prepared teeth and customized abutments. All posterior restorations were made with Procera Zirconia copings. Maxillary incisors and mandibular anterior teeth were restored with Procera Alumina.

Fig 23 Pickup impression of mandibular copings.

Fig 24 Solid master cast of the mandibular pickup impression with copings in place.

the mandibular preparations, and the pontic ridges as well as the interocclusal records. Material thickness, height, contour, and all other dimensions of the abutments, copings, and frameworks were individually designed on the computer.

All definitive copings and frameworks were tried intraorally to verify fit on the prepared teeth and customized abutments (Figs 19 to 22). Pickup impressions (Virtual VPS) were taken of all cop-

ings and frameworks to fabricate solid master casts with an accurate tissue topography (Figs 23 and 24). Sufficient space for the veneering porcelain was verified with silicone indices. The veneering ceramic was applied and the full-mouth restorations were tried in at the bisque-bake stage. The restorations were then finalized, glazed, and stained to create natural esthetics (Figs 25 to 34). The zirconia abutments were

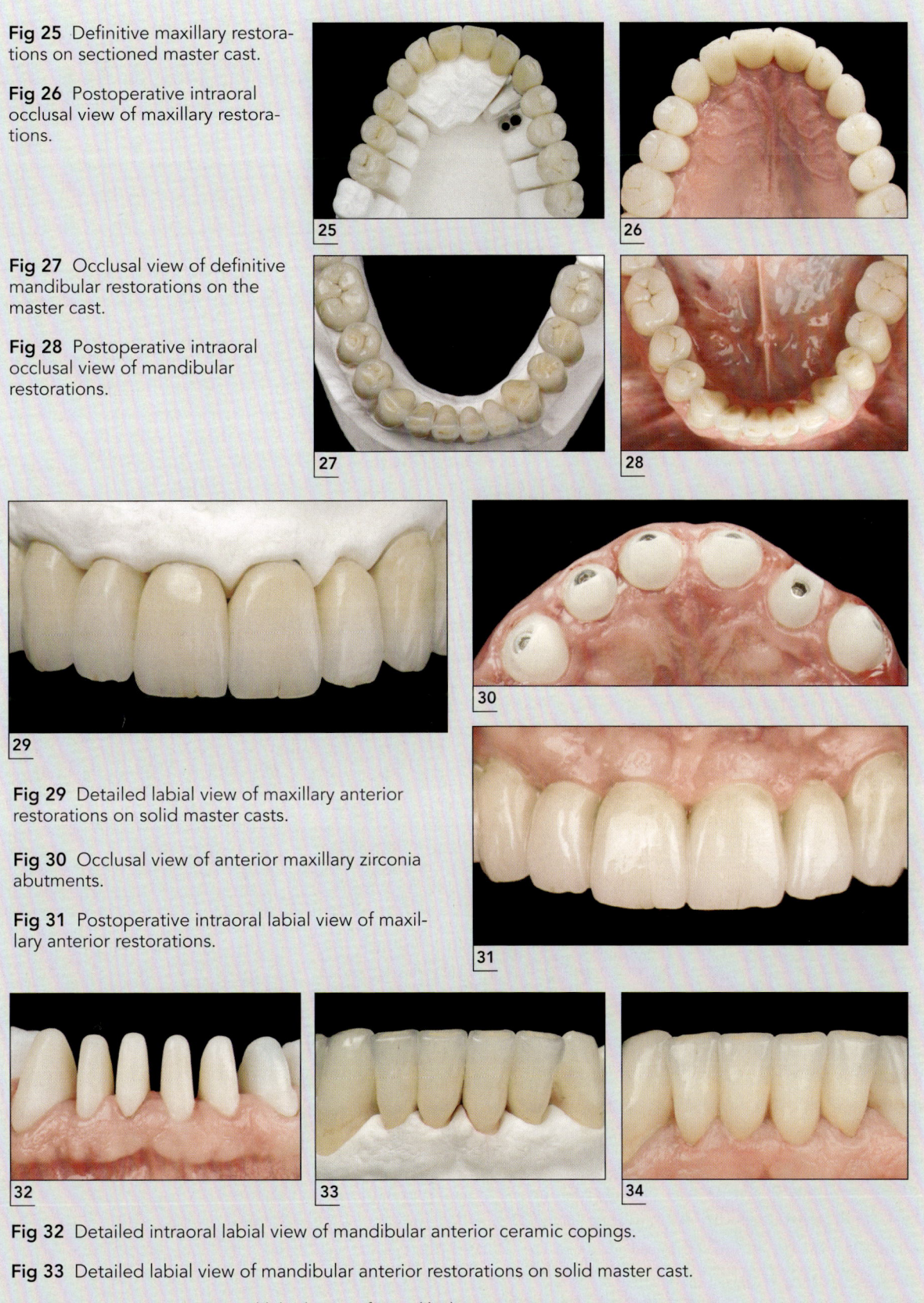

Fig 25 Definitive maxillary restorations on sectioned master cast.

Fig 26 Postoperative intraoral occlusal view of maxillary restorations.

Fig 27 Occlusal view of definitive mandibular restorations on the master cast.

Fig 28 Postoperative intraoral occlusal view of mandibular restorations.

Fig 29 Detailed labial view of maxillary anterior restorations on solid master casts.

Fig 30 Occlusal view of anterior maxillary zirconia abutments.

Fig 31 Postoperative intraoral labial view of maxillary anterior restorations.

Fig 32 Detailed intraoral labial view of mandibular anterior ceramic copings.

Fig 33 Detailed labial view of mandibular anterior restorations on solid master cast.

Fig 34 Postoperative intraoral labial view of mandibular anterior restorations.

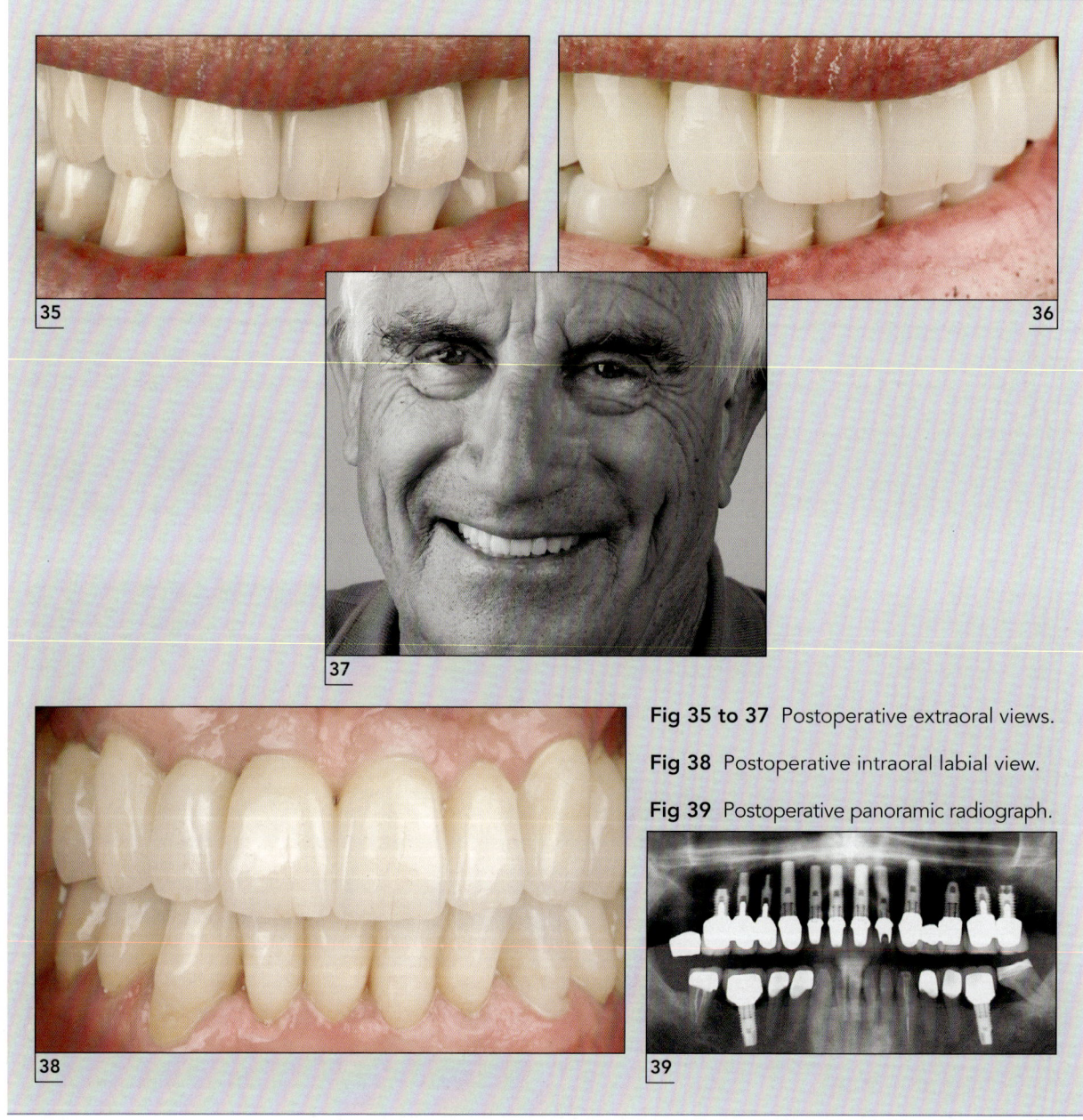

Fig 35 to 37 Postoperative extraoral views.

Fig 38 Postoperative intraoral labial view.

Fig 39 Postoperative panoramic radiograph.

tightened with a torque of 35 Ncm and screw access holes were closed with a light-cure temporary restorative material (Fermit, Ivoclar Vivadent) before final cementation. Adhesive resin (RelyX Unicem Transparent, 3M ESPE, St Paul, MN, USA) was used for definitive insertion of the implant restorations while RelyX luting (3M ESPE) was used for the mandibular natural dentition. Figures 35 to 38 show postoperative views. After definitive insertion, a panoramic radiograph was taken (Fig 39) and an occlusal splint was delivered to protect the restorations during sleep.

CONCLUSION

Scientific evidence, physical properties, and the vast clinical possibilities of the Procera CAD/CAM all-ceramic system have been discussed and illustrated in this article. While the existing evidence demonstrates excellent clinical longevity of high-strength all-ceramic restorations, further research will be necessary to fully explore their advantages and to apply them in the most favorable manner.

ACKNOWLEDGMENTS

The authors thank Dr Pedro Peña for the excellent implant surgery, Mr Iñigo Casares for the design and scanning of the copings and frameworks, and Dale Denny for the beautiful porcelain work featured in the case presentation.

REFERENCES

1. Andersson M, Oden A. A new all-ceramic crown. A dense-sintered, high-purity alumina coping with porcelain. Acta Odontol Scand 1993;51:59–64.

2. Blatz MB, Sadan A, Kern M. Ceramic restorations. Compend Contin Educ Dent 2004;25:306–312.

3. Blatz MB. Long-term clinical success of all-ceramic posterior restorations. Quintessence Int 2002,33:415–426.

4. Sadan A, Blatz MB, Lang B. Clinical considerations for densely sintered alumina and zirconia restorations: Part 1. Int J Periodontics Restorative Dent 2005;25:213–219.

5. Sadan A, Blatz MB, Lang B. Clinical considerations for densely sintered alumina and zirconia restorations: Part 2. Int J Periodontics Restorative Dent 2005;25:343–349.

6. Zeng K, Oden A, Rowcliffe D. Flexure tests on dental ceramics. Int J Prosthodont 1996;9:434–439.

7. Oden A, Andersson M, Krystek-Ondracek I, Magnusson D. Five-year clinical evaluation of Procera AllCeram crowns. J Prosthet Dent 1998;80:450–456.

8. Odman P, Andersson B. Procera AllCeram crowns followed for 5 to 10.5 years: A prospective clinical study. Int J Prosthodont 2001;14:504–509.

9. Fradeani M, D'Amelio M, Redemagni M, Corrado M. Five-year follow-up with Procera all-ceramic crowns. Quintessence Int 2005;36:105–113.

10. Galindo ML, Hagmann E, Marinello CP, Zitzmann NU. Long-term clinical results with Procera AllCeram full-ceramic crowns. Schweiz Monatsschr Zahnmed 2006;116:804–809.

11. Gamborena I, Blatz MB. A clinical guide to predictable esthetics with zirconium oxide ceramic restorations. Quintessence Dent Technol 2006;29:11–23.

12. Holst S, Bergler M, Steger E, Blatz MB, Wichmann M. The application of zirconium oxide frameworks for implant superstructures. Quintessence Dent Technol 2006;29:103–112.

13. Fischer H, Weber M, Marx R. Lifetime prediction of all-ceramic bridges by computational methods. J Dent Res 2003;82:238–242.

14. Aboushelib MN, de Jager N, Kleverlaan CJ, Feilzer AJ. Effect of loading method on the fracture mechanics of two layered all-ceramic restorative systems. Dent Mater 2006;18(Epub ahead of print).

15. Blatz MB, Chapman L, Chiche GJ, Mercante D. Shear bond strength of veneering ceramics to zirconium-oxide ceramic [abstract 0888]. J Dent Res 2006;85(special issue A).

16. Burke FJ, Fleming GJ, Nathanson D, Amrquis PM. Are adhesive technologies needed to support ceramics? An assessment of the current evidence. J Adhes Dent 2002;4:7–22.

17. Blatz MB, Sadan A, Kern M. Resin-ceramic bonding—A review of the literature. J Prosthet Dent 2003;89:268–274.

18. Blatz MB, Sadan A, Kern M. Adhesive cementation of high-strength ceramic restorations: Clinical and laboratory guidelines. Quintessence Dent Technol 2003;26:47–55.

19. Oppes S, Blatz MB, Sadan A, Chiche G, Kee E, Mercante DE. Influence of cement on microleakage and strength of ceramic crowns [abstract 2090]. J Dent Res 2006;85(special issue B).

20. Okutan M, Heydecke G, Butz F, Strub JR. Fracture load and marginal fit of shrinkage-free $ZrSiO_4$ all-ceramic crowns after chewing simulation. J Oral Rehabil 2006;33:827–832.

21. Bindl A, Luthy H, Mormann WH. Thin-wall ceramic CAD/CAM crown copings: Strength and fracture pattern. J Oral Rehabil 2006;33:520–528.

22. Yildirim M, Edelhoff D, Hanish O, Spiekermann H. Ceramic abutments—A new era in achieving optimal esthetics in implant dentistry. Int J Periodontics Restorative Dent 2000;20:81–91.

23. Glauser R, Sailer I, Wohlwend A, Studer S, Schibli M, Scharer P. Experimental zirconia abutments for implant-supported single-tooth restorations in esthetically demanding regions: 4-year results of a prospective clinical study. Int J Prosthodont 2004;17:285–290.

24. Glauser R, Wohlwend A, Studer S. Application of zirconia abutments on single-tooth implants in the maxillary esthetic zone. A 6-year clinical and radiographic follow-up report. Appl Osseointegration Res 2004;4:41–45.

25. Yildirim M, Fischer H, Marx R, Edelhoff D. In vitro fracture resistance of implant-supported all-ceramic restorations. J Prosthet Dent 2003;90:325–331.

26. Att W, Kurun S, Gerds T, Strub JR. Fracture resistance of single-tooth implant-supported all-ceramic restorations after exposure to the artificial mouth. J Oral Rehabil 2006;33:380–386.

27. Att W, Kurun S, Gerds T, Strub JR. Fracture resistance of single-tooth implant-supported all-ceramic restorations: An in vitro study. J Prosthet Dent 2006;95:111–116.

28. Studart AR, Filser F, Kocher P, Gauckler LJ. Fatigue of zirconia under cyclic loading in water and its implications for the design of dental bridges. Dent Mater 2006;10(Epub ahead of print).

29. Sailer I, Feher A, Filser F, Luthy H, Gauckler LJ, Scharer P, Franz Hammerle CH. Prospective clinical study of zirconia posterior fixed partial dentures: 3-year follow-up. Quintessence Int 2006;37:685–693.

THE 9TH INTERNATIONAL SYMPOSIUM &ON
PERIODONTICS &
RESTORATIVE DENTISTRY

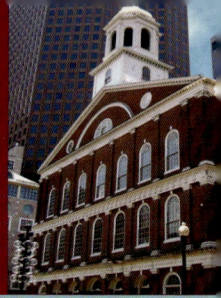

Featuring

A Critical Review of Contemporary Clinical Treatment

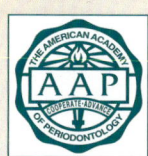

BOSTON, MA
JUNE 7–10, 2007
THE MARRIOTT HOTEL COPLEY PLACE

Chairman
Myron Nevins, DDS

Sponsored by
The International Quintessence Publishing Group, and

The American Academy of Periodontology

Thursday, June 7, 2007

Special Pre-Symposium Sessions
Visit www.quintpub.com for the detailed program

Friday, June 8, 2007

3-D Bone Augmentation for Dental Implants
Louis Rose, Moderator
Sascha Jovanovic
J. Daulton Keith
Jay Malmquist
Stefano Parma-Benfenati
Michael Pikos
Massimo Simion
Carlos Tinti

Periodontal Regeneration: Materials, Methods, and Results
Arnold Binderman, Moderator
Pamela McClain
James Mellonig
Marc Nevins
Giulio Rasperini
Maurizio Tonetti
Hom-Lay Wang

Achieving Optimal Esthetics in Challenging Cases
H.P. Weber, Moderator
David Garber
Ueli Grunder
John Kois
Burton Langer
Anthony Sclar
Masana Suzuki
Masao Yamazaki

Saturday, June 9, 2007

Maxillary Anterior Implants— A Window of Opportunity
Sergio De Paoli, Moderator
Daniel Buser
Christoph Hammerle
Jan Lindhe
Myron Nevins
Dennis Tarnow
Tiziano Testori

Prosthetic and Surgical Solutions for Problematic Cases
Morton Amsterdam, Moderator
Urs Belser
Ole Jensen
Howard Kay
Steven Lewis
Yoshihiro Ono
Stephen Parel

Finally—Clinical Application of Tissue Engineering
Samuel Lynch, Moderator
David Cochran
William Giannobile
Robert Marx
R. Gilbert Triplett

The Application of Orthodontics to Resolve Periodontal and Implant Impasses
Arnold Weisgold, Moderator
Vincent Kokich
Kevin Murphy
Robert Vanarsdall
Roger Wise

Sunday, June 10, 2007

Ceramics—The Creation of Perfection
Lloyd Miller, Moderator
Mauro Fradeani
Galip Gürel
Pascal Magne
Kenneth Malament
Konrad Meyenberg
Avishai Sadan

Recent Advances in Sinus Elevation Surgery
Mariano Sanz, Moderator
Leon Chen
Hideaki Katsuyama
Craig Misch
Tomaso Vercellotti
Stephen Wallace
Georg Watzek

Rational and Predictable Periodontal Plastic Surgery
J. Gary Maynard, Moderator
Edward P. Allen
Michael McGuire
Preston D. Miller
Yasukazu Miyamoto
Gary Reiser
Giano Ricci

For more information and registration, visit www.quintpub.com

CENTRIC RELATION AND ANTERIOR GUIDANCE: OVERCOMING ANTEROPOSTERIOR OBSTACLES

Gideon Nussbaum, DDS[1]

Centric relation is a stable, reproducible orthopedic position[1] that plays a significant role in comprehensive treatment. One diagnostic dilemma encountered when treating to centric relation is changing the relation of the maxillary anterior teeth to their mandibular counterparts. This may alter or even eliminate anterior guidance, which is also an important prerequisite for comprehensive treatment and organic occlusion.[2]

This article will address the problems regarding coupling of the anterior teeth that may occur when treating to centric relation. The discussion will use several clinical cases to illustrate a variety of diagnostic and clinical problems as well as their solutions.

[1]Private practice, Renton, Washington, USA.

Correspondence to: Dr Gideon Nussbaum, 607 SW Grady Way, Suite 300, Renton, Washington 98055, USA. E-mail: gsndds@comcast.net

This article was presented at the Meeting of the International Academy of Gnathology, Congress XXII, September 14–17, 2005, Victoria, British Columbia, Canada.

ESTABLISHING ANTERIOR GUIDANCE

Adequate anterior guidance is a complex function directly related to the form of the teeth, and thus to the vertical and horizontal overlap of the incisors and canines. Anterior guidance is influenced by the proprioception of those teeth, which provides feedback to the masticatory muscles and influences the entire stomatognathic system.[3] Unlike the posterior determinants, such as the slope of the articular eminence, the vertical and horizontal overlap of the anterior teeth are—to variable degrees—amenable to modification. However, any modifications of the anterior teeth must satisfy not only the esthetics and phonetics, but also the overall function. If the disclusive angle is too deep, restrictive symptoms and discomfort may result.[4]

Depending on the clinical situation, a determination should be made regarding three treatment choices: *(1)* restorative modification, *(2)* orthodontic modification, or *(3)* orthodontic and restorative modification.

This decision may be intuitive to a large degree, especially for clinicians who are familiar with comprehensive and multidisciplinary treatments; however, even the experienced clinician must follow specific diagnostic steps to eliminate guesswork and achieve predictable outcomes.

The following questions should be addressed during the planning stages of restorative treatment:

1. Are the lingual surfaces of the maxillary anterior teeth amenable to restorative augmentation?
2. Should the mandibular teeth be lengthened or made wider buccolingually?

Likewise, the following questions should be addressed during the planning stages of orthodontic treatment:

1. Are the maxillary teeth amenable to retraction?
2. Are the mandibular teeth amenable to proclination or extrusion?

TREATMENT PLANNING

Severe skeletal discrepancies are often a clear indication for orthognathic surgery. If the patient is dissatisfied with his or her facial appearance, and especially when the occlusion is a component of any severe facial and skeletal imbalance, orthognathic surgery should be the first choice, since the dramatic improvements in facial balance and esthetics are unparalleled in severe cases. Restorative and orthodontic methods alone may leave the patient disappointed.[5]

Some patients with skeletal discrepancies, however, are totally satisfied with their facial appearance, but have lost the coupling of their anterior teeth and thus do not have adequate anterior guidance because of the discrepancies between their habitual bite (maximum intercuspation) and their seated mandibular position (centric relation).

These types of cases, which are less extreme, will now be illustrated via four case presentations. It is the author's experience that some cases classified as surgical are in fact manageable through restorative and limited orthodontic treatment, without compromising facial esthetics or function. The cases that follow will progress from simple to more complex.

CASE 1

This case illustrates the decision-making process when the diagnostic and treatment planning stages reveal a loss of coupling of the anterior teeth. When the teeth are restored with veneers, coupling with a proper disclusive angle should be achieved.

Figures 1 to 3 show the preoperative condition of the patient. Note the high smile line (ie, a gummy smile). The exact esthetic restorative procedures are not the focus of this article; however, it should be noted that the crown length of the maxillary anterior teeth was increased to its maximum in the apical direction to improve the smile. In excursive movements (Figs 2 and 3), the posterior teeth rubbed against each other, interfering with an organic gnathologic occlusion.

A full diagnostic process was carried out to determine the slope of the articular eminence (Fig 4), including a full-mouth waxup of the teeth involved in treatment (Fig 5). The waxup showed that the lateral incisors and canines were uncoupled. It was decided that restorative treatment of these teeth would achieve the desired anterior guidance.

The diagnostic waxup was transferred to the mandibular arch, which was not treated in this stage of treatment.

To decide if the uncoupled canines and lateral incisors should be veneered or crowned, the restoration of the mandibular anterior teeth was simulated via a putty matrix directly from the waxup. This way, it was clearly seen if the lingual surfaces of the maxillary teeth, which were addressed in this treatment segment, required augmentation with a restoration.

Figure 6 shows the teeth following placement of the veneers and crowns. The central incisors had existing crowns, which were replaced. Next, the mandibular anterior teeth were restored (Figs 7 and 8). Crown lengthening was performed on the maxillary teeth to reduce the excessive gingival display, after which the maxillary anterior restoration was completed (Fig 9). The final result is shown in Fig 10.

CASE 1 (Figs 1 to 10)

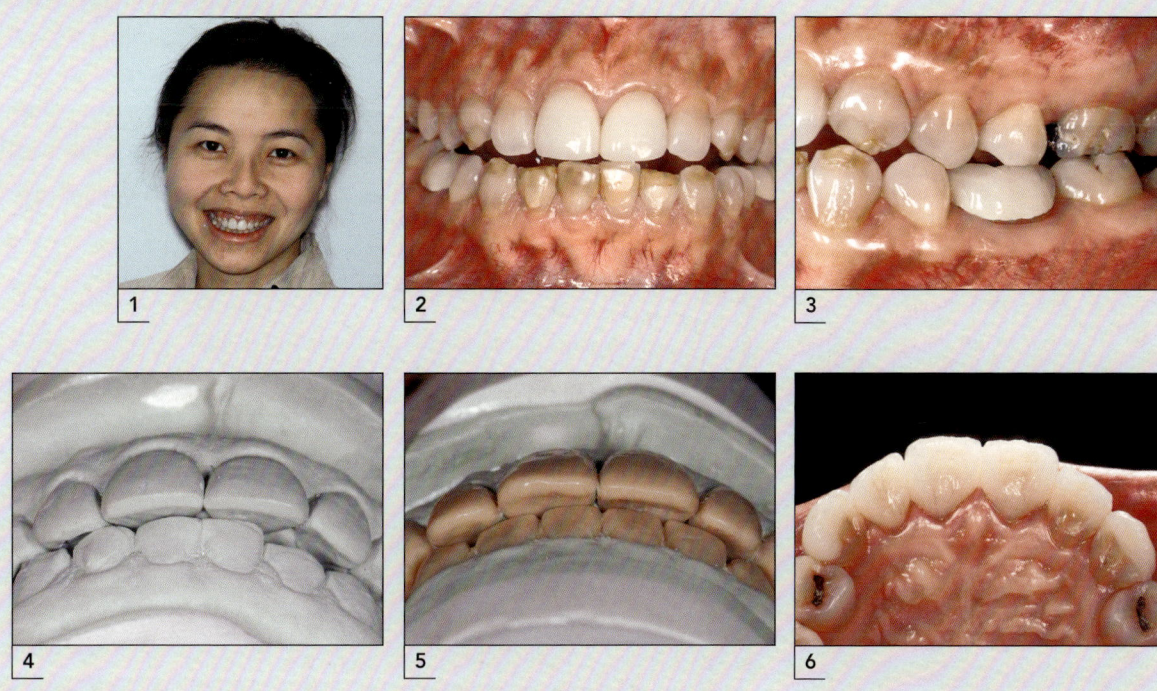

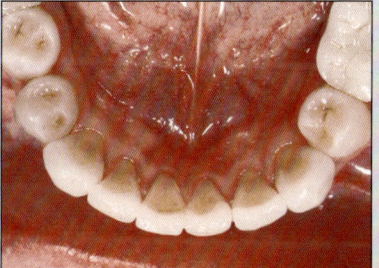

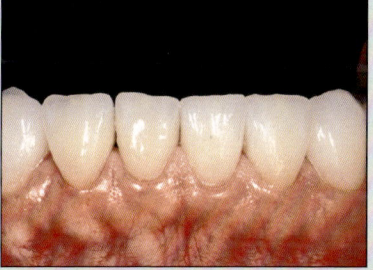

Figs 1 to 3 The initial situation.

Fig 4 Diagnostic casts revealed that the lateral incisors and canines were uncoupled.

Fig 5 The pretreatment waxup.

Fig 6 The maxillary anterior teeth following placement of the veneers and crowns. The central incisors had existing crowns, which were replaced.

Figs 7 and 8 The restored mandibular anterior teeth.

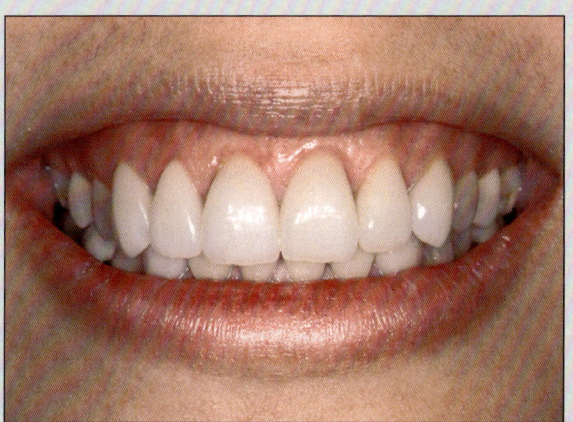

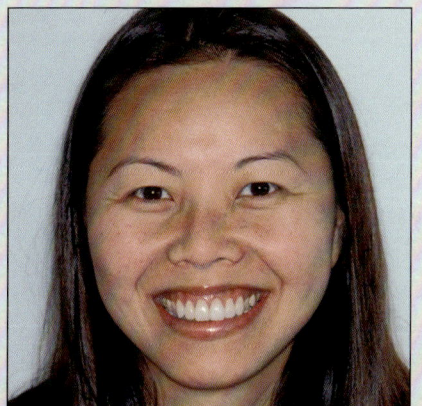

Figs 9 and 10 The final result.

CASE 2 (Figs 11 to 22)

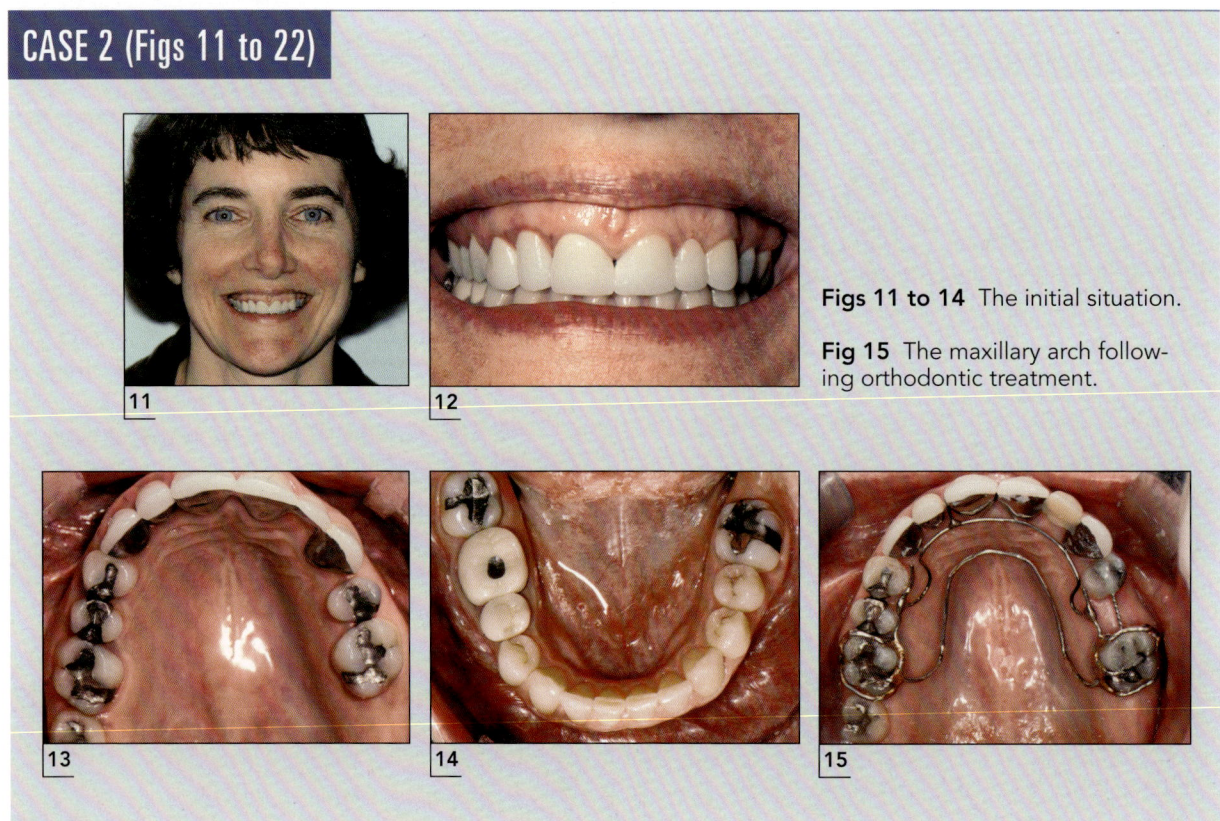

Figs 11 to 14 The initial situation.

Fig 15 The maxillary arch following orthodontic treatment.

CASE 2

This case involved a patient with a history of partial anodontia. The multidisciplinary treatment plan included crown lengthening and orthodontic treatment to procline the retruded maxillary anterior teeth and improve the facial esthetics, as well as to correct the lack of a sufficient overjet and an overly steep anterior guidance, which was restrictive.

The case was complicated by the loss of coupling of the anterior teeth, caused by a centric slide and a seating of the joint, and worsened further by the orthodontic treatment.

The anterior guidance was managed via lengthening and labial thickening of the mandibular anterior teeth, and by accentuating the lingual marginal ridges of the maxillary teeth.

The initial situation showed excessive gingival display, a retruded premaxillary region, and tight anterior coupling with insufficient and restrictive horizontal overlap (overjet) (Figs 11 to 14).

During the diagnostic phase, it became clear that this was a Class II relation, not Class I as it appeared in maximum intercuspation. This "closet" Class II situation is not uncommon, because the true relation often reveals itself once the occlusion "unlocks" following treatment or joint stabilization procedures such as equilibration, or following the use of an orthotic.[6]

Figure 15 shows the maxillary arch following orthodontic treatment. Note the proclination of the anterior teeth. A diagnostic waxup was performed after orthodontic treatment but before crown lengthening (Fig 16).

Most important to this discussion, the lack of coupling in centric relation (Fig 17) was corrected following crown lengthening and thickening (via the placement of labial porcelain veneers on the mandibular teeth). The provisional stage of the treatment is shown in Fig 18.

The final results are shown in Figs 19 to 22.

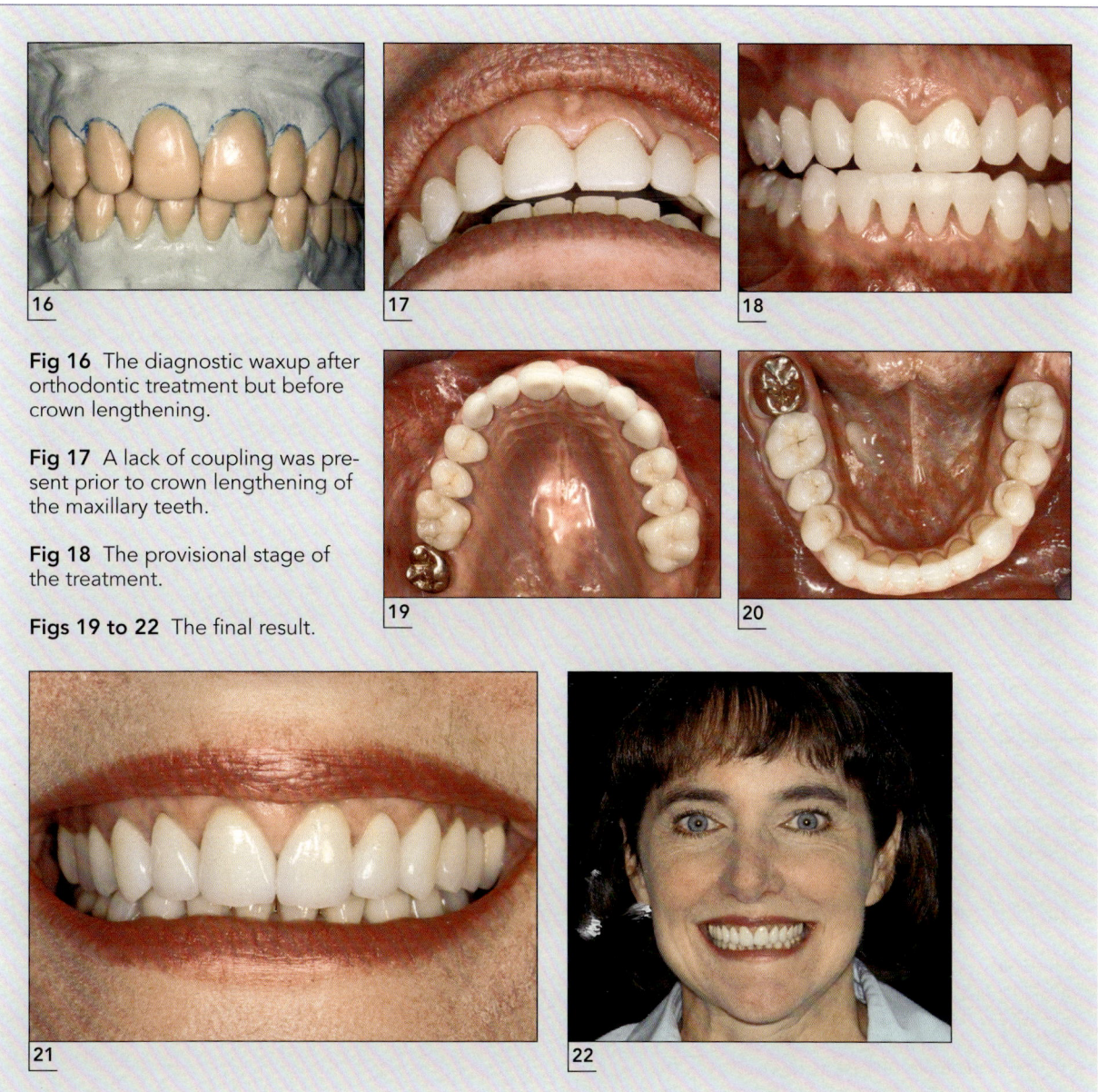

Fig 16 The diagnostic waxup after orthodontic treatment but before crown lengthening.

Fig 17 A lack of coupling was present prior to crown lengthening of the maxillary teeth.

Fig 18 The provisional stage of the treatment.

Figs 19 to 22 The final result.

CASE 3

This case involved the orthodontic and restorative treatment of a patient who also showed severe caries. The orthodontic treatment was complicated by the need for decay control, which required ongoing temporization. The decay was finally brought under control during the provisional stage.

In this case, the anterior guidance was managed by altering the vertical dimension of occlusion (VDO). Often, dental treatment involves increasing the VDO to provide more space for the restorative material; however, in this case, the VDO was decreased to provide coupling and counteract the centric slide and joint resolution, which caused the loss of coupling. It is the author's experience that a small (less than 1 mm) decrease of the VDO in the molar region will make enough of a difference in the anterior region to obtain coupling without any adverse effect on muscle function or chewing efficiency.

CASE 3 (Figs 23 to 33)

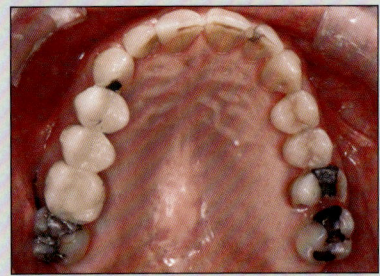 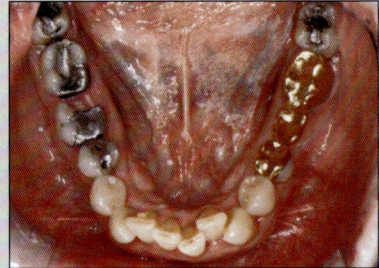 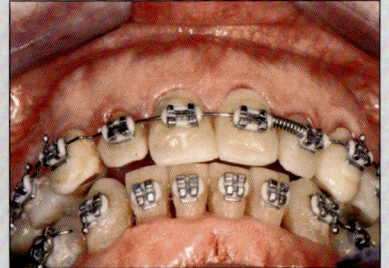

Figs 23 and 24 The initial situation

Fig 25 A lack of coupling was present throughout the disease control and orthodontic treatments.

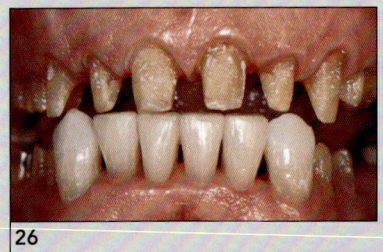 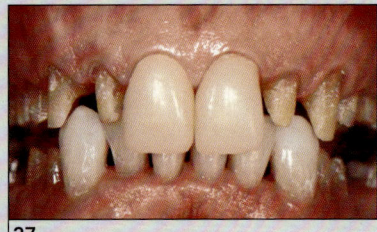

Fig 26 Complete control of the VDO was achieved once the teeth were prepared.

Fig 27 The provisionals of the central incisors placed on the maxillary preparations.

26

27

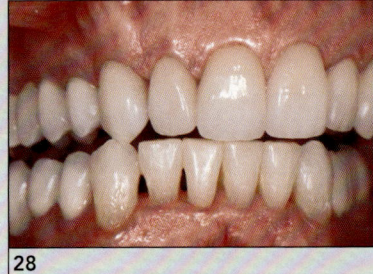 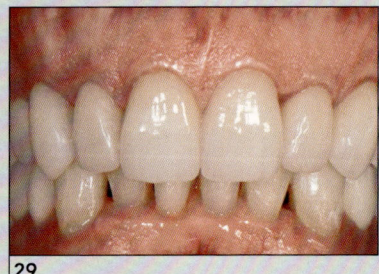 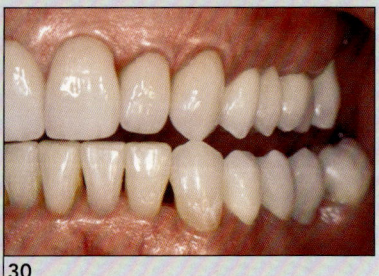

28

29

30

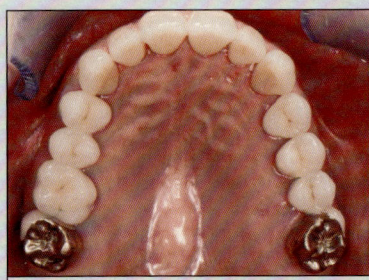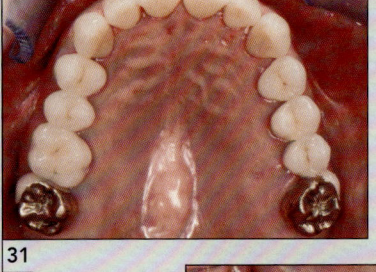

Figs 28 to 33 The final result.

31

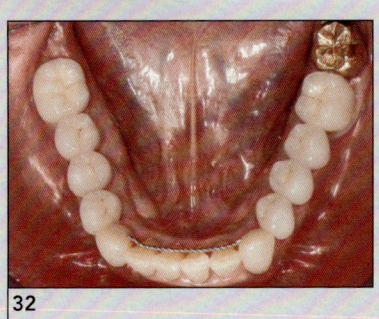

32

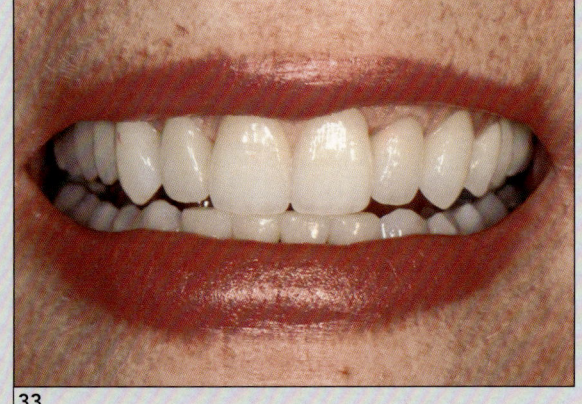

33

CASE 4 (Figs 34 to 44)

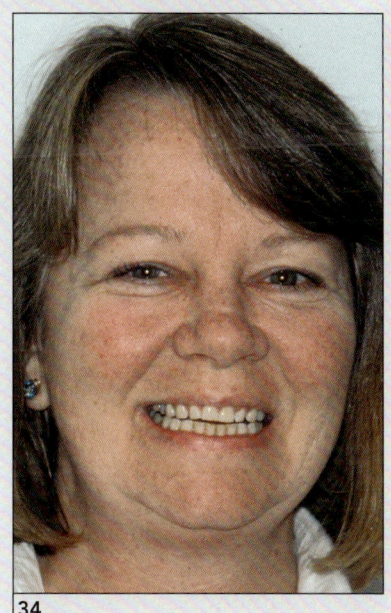

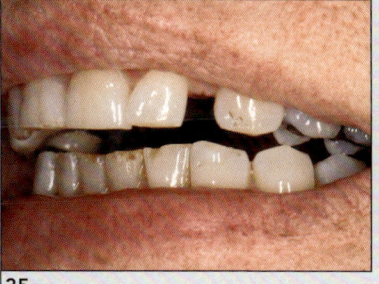

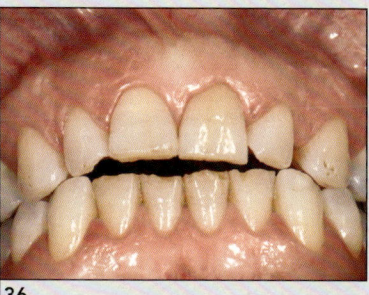

Figs 34 to 36 The initial situation.

Fig 37 A 5-mm discrepancy was noted, in conjunction with upright mandibular teeth and a lack of excessive proclination of the maxillary teeth.

Figures 23 and 24 show the initial situation. Severe decay was present in every quadrant.

A lack of coupling was present throughout the disease control and orthodontic treatments (Fig 25). As with the previous case, a hidden Class II relation was noted during the diagnostic phase, which included mounted casts in centric relation.

Once the teeth were prepared and thus taken out of the equation, the mandible was free to be influenced by the posterior determinants, and total control of the VDO was achieved (Fig 26).

The maxillary provisionals were placed onto the preparations opposing the vitally bleached mandibular teeth. It is also useful to place only the provisional restorations for the maxillary central incisors (Fig 27). This joint loading procedure is similar to the use of a leaf gauge and facilitates treatment to centric relation and control of the VDO.

The final result is shown in Figs 28 to 33. Note that anterior and canine guidance was adequately obtained because of the increased overbite, which was achieved without retraction of the maxillary posterior teeth into an ideal Class I relation.

CASE 4

In this case, orthodontic and restorative treatments were used to camouflage a skeletal discrepancy. Orthognathic surgery was ruled out immediately, because the patient was content with her facial appearance.

The difficulty in establishing anterior guidance was compounded by a centric relation–maximum intercuspation discrepancy and the seating of the condyles, as well as a horizontal open bite of 5 mm in the incisor region.

Although the diastemas could have been treated with restorative means alone, orthodontic and restorative treatments were used to establish adequate anterior guidance.

The diagnostic phase included cast articulation in centric relation and an orthodontic setup, in conjunction with a diagnostic waxup and occlusal equilibration.

Figures 34 to 36 show the preoperative condition. The patient had a slightly retrognathic facial structure, but was not interested in orthognathic surgery, because her primary goals were to have

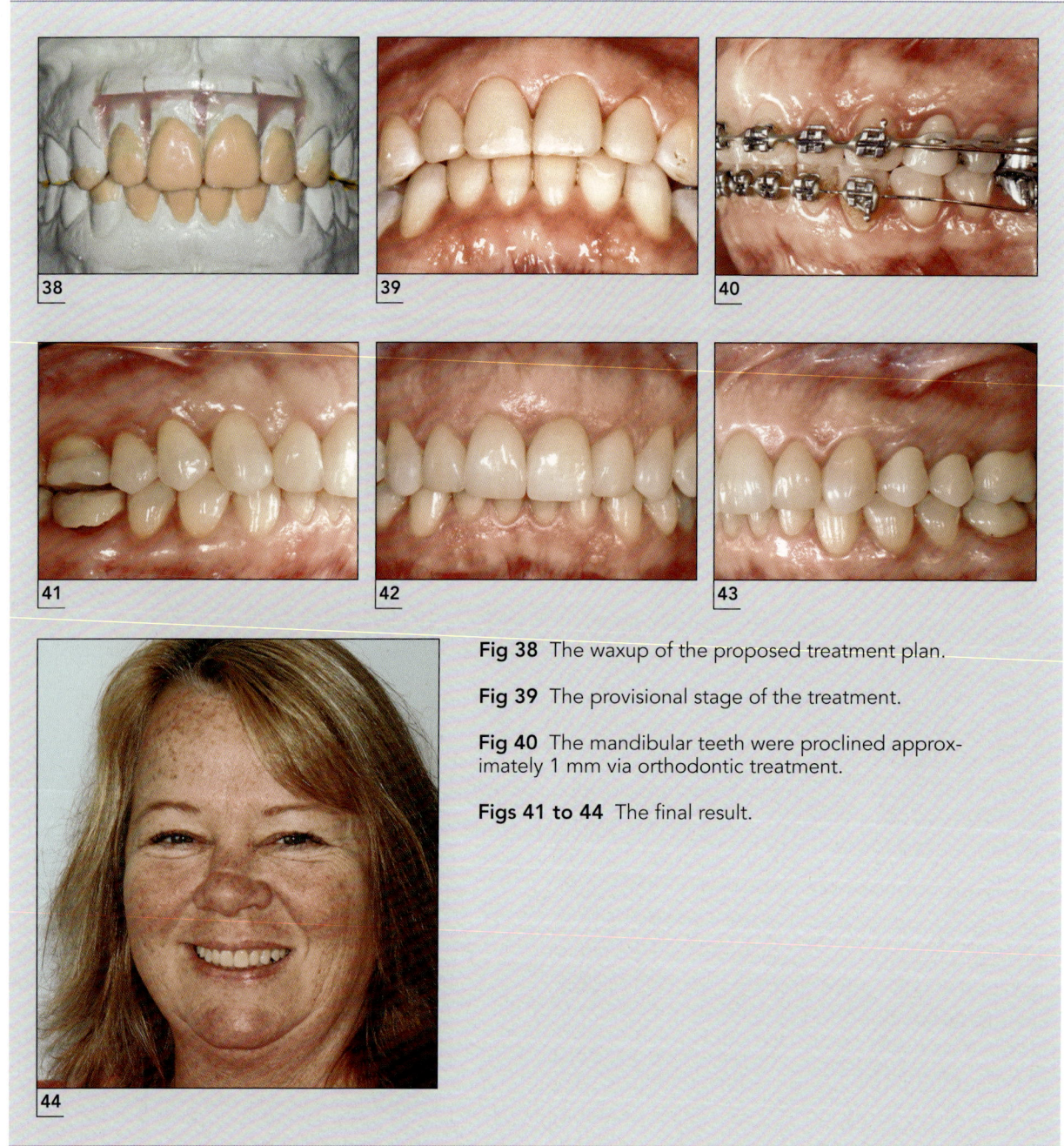

Fig 38 The waxup of the proposed treatment plan.

Fig 39 The provisional stage of the treatment.

Fig 40 The mandibular teeth were proclined approximately 1 mm via orthodontic treatment.

Figs 41 to 44 The final result.

the gaps in her teeth corrected and to have a more esthetic smile.

From a clinical diagnostic perspective, it may seem that because of the 5-mm discrepancy (Fig 37), fairly upright mandibular teeth, and lack of excessive proclination of the maxillary anterior teeth, it will not be possible to provide coupling and still maintain a good appearance with an acceptable interincisal angle.

However, this goal becomes more realistic after equilibrating the casts to bring the VDO back down to the original maximum intercuspation, performing the orthodontic treatment of the diastemas, and creating a waxup of the proposed restorative treatment (Fig 38).

During the provisional stage (Fig 39), the marginal ridges on the crowns of the maxillary anterior teeth were accentuated to reach toward the opposing dentition, which was orthodontically proclined (Fig 40) by approximately 1 mm and lengthened with resin composite.

Figures 41 to 43 show the nearly completed restored mouth. A few of the remaining molars will be restored in the future. Overall, the treatment goals were achieved: the patient's smile was improved and the anterior guidance was restored (Fig 44).

CONCLUSION

Since comprehensive treatment must include consideration of the temporomandibular joint (TMJ), the diagnosis and treatment of the TMJ should be intimately related to any treatment that involves significant occlusal changes. After all, the teeth and dental arches are not free floating in the face, but rather are continuous with the jaw and are connected to the TMJ in a very clear manner. Therefore, if changes to the occlusion affect the joints, the reverse is true as well.

This article discussed and presented cases dealing with the adverse effect of losing the coupling of the anterior teeth as a consequence of changes at the TMJ.

Considering that the normal range of centric relation is much larger than the ideal—be it the cephalometric ideal seen in orthodontics or the golden proportional ideal seen in restorative/esthetic dentistry—it is possible to make large dental changes that still fall within the normal range. Therefore, when dealing with cases that seem too complex to treat during clinical examination, it is incumbent on clinicians to truly diagnose the situation via casts, equilibrations, and waxups to discover what is truly possible.

ACKNOWLEDGMENT

The author would like to acknowledge Uwe Brosamle, CA, USA, for the fabrication of the restorations.

REFERENCES

1. Okeson J. Management of Temporomandibular Disorders and Occlusion. St Louis: Mosby, 1998.
2. Hockel J. Orthopedic Gnathology. Chicago: Quintessence, 1983.
3. Rufenacht C, Lee R. Fundamentals of Esthetics. Chicago: Quintessence, 1990.
4. McHorris WH. Focus on anterior guidance. J Gnathol 1989;8:3–13.
5. McLaughlin R, Bennet J, Trevisi H. Systemized Orthodontic Treatment Mechanics. St Louis: Mosby, 2004.
6. Roth R. Gnathological concepts and orthdontic treatment goals. In: Jarabak J, Fizzell J (eds). Technique and Treatment with Light Wire Appliances, ed 2. St Louis: Mosby, 1972:1160–1223.

PRECISION IN DENTAL ESTHETICS

CLINICAL AND LABORATORY PROCEDURES

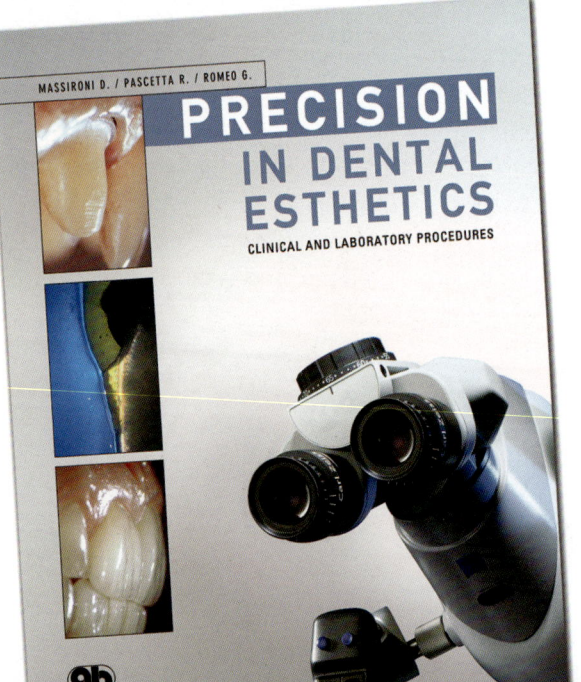

Domenico Massironi, Romeo Pascetta, Giuseppe Romeo

Achieving a favorable esthetic and functional prosthetic outcome requires progression through an intricate sequence of clinical steps. The first section of this beautifully illustrated, highly practical book guides the dental practitioner through each of these steps in the treatment of various common clinical situations. The second part addresses the technical and esthetic aspects of dental laboratory techniques, covering precision in metals and new and conventional ceramics as well as the esthetic realization of prosthetic devices, including diagnostic waxups, communication with patients and clinicians, color matching, and the fabrication of ceramic restorations. Throughout the book, the authors advocate a philosophy emphasizing close clinician-technician collaboration and cooperation, and they are strong proponents of the use of the microscope in most dental procedures.

CONTENTS

1. Managing the Treatment Plan with the Prosthetic Team
2. Magnification Systems Used in Dentistry
3. Tooth Preparation for Complete Crowns
4. Finish Line Designs for Complete Crown Preparations
5. Repositioning and Completing the Finish Line with Oscillating Instruments
6. Technical Considerations for Soft Tissue Retraction
7. Clinical Considerations for Provisional Prostheses
8. Technical Considerations for Provisional Prostheses
9. Custom Impression Trays and Impression Materials
10. Laboratory Procedures
11. Using Ceramic in Prosthetic Restoration
12. Esthetic Considerations for Ceramic Restorations
13. Cementation *(with Federico Ferraris)*

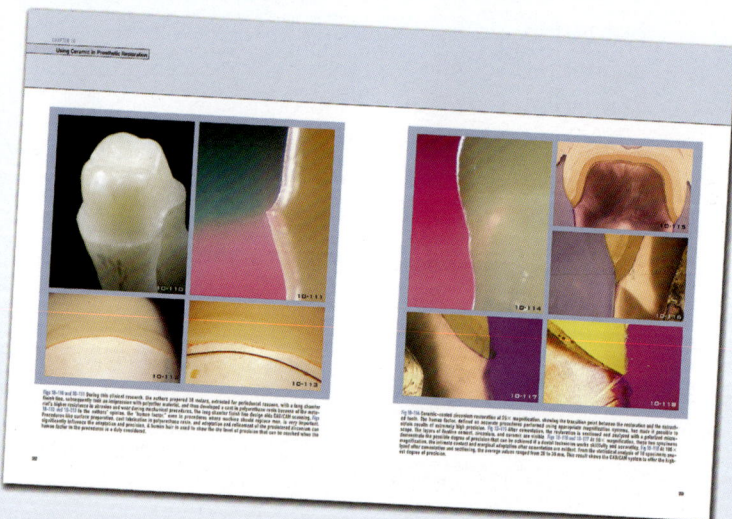

464 pp; 1,331 illus (mostly color); ISBN 1-85097-163-3; US $278

Quintessence Publishing Co, Inc 4350 Chandler Drive, Hanover Park, IL 60133

Website: www.quintpub.com • E-mail: service@quintbook.com • Tel: (630) 736-3600 • Fax: (630) 736-3633

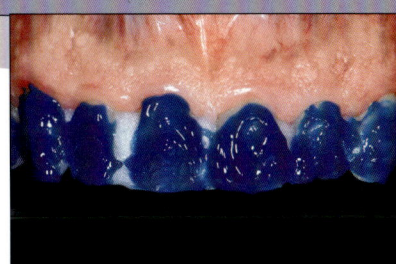

PERMANENT DIAGNOSTIC PROVISIONALS: PREDICTABLE OUTCOMES USING PORCELAIN LAMINATE VENEERS

Galip Gürel, MSc[1]

Porcelain laminate veneers are conservative and esthetic dental restorations that offer both longevity and durability when used correctly and in appropriate clinical situations.[1]

In a retrospective study, Friedman[2] showed that the success rate of porcelain laminate veneers is as high as 94%. In other words, only 7 of 100 veneers are likely to fail over a 15-year period, as long as there is no presence of bruxing or parafunction. Most failures will be either fractures (67%), microleakage (22%), or delamination or debonding (11%).

It should be noted that veneers are bonded on minimally invasive preparations, usually on enamel. Of course, failure can and will occur from time to time; therefore, extra attention must be paid to the tooth structure. It has been established that bonding veneers to enamel provides the best bond strength.[3–5] It is unlikely that microleakage or debonding will occur when the entire tooth is surrounded with enamel; however, one potential problem is porcelain fracture caused by external forces, such as the occlusal force.

DENTINOENAMEL JUNCTION

The dentinoenamel junction (DEJ) is an important part of the tooth's overall structural strength. This is because of a fascinating feature of the

[1]Private practice, Istanbul, Turkey.

Correspondence to: Dr Galip Gürel, Tesvikiye cad. Bayer apt. 143/6, Nisantasi, 80200 Istanbul, Turkey. E-mail: galipgurel@galipgurel.com

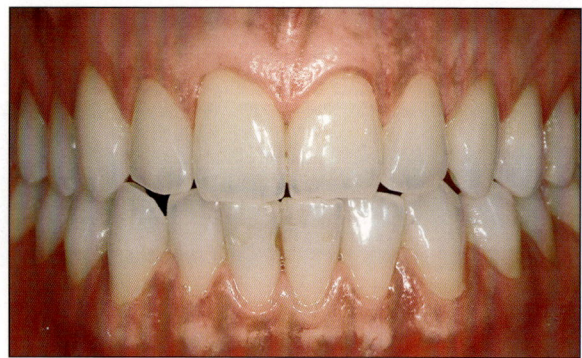

Fig 1 Short maxillary teeth with an edge-to-edge occlusion.

natural tooth—a complex fusion at the DEJ that can be regarded as a fibril-reinforced bond.[6] If the preparations are limited, there will be no flexibility because of the tooth's natural rigidity. Even if the preparation line passes through the DEJ margin and enters into the dentin, it will not create a significant problem for minor invasions. However, overdoing the rotated or aggressive preparation of protrusively placed teeth will lead to larger areas of exposed dentin structure, which will lower the bonding values and cause flexing of the tooth structure.[7] When an aggressively prepared tooth starts flexing, especially in conjunction with a very rigid porcelain veneer, the adhesive luting resin absorbs all of the stresses. When the tooth receives occlusal forces and flexes, the luting resin at the margin will start to peel off. Because of this, some microleakage/ delamination is likely to occur.

To minimize these problems, it is important to be very precise during tooth preparation.[8] The ideal indication for the use of porcelain laminate veneers is teeth that are perfectly aligned but require some additive restorations to obtain lip support or length (Fig 1). The amount of tooth structure that is removed should be equivalent to the thickness of the veneer that will be placed.

STANDARD PREPARATION

After placing an amount of resin composite on the tooth surface that is equivalent to the thickness of the porcelain laminate veneer and is of the necessary length (Figs 2a to 2c), the tooth preparation can begin with the use of a depth cutter (Figs 3a to 3c).[9–11] The amount of tooth preparation depends on the restorative material and the color of the tooth. Once the amount is established, the surface of the tooth is painted in a different color and a round-ended fissure bur is used to finalize the facial reduction. It is important to hold the bur at three different angles to respect the facial convexity of the tooth structure. This makes it possible to achieve a uniform thickness throughout the porcelain material, or as it should now be called, the porcelain buildup.

Once this major reduction is accomplished, the preparation should be finished on the gingival margins and extended toward the papilla to finish the interproximal elbow preparation, which is very important, especially when the case involves discolorations. If the depth is not correctly prepared, the joint between the dark-colored tooth and the light-colored porcelain will be visible when the teeth are viewed from an angle. To prepare this elbow-like extension, the bur should be held almost 60 degrees toward the palate until the exact depth has been achieved, and then held upright to finish the interproximal preparation.[12] Finally, the butt-joint preparation of the incisal edge must provide enough room for the lab technician to build up the necessary esthetic effects, eg, translucence, opalescence, and the incisal silhouette.

In situations in which the shape, volume, and contours of the tooth will mostly remain unchanged, a standard preparation will be the easiest to execute (Figs 4a to 4c).[13] The amount of the preparation should be equivalent to the amount of porcelain buildup that is required (Figs 5a to 5d).

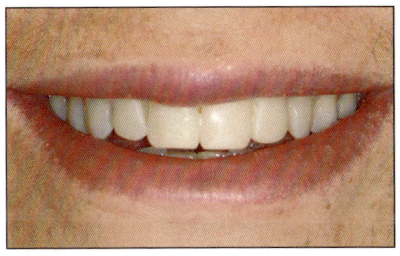 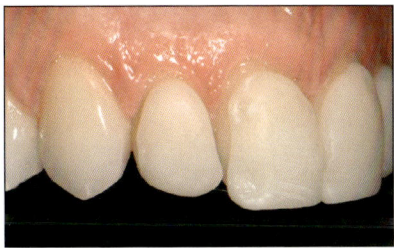 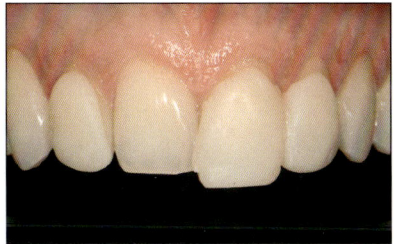

Figs 2a to 2c The short and lingually positioned teeth were lengthened and an additive facial resin composite mockup was placed to evaluate the lip support.

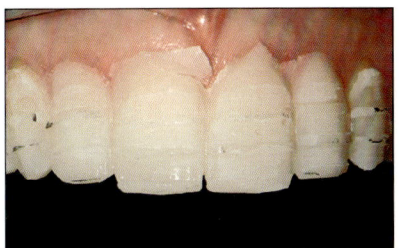 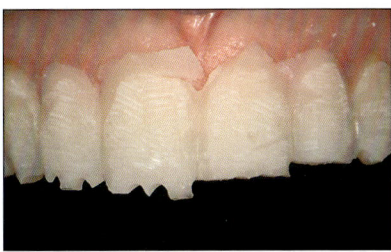 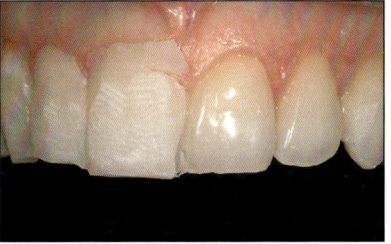

Figs 3a to 3c The tooth preparation should follow the mockup that was placed on the unprepared teeth. Note the untouched enamel surface even after the facial preparation is finished.

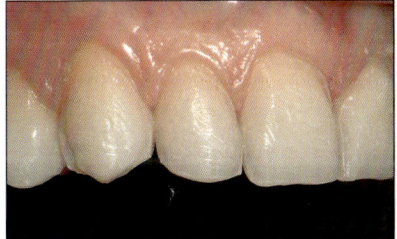 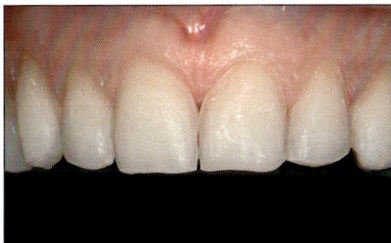 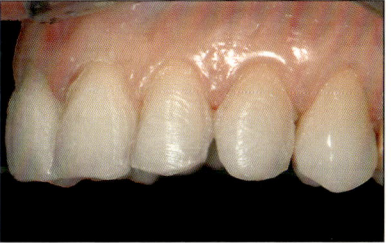

Figs 4a to 4c For better bonding, the aprismatic enamel layer must be removed. Note the minimally invasive preparation.

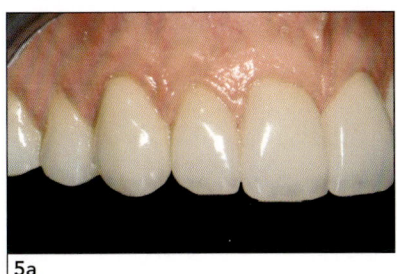 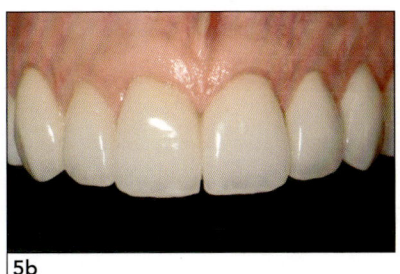 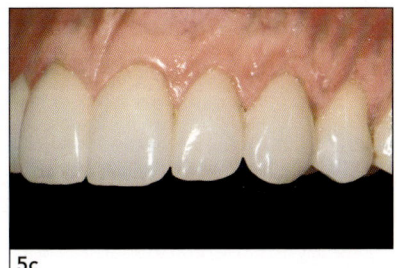

5a 5b 5c

Figs 5a to 5d The finished and bonded veneers. Note that the edge-to-edge position was changed to a reasonable overjet-overbite relationship by building up the veneers labially.

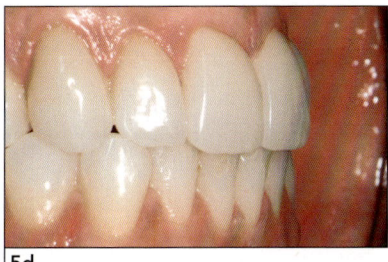

5d

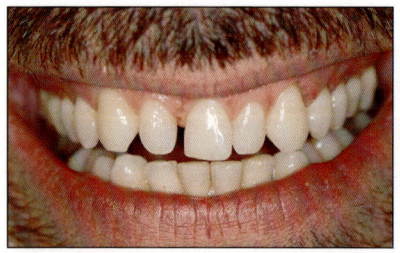

Fig 6 A shifted left central incisor caused by the loss of the right central incisor.

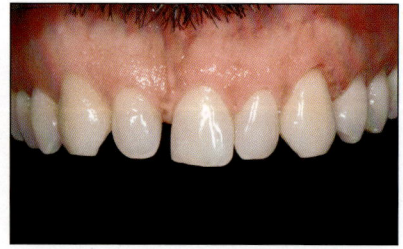

Fig 7 The mesially shifted midline created obvious esthetic problems.

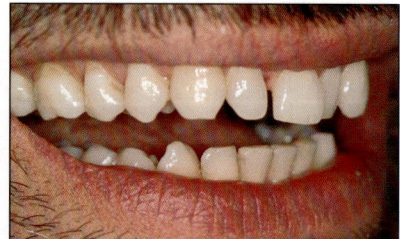

Fig 8 Some crowding was evident.

IMPROPERLY ALIGNED TEETH

A major concern when using porcelain laminate veneers is space management. Both spaced dentitions and crowded teeth can present problems. Treatment will be more difficult if the spaced teeth are not properly aligned in the dental arch. In these cases, it may be unclear how to plan the treatment and prepare the teeth.

The first goal should be meeting the esthetic desires of the patient. Because a new smile design will be created, all changes must be clearly communicated to the patient.

This communication between the patient and clinician will determine the success or failure of the treatment. The clinician must be completely in tune with the attitude of the patient, including both verbal requests and the less obvious nonverbal cues. The clinician who presents a confident, competent, and observant attitude will make the patient feel relaxed and positive about the treatment. The planned smile design should be discussed with the patient and modified to fit his or her opinions.

However, the patient may request an alteration that is unrealistic for his or her face. The ability to say "no" will save the clinician many sleepless nights, as one setback can easily erase many brilliant and successful procedures. If the esthetic dentist and patient find it difficult to agree on the objectives, it is in the best interests of both parties to not begin the treatment.

Treatment Planning

In this case of an improperly aligned dentition, the midline showed a large shift to the right caused by a loss of the right central incisor when the patient was 12 years old (Fig 6). The left central incisor had shifted towards the right and the right lateral incisor had shifted mesially (Fig 7).

Research shows that a midline shift is not noticeable until it is almost 4 mm to one side. However, if the midline is canted more than 1 to 1.5 mm, it will be readily noticeable.[14] With that in mind, if the midline is kept perpendicular to the papillary line, a move less than 1 to 2 mm to one side will not be visible to the untrained eye.

However, when the mouth was viewed from an angle, another problem was visible in the palatal and lingual direction (Fig 8). Some teeth were aligned lingually, such as the left lateral incisor, and some teeth were aligned buccally, such as the left canine. The question was how to prepare these teeth—should the protruded teeth be prepared aggressively, and should resin composite or porcelain be used on the lateral incisor?

Another aspect that must be evaluated is the occlusal plane. In this case, the anterior teeth were slightly shorter than the posterior teeth.

There are many different options for treatment planning. For example, in this patient, orthodontic treatment could be used to push the maxillary left and right quadrants toward the posterior, thus providing space for implant treatment at the right central incisor site. Another option would be to

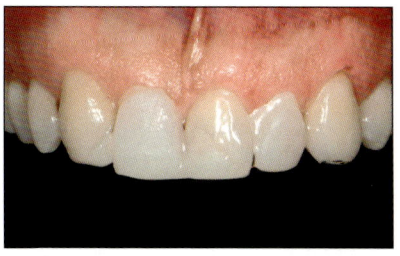 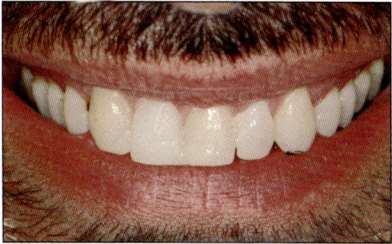 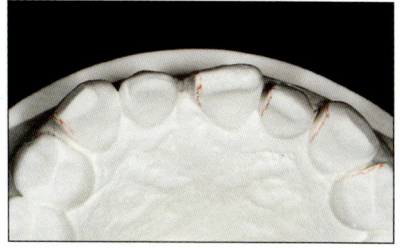

Figs 9a and 9b The easiest way to predict the final outcome is to prepare a new smile design with a mockup and check it against the frame of the teeth, ie, the lips.

Fig 10 Occlusal view of the cast. Note the slicing performed on the mesial aspects of the left incisors and canine.

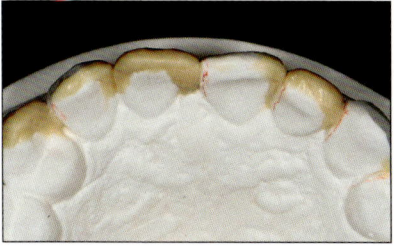 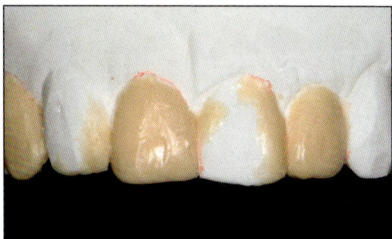 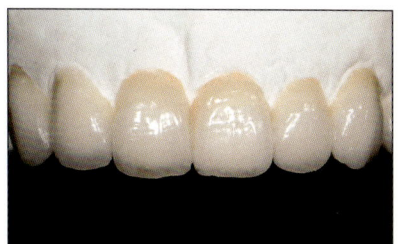

Figs 11a and 11b A rough waxup was fabricated to evaluate the correct proportions and functional relation of the maxilla and mandible.

Fig 12 The final waxup, built with the layering technique. Note that all details, such as the dentin, enamel, and incisal translucencies, are delicately layered.

shift the midline toward the left, bringing the lateral incisor mesially to the central incisor site and then restoring the necessary teeth with porcelain laminate veneers. A third option would be restoring the teeth with veneers without using orthodontics.

However, success would not be guaranteed because of the large midline shift. In fact, at this stage, it is impossible to be sure of any outcome through intraoral and extraoral examinations alone.

Resin Composite Mockup

In complex cases such as this, a resin composite mockup is necessary before the situation can be explained to the patient (Figs 9a to 9b).[15–17] A hand-carved resin composite can be used to visualize the final outcome of the veneer treatment. At this stage, the mockup can be less precise than a waxup; it is needed to estimate the necessary changes and their effect on the lip structure, pho-

netics, and occlusion.[18–20] Further, the mockup will serve as a guide for the lab technician to build the waxup. Eventually, all information will be shared with the patient, so the first step of treatment will be approved by both the clinician and patient.[21]

Next, two impressions of the dental arch should be taken: one of the original tooth structure and another of the mockup.

Waxup

The lab technician should use the two impressions along with a silicone index to fabricate the final waxup. The technician is now free to slice the cast, as long as any cuts stay within the limits of the enamel (Fig 10). Thus, the soft tissue can be recontoured and the first, rough waxup used to evaluate the esthetics and function of the expected outcome (Figs 11a and 11b). If accepted, the layering waxup technique is used to simulate the translucency and texture of dentin and enamel (Fig 12).

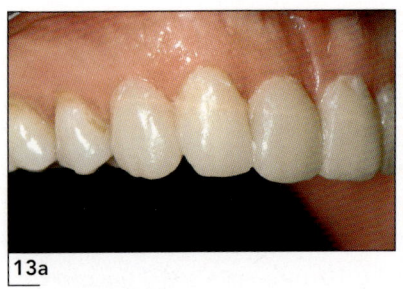

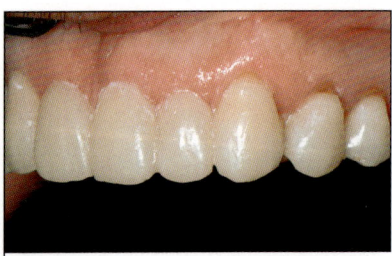

13a

13b

Figs 13a and 13b The waxup was transferred to the mouth. The impression taken from the waxup was filled with a flowable resin composite and polymerized in the mouth as the esthetic pre-evaluative temporary.

Esthetic Pre-recontouring

At this stage, a silicone index was fabricated from the final waxup to indicate the final contours of the teeth. The index was then placed over the dental arch to help visualize the existing situation relative to the final outcome of the waxup and veneers. One or more of the teeth may touch or push the silicone index buccally, indicating that those teeth are either rotated or positioned more labially than the expected final outcome. Any such teeth should be trimmed. This process is known as *esthetic pre-recontouring* (EPR).[22]

Esthetic Pre-evaluative Temporaries

Next, the waxup was applied on the tooth structure (Figs 13a and 13b). A transparent silicone impression was fabricated from the waxup and filled with the flowable resin composite. It was then placed on the unprepared teeth and light cured, and the translucent impression material was removed from the mouth. Note that this would not have been possible if the teeth had been rotated or positioned buccally, or if EPR had not been performed, because the impression would not have fit over the teeth. Next, the gingival margins were trimmed slightly. At this stage, the exact final outcome of the treatment has been achieved, only in plastic instead of porcelain. Because the patient is not anesthetized, it is very easy to evaluate the esthetic outcome, since the lip support and coronally extended length can be easily observed and approved by the patient. Further, the functional movements should be evaluated to ensure that an anterior constriction is not present and that the phonetics are acceptable.

These plastic teeth are known as *esthetic pre-evaluative temporaries* (EPTs), which simply means they were fabricated before preparing the teeth.[22-24] The EPTs can then be checked with the silicone index to ensure that they are placed correctly in the mouth.

Tooth Preparation Using EPTs

An important question remains: Is this technique still applicable when the teeth are not properly aligned? In other words, can the final outcome of such cases be precisely and predictably achieved using this method?

The benefit of EPTs, besides the ability to evaluate the esthetics and function of a given treatment, is that they provide an excellent guideline for preparing the teeth. Because the EPT represents the exact final contours of the treatment, the teeth can be prepared in the same way as in a very simple case in which the teeth are properly aligned (Fig 14).[22-24] In some situations, the tooth surface may not be prepared at all; if, for example, the tooth is placed too palatally (ie, more than 0.6 mm from the facial contours of the EPT) (Fig 15). Once any major reductions are made with the depth cutters followed by the round fissure burs, the gingival margins and interproximal lines can be finished (Fig 16).

A similar amount of reduction of the incisal edge will be necessary in most cases, and usually, very little healthy incisal tooth structure will require preparation (Figs 17a and 17b).

After making the necessary reductions, the butt joint margins should be finished.[25] The reduction can then be checked against the silicone index.

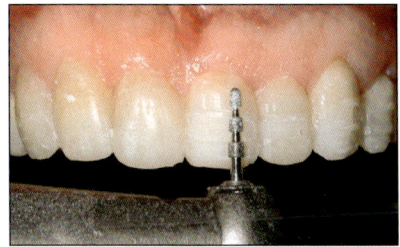

Fig 14 Once the restoration is approved by the patient and clinician, the teeth can be prepared through the EPT.

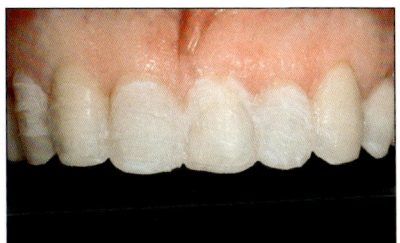

Fig 15 A round diamond fissure bur was used to make the necessary facial reduction. Note the untouched enamel surface of the left lateral incisor.

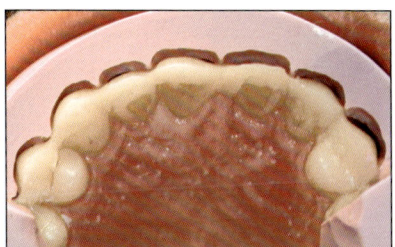

Fig 16 This precise preparation depth can be checked against the silicone index.

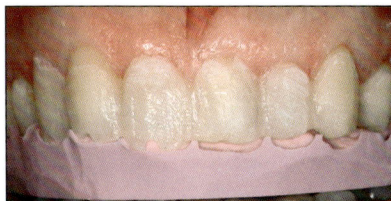

Figs 17a and 17b The incisal edge position with the EPT in place was checked against the silicone index. Note the almost untouched incisal edges.

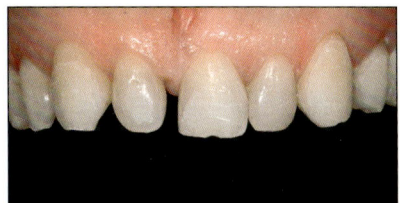

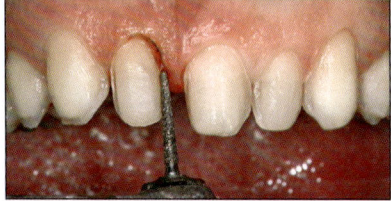

Fig 18 The soft tissue mesial to the right lateral incisor was recontoured and the preparation was peformed subgingivally.

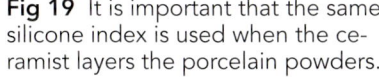

Fig 19 It is important that the same silicone index is used when the ceramist layers the porcelain powders.

Fig 20 The finished and polished porcelain laminate veneers on the cast.

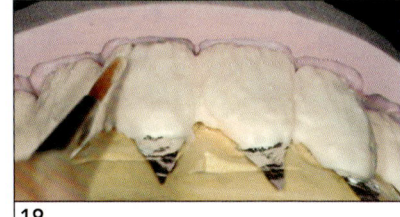

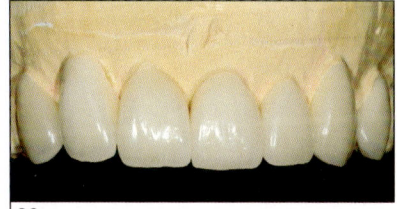

When treating with porcelain laminate veneers, the gingival chamfer should be finished supragingivally in most cases, unless severe discoloration or a spaced dentition are present. In such cases, the gingival and elbow-like extension preparations should be subgingival in that region in order to build up an emergence profile with the porcelain laminate veneers that will push the papilla slightly coronally, thus creating a clear triangular shape. In this case, the mesial, gingival portion of the right lateral incisor was prepared slightly subgingivally so that the ceramist would have more control over the emergence profile of the porcelain laminate veneers, which helped the papilla fill the gap between the two veneers (Fig 18).

Once the preparation was finished, an impression was taken and the provisionals were fabricated. The provisionals should be exactly the same as the EPT. This provides the patient a second chance to evaluate the final outcome.

Laboratory Procedures

The veneers can be fabricated with feldspathic porcelain on a refractory die or platinium foil. Other options include pressable ceramics with external staining or layering techniques.

In this case, the feldspathic porcelain was fabricated using the platinium foil technique. Whichever method is used, it is important that the ceramist uses the same silicone index (Fig 19) that has already been approved by the patient. The rest of the procedures depend on the ceramist's knowledge and ability regarding the integration of color, form, shape, and texture (Fig 20).

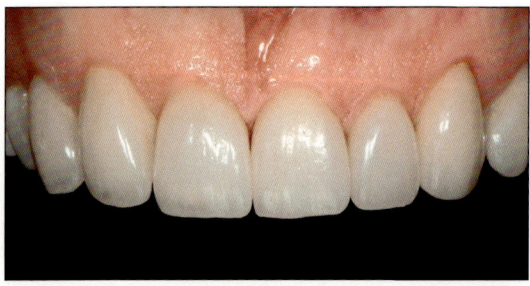
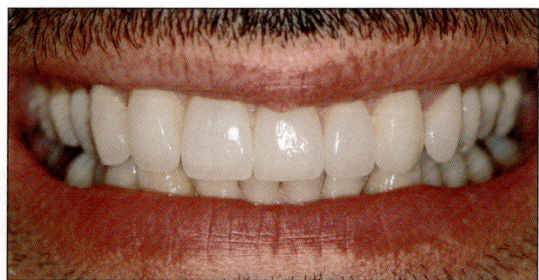

Figs 21a and 21b The finished and polished veneers in the mouth. Note the slight gingival irregularity. Since the lips completely covered this area, there was no need for overengineering.

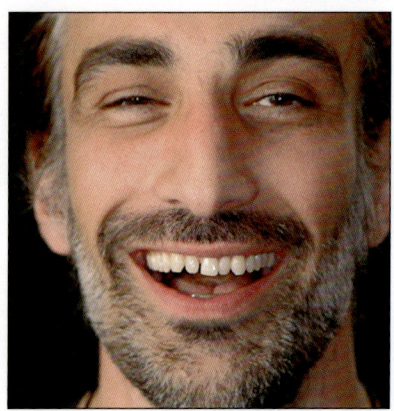
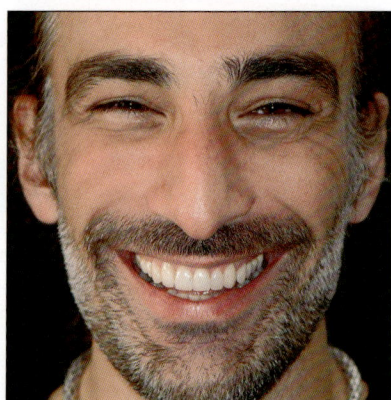

Figs 21c and 21d Before *(left)* and after *(right)* photographs.

Try-in

Once the veneers are completed, a try-in should be scheduled. Preferably, the provisionals should be removed and the veneers tried in without anesthesia.

The veneers should be tried in one at a time to check the marginal fit, and then all together to check the color and overall integration with the lips and face.

Bonding

For the bonding procedure, the author suggests using a sectional rubber dam placed in the mouth. Preferably, the bonding should start with the central incisors, proceed to the lateral incisor and canine on one side, and then finish with the lateral incisor and canine on the remaining side.

The soft tissues should be handled very gently. Once the veneer has been placed and is completely seated, the author suggests spot-tacking it with a 2-mm turbo tip. This will hold the veneer in place. Next, switch the tip of the light source to a larger diameter, such as 13 mm. Light cure the excess flesh around the gingiva for only 1 or 2 seconds. This will not fully polymerize the luting resin; instead, it will produce a jelly-like consistency that is very easy to clean using an explorer dipped in adhesive liquid. Finally, use dental floss to clean the interproximal contacts.

At this stage, the luting resin can be fully polymerized. To finalize the bonding procedure, a no. 12 blade should be used to clean any remaining resin composite on the margins. If necessary, the margins can be polished with a rubber cup. Do not use a diamond bur, which will ruin the glaze and polish of the porcelain.

The final position, form, phonetics, and lip support of porcelain laminate veneers should never be a matter of guesswork. The same esthetic, functional, and phonetic results that are established during the EPT and provisionalization phases will be present in the final outcome (Figs 21a to 21d).

Fig 22a Discolored teeth with a short crown length, along with some missing molars and unesthetic crowns in the posterior.

Fig 22b The teeth after periodontal therapy and bleaching.

Figs 23a to 23d The waxup was fabricated using the layering technique. The esthetics and functional integration were clearly improved.

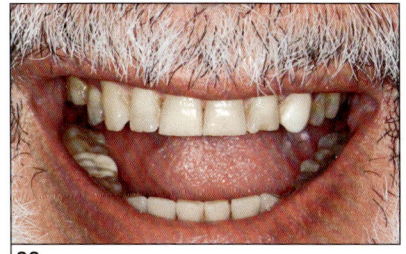

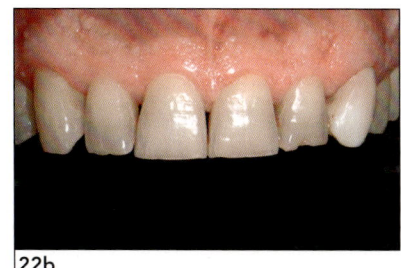

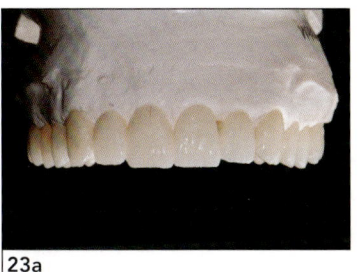

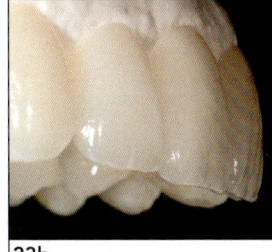

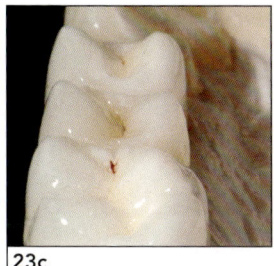

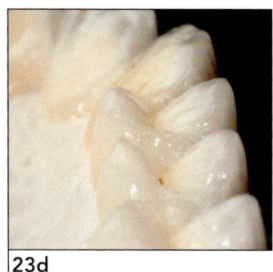

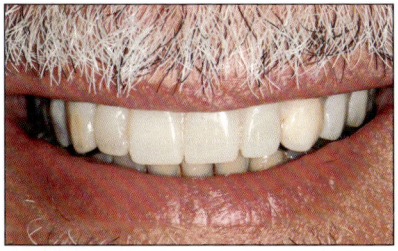

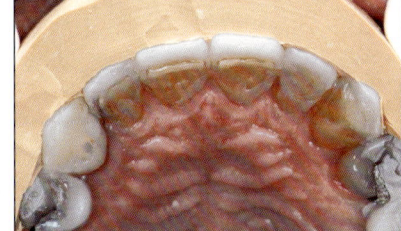

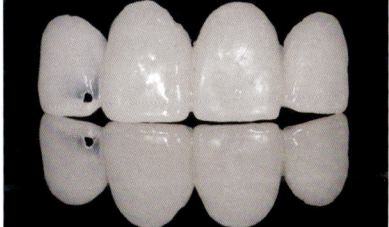

Fig 24a The waxup was transferred to the mouth to create the EPT, as described previously.

Fig 24b The silicone index was used to check the position of the EPT.

Fig 25 The EPT was removed from the mouth so that the margins could be trimmed.

LATEST CONCEPTS: PERMANENT DIAGNOSTIC PROVISIONALS

It is important to note that no amount of planning can guarantee patient satisfaction. Even if the patient approves the final outcome, there are many factors, such as feedback from friends and family or self-confidence issues, that may influence and change the patient's opinion of the restoration. In hindsight, some patients may claim that the provisional period was too short for them to form an adequate opinion of the esthetics and function. Therefore, in particularly complex cases, and when the occlusion requires extra, long-term at-

tention, the trial period of the EPTs can be extended. Such a case will now be presented (Figs 22a and 22b).

As with the other procedures, a delicate waxup was prepared (Figs 23a to 23d). The EPTs were fabricated and fully polymerized as described above (Figs 24a and 24b), and then removed so that the gingival margins could be trimmed (Fig 25). At this stage, the EPTs are indirect resin composite or acrylic restorations.

Next, the tooth surface was fully acid etched, the adhesive was applied, and the EPT was bonded permanently. The result can be called a *permanent diagnostic provisional* (PDP). This ap-

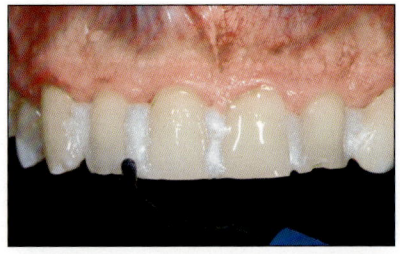

Fig 26a The interproximal contours of the teeth were blocked out with an opal dam.

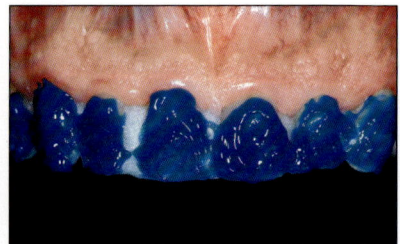

Fig 26b Total acid etching was performed.

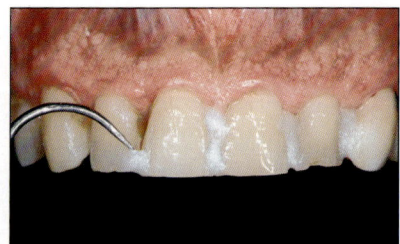

Fig 26c The teeth were rinsed and the blockout material was removed.

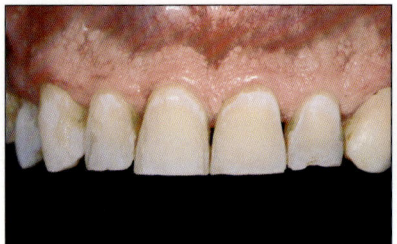

Fig 26d The margins were unetched in order to achieve low bond values, thus making it easier to prepare these margins later in the process. Note the etched and unetched enamel surfaces.

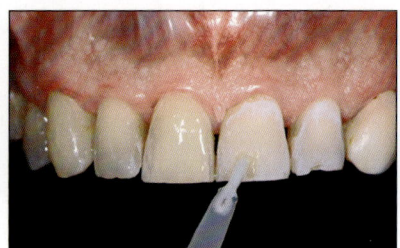

Fig 26e The bonding agent was applied to the enamel surfaces.

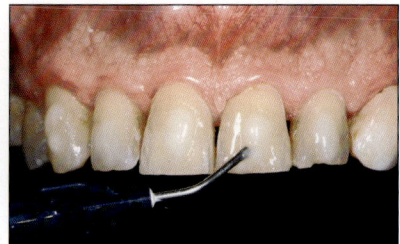

Fig 26f Flowable resin composite was placed on the tooth surfaces and the PDPs were fully bonded.

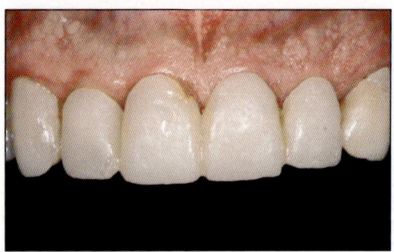

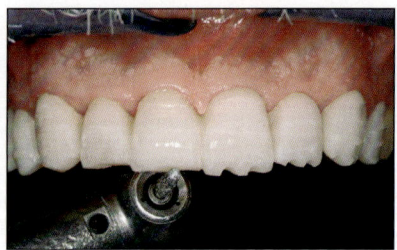

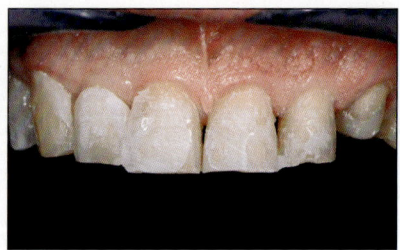

Figs 27a to 27c Six weeks after delivering the PDP, the esthetic and functional outcome was approved by the patient and tooth preparation proceeded as follows: (a) facial preparation with the depth cutter, (b) incisal reduction, (c) preparation to accommodate the thickness of the veneers.

proach allows for an extensive try-in and evaluation of the restorations before the teeth have even been prepared.[26]

However, there are some drawbacks to this approach. In the author's experience, when the PDPs are fully bonded, there may be problems with the preparation of the gingival and interproximal margins. Therefore, to avoid acid etching these areas (thus producing a lower bond value), the interproximal margins should be isolated (eg, with an opal dam, as used for bleaching) and the adhesive should be fully applied to prevent microleakage at the margins (Figs 26a to 26f).

Because the PDP is fully bonded, the patient can wear the restoration for as long as he or she needs to evaluate and approve the overall performance, including the occlusion, esthetics, and phonetics (Fig 27a to 27c).

When the patient returned for the final restoration, the preparation and proceeding steps were exactly the same as described above (Figs 28 to 31).

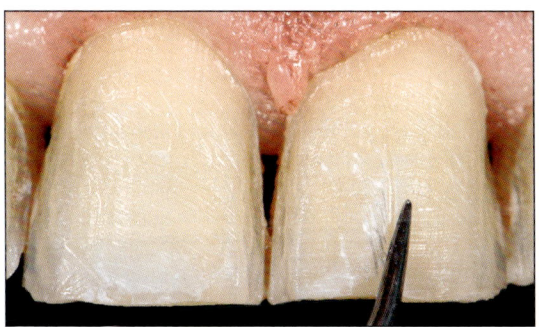

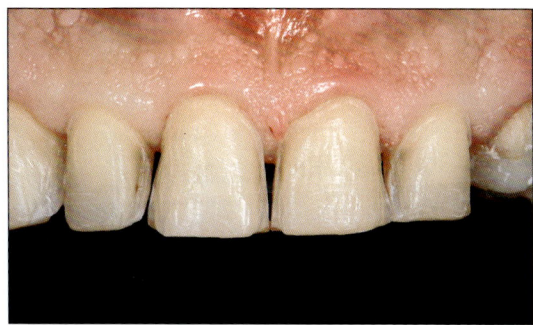

Fig 28a An explorer was used to check for any remaining resin composite. If any resin composite is still bonded on the enamel, it will leave a dark scratch mark.

Fig 28b The finished, minimally invasive preparations.

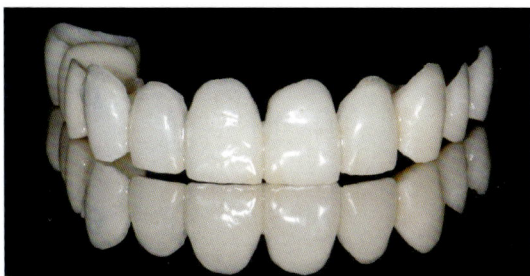

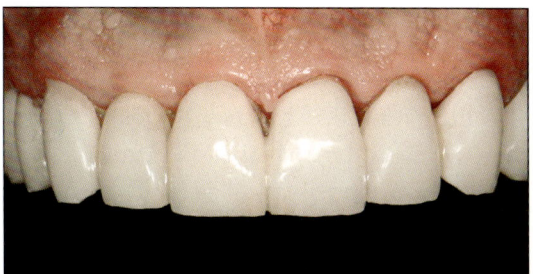

Figs 29a and 29b After taking the impressions, the prefabricated provisionals were placed on the prepared teeth.

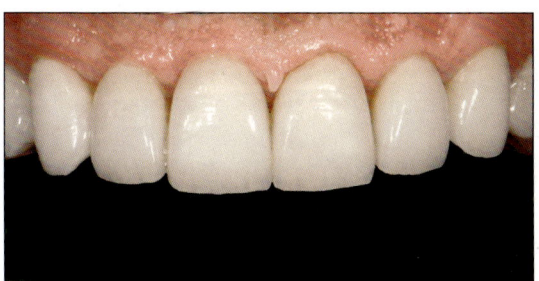

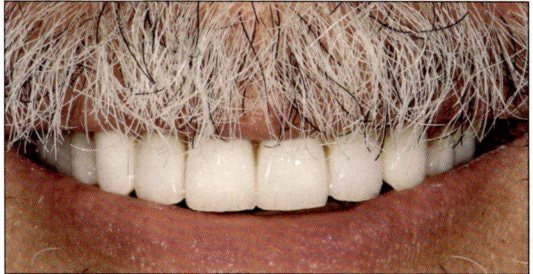

Figs 30a and 30b The final porcelain laminate veneers in the mouth.

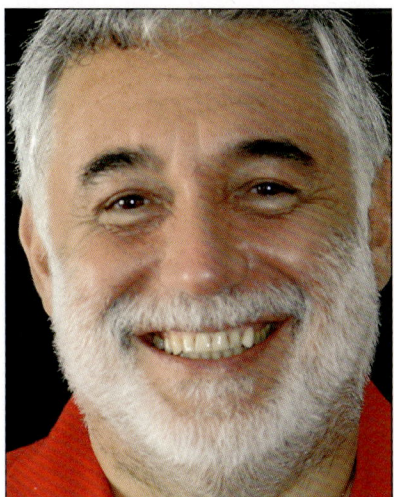

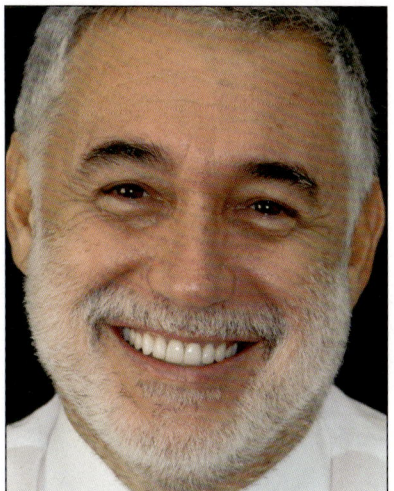

Figs 31a and 31b Before *(left)* and after *(right)* photographs.

CONCLUSIONS

Porcelain laminate veneers have a well-established record of success as esthetic and functional restorations. However, even though it is a very conservative treatment option, some basic rules should be followed. The case must be carefully selected, and thorough treatment planning must be practiced. The use of the mockup, waxup, EPT, and silicone index provides the best esthetic, phonetic, and functional outcomes, allows for easy communication with the patient, and requires minimal invasion of the recipient tooth.

Esthetics is a subjective issue, and requires excellent communication between the clinician, patient, and technician. The techniques described in this article aid in communication and provide excellent, reliable outcomes. By allowing the patient to evaluate the performance of the restoration over a long period, better results and increased satisfaction are ensured.

ACKNOWLEDGMENTS

Special thanks to Gerald Ubassy, CDT for his work on the first case, Jason J. Kim, CDT MDT for the second case, and Yi-Yuan Chang, MDC for the third case.

REFERENCES

1. Horn HR. Porcelain laminate veneers bonded to etched enamel. Dent Clin North Am 1983;27:671–684.
2. Friedman MJ. A 15 year review of porcelain veneer failure—A clinician's observations. Compend Contin Educ Dent 1998;19:625–636.
3. Noack MJ, Roulet J-F. Rasterelelektronenmikroskopische Beurteilung der Atzwirkung verschiedener Atzgele auf Schmelz. Dtsch Zahnarztl Z 1987;42:953–959.
4. Van Meerbeek B, Peumans M, Gladys S, et al. Three-year clinical effectiveness of four total-etch dentinal adhesive systems in cervical lesions. Quintessence Int 1996;27:775–784.
5. Van Meerbeek B, Perdigao J, Lambrechts P, et al. The clinical performance of adhesives. J Dent 1998;26:1–20.
6. Lin CP, Douglas WH, Erlandsen SL. Scanning electron microscopy of type I collagen at the dentin-enamel junction of human teeth. J Histochem Cytochem 1993;41:381–388.
7. Magne P. Douglas WH. Porcelain veneers: Dentin bonding optimization and biomimetic recovery of the crown. Int J Prosthodont 1999;12:111–121.
8. Belser UC, Magne P, Magne M. Ceramic laminate veneers: Continuous evolution of indications. J Esthet Dent 1997;9:197–207.
9. Garber DA, Goldstein RE, Feinman RA. Porcelain Laminate Veneers. Chicago: Quintessence, 1988.
10. Nixon RL. Porcelain veneers. An esthetic therapeutic alternative. In: Rufenacht CR. Fundamentals of Esthetics. Chicago: Quintessence, 1990:329–368.
11. Garber DA. Porcelain laminate veneers: Ten years later. Part 1. Tooth preparation. J Esthet Dent 1993;5:56–62.
12. Morley J. The role of cosmetic dentistry in restoring a youthful appearance. J Am Dent Assoc 1999;130: 1166–1172.
13. Strub JR, Turp JC. Esthetics in dental prosthetics. In: Fischer J. Esthetics and Prosthetics. Chicago: Quintessence, 1999:11.
14. Kokich VO Jr, Kiyak HA, Shapiro PA. Comparing the perception of dentists and lay people to altered dental esthetics. J Esthet Dent 1999;11:311–324.
15. Dietschi D. Free-hand composite resin restorations: A key to anterior aesthetics. Pract Periodont Aesthet Dent 1995;7:15–25.
16. Vanini L. Light and color in anterior composite restorations. Pract Periodont Aesthet Dent 1996;8:673–682.
17. Baratieri LN. Esthetics: Direct Adhesive Restorations on Fractured Anterior Teeth. Chicago: Quintessence, 1998:135–205.
18. Peumans M, Van Meerbeek B, Lambrechts P, Vanherle G, Quirynen M. The influence of direct composite additions for the correction of tooth form and/or position on periodontal health: A retrospective study. J Periodontal 1998;69:422–427.
19. Chiche GJ, Pinault A. Esthetics of Anterior Fixed Prosthodontics. Chicago: Quintessence, 1994:33–52.
20. Romano R, Bichacho N, Touati B (eds). The Art of the Smile. Chicago: Quintessence, 2005:7–24.
21. Dawson PE. Evaluation, Diagnosis and Treatment of Occlusal Problems, ed 2. St Louis: Mosby, 1989:274–297.
22. Gürel G. The Science and Art of Porcelain Laminate Veneers. Chicago: Quintessence, 2003.
23. Gürel G. Predictable, precise and repeatable preparation for porcelain laminate veneers. Pract Proced Aesthet Dent 2003;151:17–24.
24. Gürel G. Predictable tooth preparation for porcelain laminate veneers in complicated cases. Quintessence Dent Technol 2003;26:99–111.
25. Castelnuovo J, Tjan AH, Phillips K, Nicholls JI, Kois JC. Fracture load and mode of failure of ceramic veneers with different preparations. J Prosthet Dent 2000;83:171–180.
26. Gürel G, Bichacho N. PPAD. Permanent diagnostic provisional restorations for predictable results when redesigning the smile. Pract Proced Aesthet Dent 2006;18:281–290.

TRANSFER OF INFORMATION FOR ESTHETIC AND FUNCTIONAL PREDICTABILITY IN SEVERE WEAR CASES

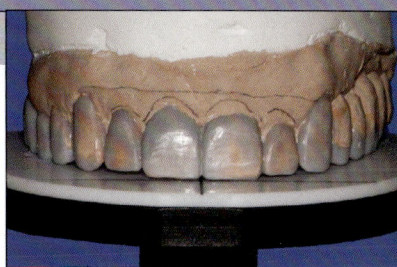

Tal Morr, DMD, MSD[1]

Prosthodontists are often called upon to reconstruct the occlusion in patients with severe wear. There may be a multitude of issues to address in such cases, including attrition, abrasion, and erosion, all of which contribute to uneven wear and compensatory eruption throughout the arches. There may also be incisal wear and/or interproximal wear, and as a result, the occlusal plane may need leveling and lengthening for enhanced esthetics and to allow correction and control of the occlusal relationship.

Treating the edentulous patient requires the fabrication of occlusion rims to allow evaluation of critical esthetic and functional information, mounting of the final casts, and fabrication of esthetic and functional complete dentures.[1–8] The esthetic and functional information includes determination of the incisal edge position at rest, the occlusal plane, midline and angulation of the midline, lip support, facial plane of the incisors, arch form, and buccal corridors. In addition, the clinician can evaluate the vertical dimension of occlusion, check phonetics, and take a centric record.

CRITICAL ESTHETIC DETERMINANTS

All comprehensive treatment planning should begin with an esthetic evaluation. Evaluation of the face is essential in determining the ideal esthetic orientation of the teeth from a horizontal perspective. The horizontal reference planes will help the clinician align the occlusal plane and the soft tissue levels along with other related esthetic determinants. The horizontal reference planes should be evaluated from two perspectives: the frontal and the sagittal. The frontal perspective is assessed by having the patient look out into the horizon and choosing the ideally leveled plane. The most commonly used horizontal reference

[1]Private practice, Aventura, Florida, USA.

Correspondence to: Dr Tal Morr, 20760 West Dixie Hwy, Aventura, FL 33019, USA. E-mail: tmprostho@yahoo.com

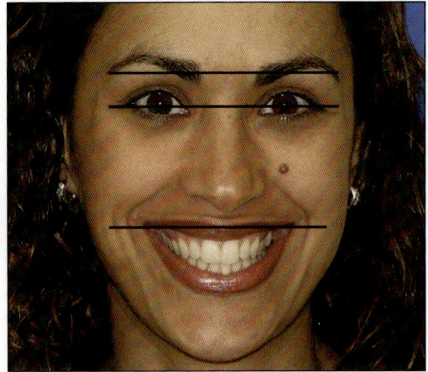

Fig 1 Horizontal reference planes: ophriac, interpupillary, and commisural planes respectively.

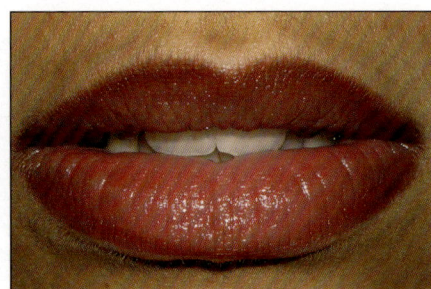

Fig 2 Sample incisal edge at rest.

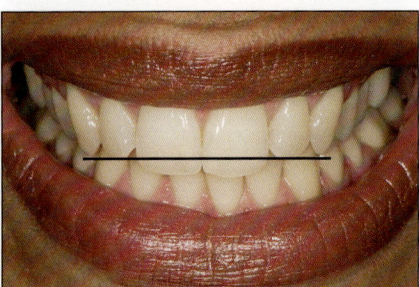

Fig 3 Sample incisal plane.

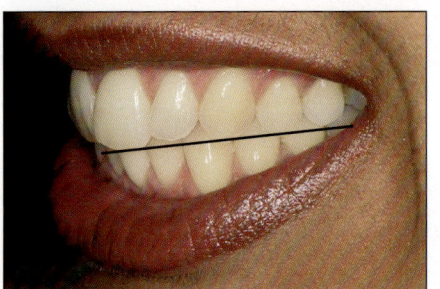

Fig 4 Sample occlusal plane.

planes include the ophriac line, interpupillary line, and commissural line (Fig 1).[5,9–10] Most people are slightly asymmetric in these planes, and in these cases, the floor is used as the horizontal reference plane. From a lateral (sagittal) perspective, the patient holds his or her head erect, again looking out to the horizon. From the saggital perspective, the horizontal reference plane should again be leveled with the floor. Once the horizontal reference plane is established, the critical esthetic determinants are established in relationship to the horizontal reference plane.

The incisal edge position, incisal plane, and occlusal plane are the three most important esthetic determinants in the development of the treatment plan. These determinants enable the clinician to transfer information throughout the treatment, and are related in specific ways to other esthetic criteria. The first step in determining the position of the teeth is evaluation of the incisal edge position at rest (Fig 2). Tooth exposure is considered to be esthetic in the 1- to 5-mm range.[8,11] To achieve this range, tooth proportions can be adjusted by either shortening or lengthening the anterior teeth. For example, if crown lengthening is indicated on teeth that were previously ideally proportioned, the incisal edge length can be reduced. Maintaining a minimum of 1 mm of tooth exposure at rest should be the goal. Once the final incisal edge position is determined, the incisal plane (a line from canine to canine in the anterior portion of the occlusal plane) is evaluated (Fig 3). The incisal plane should be leveled to the chosen horizontal reference plane (the floor, interpupillary line, etc), and evaluated from the frontal perspective while the patient is smiling. The next step is to evaluate the occlusal plane from a sagittal view of the patient's smile. The occlusal plane should be flat from the incisal edge of the central incisor back to approximately the mesial of the first molar (Fig 4). The illusion of a radial relationship of the smile line to the lower lip derives from the cant of the maxilla in the frontal perspective (see Fig 3).

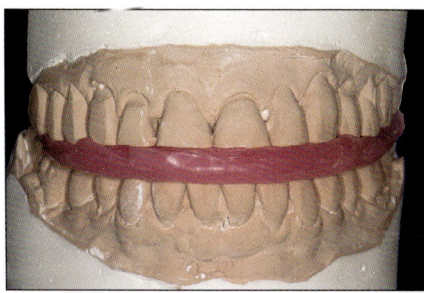

Fig 5 Casts mounted using the occlusal plane guide.

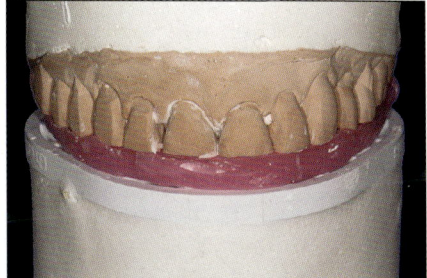

Fig 6 Mounting plate mounted against the occlusal plane guide.

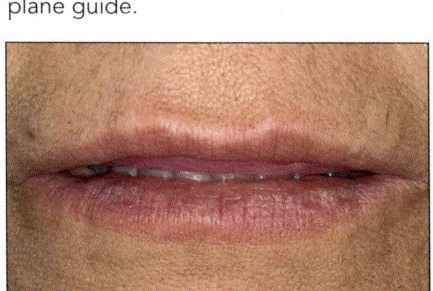

Fig 7 Evaluation of the incisal edge at rest with the occlusal plane guide.

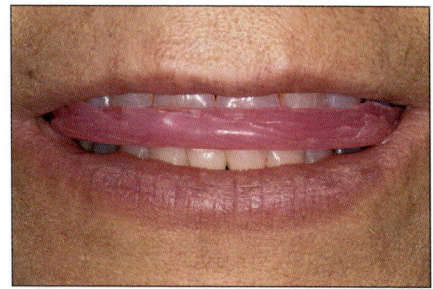

Fig 8 Evaluation of the occlusal plane using the occlusal plane guide with the patient smiling.

The original occlusal plane guide technique

As with the edentulous patient, a method of transferring critical esthetic and functional information is needed to allow the technician to predictably achieve the ideal esthetic orientation and occlusal relationship of the teeth in the waxup. The original occlusal plane guide technique[12] employed a vacuform machine and acrylic resin to evaluate the ideal esthetic determinants in the patient's mouth. The maxillary cast was mounted to the articulator with the occlusal plane guide using a facebow, an earbow, or a dentofacial analyzer. The mandibular cast was mounted at the evaluated vertical dimension using the occlusal plane guide (Fig 5). The mandibular cast was removed, and a flat mounting plate was placed against the acrylic resin and mounted to the lower member of the articulator (Fig 6). When the occlusal plane guide was removed, the space between the original cast and the flat plane indicated the exact amount the teeth needed to be lengthened. Unfortunately, there were problems with delamination of the acrylic

resin from the vacuform material, and the acrylic resin was difficult to trim and shape. Wax is a more suitable material for this technique due to its ease of trimming and shaping, and its ability to take a centric record at the appropriate vertical dimension (Figs 7 and 8). The centric record should be taken at the appropriate vertical dimension with both the ideal overjet and overbite relationship. This will minimize the negative effect of the arc of closure if the casts are not mounted in a direct relationship to the hinge axis of the articulator and the vertical dimension is modified.

Diagnostic waxup fabrication

Step 1: Develop the occlusal plane

Mount the casts on the articulator at the correct vertical dimension and relative to the mounting plate, and remove the maxillary wax occlusal plane guide. The resulting space indicates the amount of wax to be added to reach the ideal occlusal plane (Fig 9). First, add wax to the incisal edges of the anterior teeth and the buccal cusp

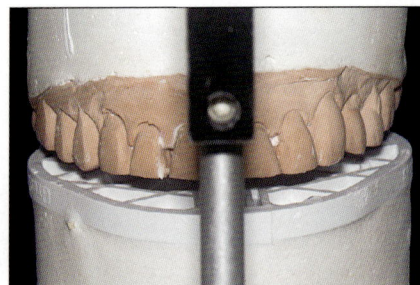

Fig 9 Maxillary cast without the occlusal plane guide.

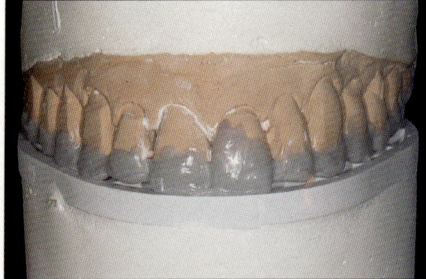

Fig 10 Wax is added to incisal edges of anterior teeth and buccal cusp tips of posterior teeth.

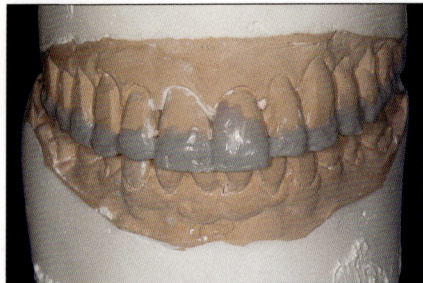

Fig 11 Evaluation of vertical dimension with the casts together.

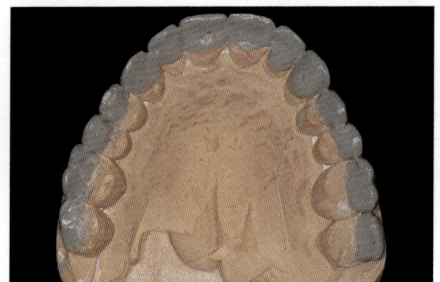

Fig 12 Lingual view of waxup creating anterior guidance.

tips of the posterior teeth (Fig 10). If wax is added to fill the space from the mounting plate distal to the mesial cusp of the first molar, it will be impossible to close the casts together in the posterior area due to the axis of closure of the hinge. Therefore, the length of the wax distal to the first molar should be short of the mounting plate, but equal in distance from the flat plane on both sides.

Step 2: Alter the vertical dimension of occlusion (if needed)

Ideally, the casts should be mounted at or close to the correct vertical dimension of occlusion based on the restorative space needed to develop the ideal anterior relationship, including the anterior guidance and room for the envelope of function. If the casts are mounted at the ideal vertical dimension of occlusion, the effect of the arc of rotation will be insignificant. If the casts are not mounted at the ideal vertical dimension, open or close the articulator pin to develop the ideal space needed for the restorative material (Fig 11). If the casts do not close to the ideal position, ei-

ther shorten the maxillary posterior teeth, move the maxillary buccal cusps facially, or move the mandibular buccal cusps lingually. This is a purely subjective process and can be refined during the next step.

Step 3: Develop the anterior guidance

If the mandibular anterior incisal plane is irregular and the treatment plan calls for restoration of the mandibular anterior teeth, level the mandibular incisal plane with wax, followed by the lingual aspect of the maxillary anterior teeth, to develop the correct anterior guidance relationship. If only one arch will be restored, add wax to the appropriate teeth (Fig 12).

Step 4: Level the mandibular posterior plane

If the mandibular occlusal plane requires leveling, add wax to the mandibular occlusal surfaces to level the mandibular arch (Fig 13). It may not be possible to level the mandibular posterior plane with the mandibular anterior plane because this may require opening the vertical dimension too much. If this is the case, level as much as possible.

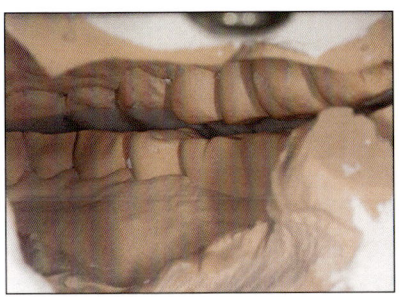

Fig 13 Evaluation of space to wax the mandibular occlusal surfaces.

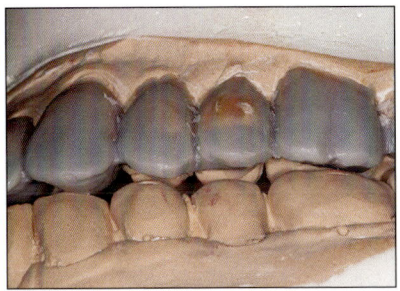

Fig 14 Evaluation of space to wax the maxillary occlusal surfaces.

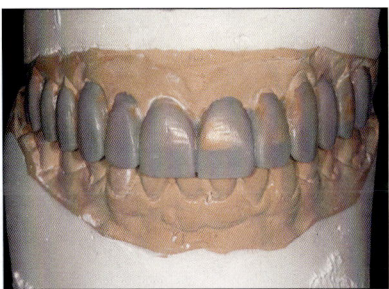

Fig 15 Final waxup.

The level of the lower posterior plane can be evaluated by opening the pin slightly and assessing the space between the maxillary and mandibular posterior cusp tips. There should be equal space on either side of the arch.

Step 5: Add wax to the maxillary occlusal surfaces to develop the occlusal contacts

Once the mandibular teeth are ideal, add wax to the maxillary posterior occlusal surfaces to fit into the mandibular occlusal surfaces in the correct relationship (Fig 14).

Step 6: Refine the occlusion and perfect the contours

Add to or modify the occlusal surfaces to perfect the occlusal relationship and to idealize the esthetic contours (Fig 15). The final contours of the central incisors should be determined first, followed by the lateral incisors and canines, since the symmetry of these teeth is not as critical as the central incisors.

Relationships to the critical esthetic determinants

There are certain relationships that can be developed regarding the critical esthetic determinants. It has been established that the midline position is not as critical as the midline verticality.[13] If the incisal plane has been idealized in the waxup, the midline should be perfectly *perpendicular* to the incisal plane. Ideally, the facial plane of the in-

cisors should be *perpendicular* or slightly acute relative to the occlusal plane from a sagittal perspective. The gingival plane should be *parallel* to the incisal plane.

CASE PRESENTATION

An 82-year-old man presented to the office in need of a complex rehabilitation. He had noticed rapid wear on his anterior mandibular teeth in the last couple of years, and that his maxillary and mandibular anterior teeth were "on top of each other." Considering the severe occlusal wear and Class III malocclusion, a thorough esthetic evaluation was done to formulate a treatment plan. The incisal edge position at rest was evaluated first. The patient showed approximately 2 to 3 mm of tooth structure with the lips in repose (Fig 16). According to esthetic principles, this fell within the desired range. When the patient smiled, the incisal plane also seemed adequate; however, a distinct step between the anterior and posterior planes existed, indicating an esthetic need to lengthen the maxillary posterior teeth (Fig 17). Opening the vertical dimension of occlusion would be beneficial in this case because this patient was in need of a dramatic leveling of the maxillary occlusal plane and the mandibular incisal and occlusal planes to create room for development of a better functional relationship of the anterior teeth (Figs 18 to 20).

CASE PRESENTATION

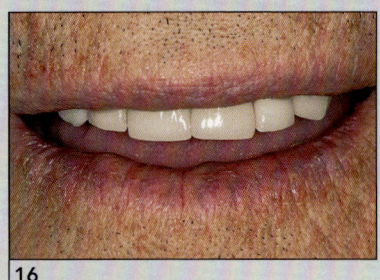
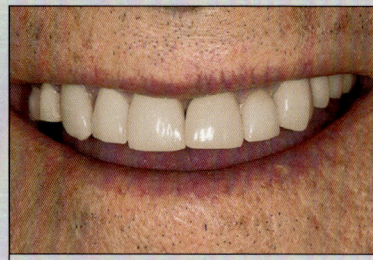

Fig 16 Initial incisal edge at rest. Note the good position of incisal edges and incisal plane.

Fig 17 Initial smile. Note the discrepancy in the posterior occlusal plane.

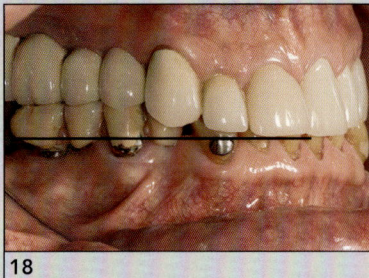
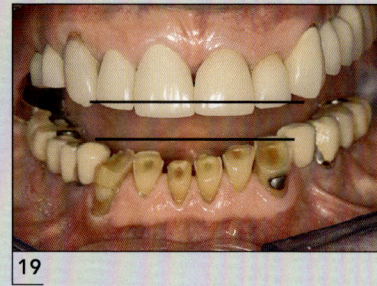
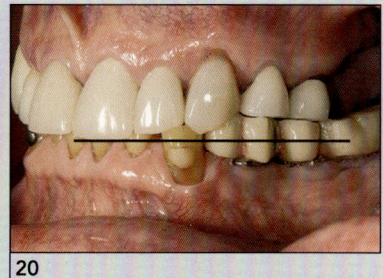

Fig 18 Initial right lateral view. Note the discrepancy between the anterior and posterior occlusal planes.

Fig 19 Initial intraoral view. Note the discrepancy of the mandibular anterior incisal plane.

Fig 20 Initial left lateral view. Note the discrepancy between the anterior and posterior occlusal planes.

Modified occlusal plane guide technique

In this case, the anterior occlusal plane was deemed adequate at the esthetic evaluation, so the wax was added to the posterior occlusal plane. This occlusal plane guide was tried in the mouth and shaped to the correct length corresponding to the ideal esthetic plane. A centric record was taken at the anticipated vertical dimension to aid in creating a better relationship in the anterior region, as well as room to level both the maxillary and mandibular occlusal planes.

Mounting the casts

Once the wax of the occlusal plane guide was idealized, the maxillary cast with the occlusal plane guide was mounted on the Kois dentofacial analyzer mounting plate (Panadent, Grand Terrace,

CA, USA) by aligning the facial aspect of the incisors with the line drawn on the platform (Fig 21). The midline on the maxillary diagnostic cast was aligned with the midline drawn on the platform. The Panadent system mounting platform was developed using scientific data (unpublished research, 2006), so there is no need to use the dentofacial analyzer or an earbow leveled to the horizontal plane with this technique (Figs 22 and 23). The incisal edge position on the mounting platform that was used to align the cast is based on a 100-mm measurement from the hinge axis of the articulator (Fig 24). According to Kois and Kois and others,[14–18] this measurement is the average in the population from the hinge axis to the incisal edge position, with 80% of the population falling within 1 standard deviation of the mean. The maxillary cast was mounted relative to the hinge axis using the mounting plate. By using the wax to mount the cast, there was an ideal esthetic relationship of the cast to the mounting plate. Once

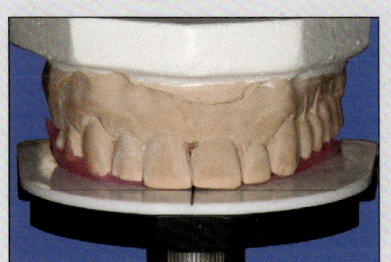

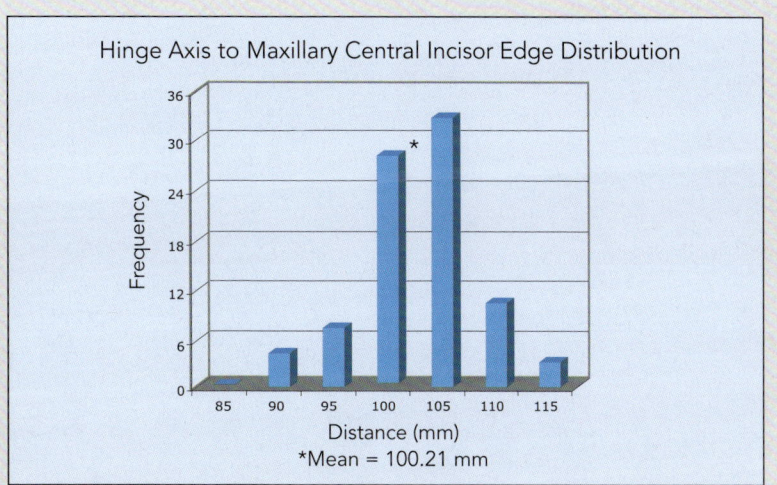

Fig 21 Diagnostic cast mounted on the dentofacial analyzer mounting platform using the occlusal plane guide.

Fig 22 Diagram of findings in research conducted by Kois and Kois.[14]

Fig 23 Illustration of measurement in research conducted by Kois and Kois.[14]

Fig 24 Articulator with dentofacial analyzer mounting platform.

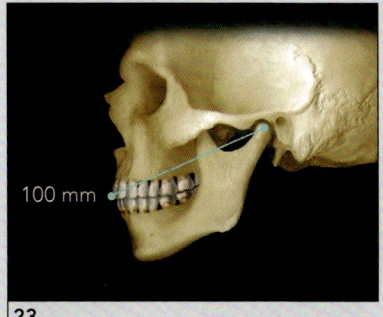

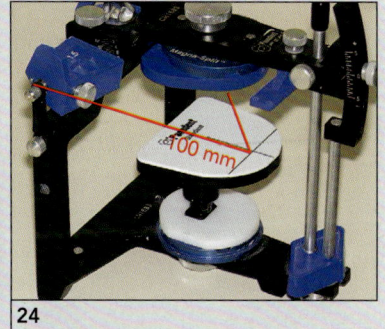

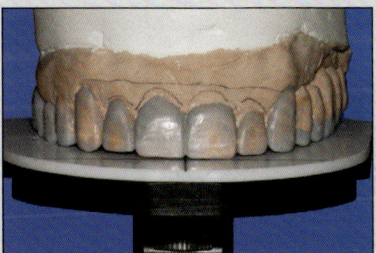

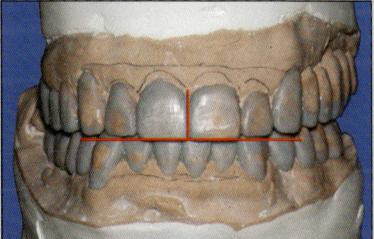

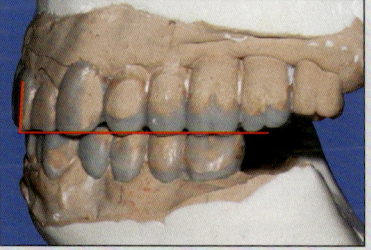

Fig 25 Maxillary waxup on the dentofacial analyzer mounting platform.

Fig 26 Final waxup. Note the perpendicular relationship of the incisal plane to the interincisal angle.

Fig 27 Lateral view of final waxup. Note the perpendicular relationship of the facial plane of the incisors to the occlusal plane.

the maxillary cast was mounted, the mounting plate was removed and the mandibular cast was mounted using the occlusal plane guide at the appropriate vertical dimension. The wax occlusal plane guide was removed and the diagnostic waxup was fabricated as previously described, although the maxillary cast was waxed against the dentofacial analyzer mounting plate rather than a standard mounting plate (Fig 25). Both arches were leveled and aligned to the horizontal reference plane, and other relationships, such as the interincisal angle and the facial plane of the incisors, were also incorporated in the waxup (Figs 26 and 27).

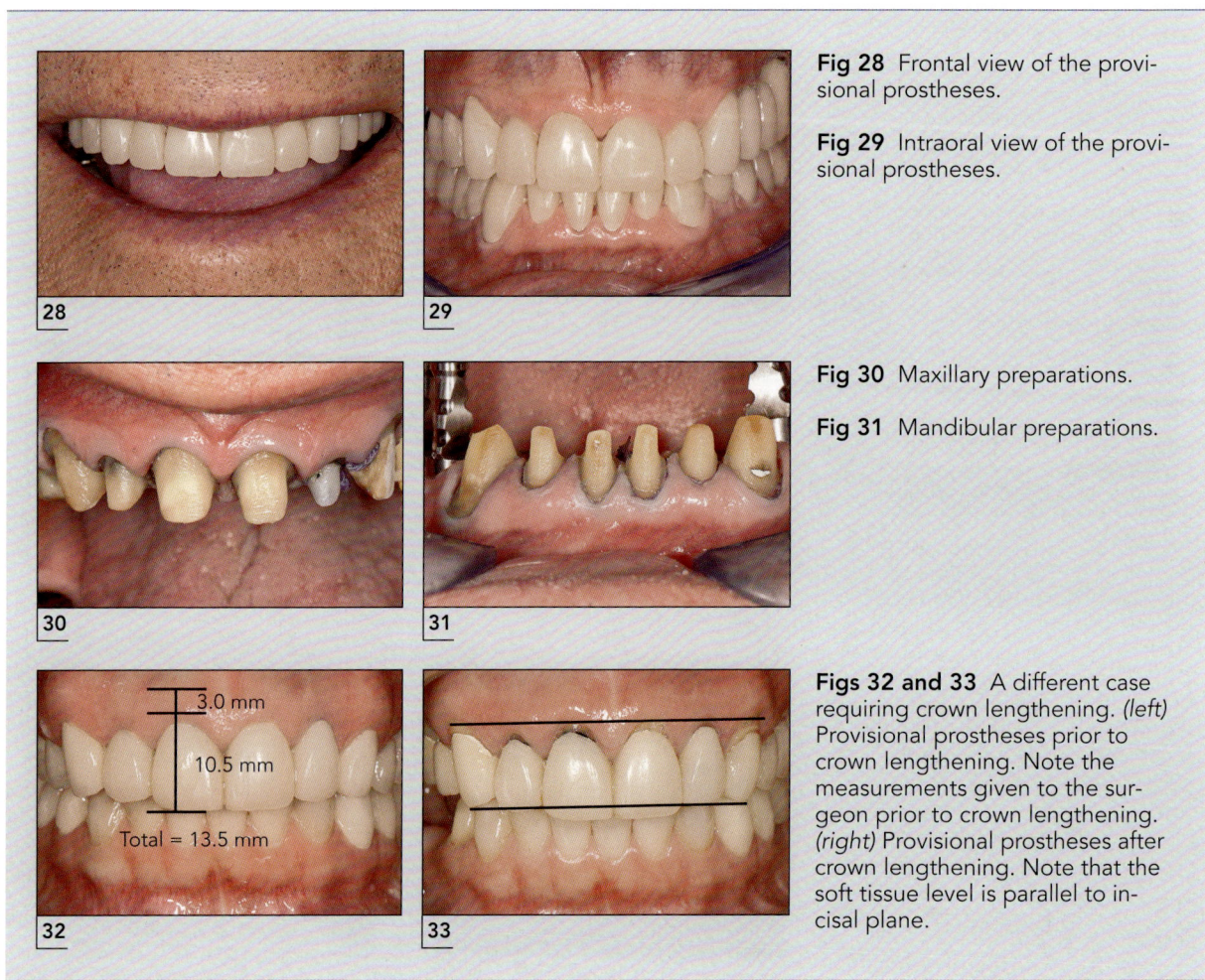

Fig 28 Frontal view of the provisional prostheses.

Fig 29 Intraoral view of the provisional prostheses.

Fig 30 Maxillary preparations.

Fig 31 Mandibular preparations.

Figs 32 and 33 A different case requiring crown lengthening. *(left)* Provisional prostheses prior to crown lengthening. Note the measurements given to the surgeon prior to crown lengthening. *(right)* Provisional prostheses after crown lengthening. Note that the soft tissue level is parallel to incisal plane.

Making the provisional prostheses

Once the waxup was complete, a provisional shell was made by fabricating a matrix and painting in both incisal- and dentin-colored cold-cure acrylic resin. These prostheses were filled with acrylic resin, relined in the mouth, trimmed, and equilibrated slightly. It was difficult to visualize the esthetic aspect of the provisional prostheses while the patient was anesthetized, so he was allowed to leave and return 1 week later for further refinement. There will almost always be a need to slightly recontour the provisional prostheses to achieve the desired esthetic outcome, but modification of the incisal edge position and occlusal plane is rarely needed when this technique is used (Figs 28 and 29).

Crown lengthening

This patient refused crown lengthening, but after preparation there was enough tooth structure for retention of the final restorations (Figs 30 and 31). In a complex wear case, a surgical procedure is often needed to level the soft tissue for esthetic and/or structural reasons. Because the ideal incisal edge position and incisal plane are developed in the provisional stage based on the horizontal reference plane, it is easy to develop ideal soft tissue levels. If the clinician has determined the proper esthetic and structural length for the teeth, he or she can ask the surgeon to measure from the incisal edge up to the desired soft tissue height and add 2.5 to 3.0 mm of length for the biologic width to achieve the new bone level (Fig 32). Once the

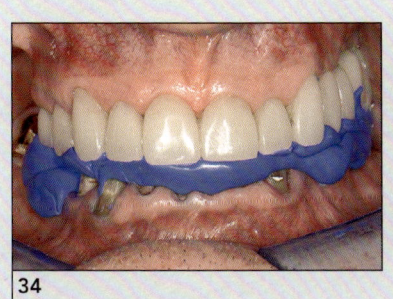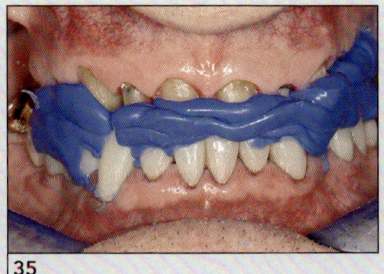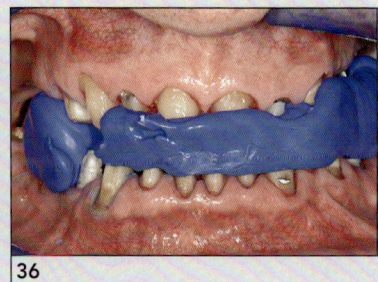

Fig 34 Centric record of the maxillary provisional prosthesis to the mandibular preparations.

Fig 35 Centric record of the maxillary preparations to the mandibular provisional prosthesis.

Fig 36 Centric record of the maxillary preparations to the mandibular preparations.

bone level is idealized, the soft tissue is positioned and sutured 2 to 3 mm more coronal than the bone. If the ideal tooth width has been developed in the provisional prosthesis, the surgeon also has the information necessary to scallop the bone so the gingival zenith will be in the correct position (the height of the contour of the soft tissue, distal to the center of the tooth) (Fig 33).

Centric record and cross-mounting

Once the biologic width is redeveloped and the provisional prostheses are relined, a final impression is taken of at least one arch. This is then mounted on the articulator using the dentofacial analyzer to develop the correct relationship with the face. The various centric records allow the technician to mount the casts of the provisional prostheses and the preparations in identical 3-dimensional positions. Four critical relationships (centric records) need to be taken if both arches are to be fabricated at the same time. The first is a provisional prosthesis–to–provisional prosthesis relationship (see Fig 29). There is no need to take an occlusion rim for this relationship if there is an ideally generated occlusal relationship that shows bilateral simultaneous contacts in centric occlusion. The second and third centric records are

those of the preparations against the opposing provisional prostheses in both arches (Figs 34 and 35). The final relationship needed is the centric record of the preparations to preparations (Fig 36).

If only one arch is undergoing restoration, the provisional-to-provisional and provisional-to-preparation relationships need to be taken only for that arch. These 3-dimensional relationships of the preparation casts to the provisional casts are essential in allowing the technician to duplicate both the esthetic and functional relationships that were developed in the provisional prostheses.

Transferring information in the laboratory

Once the casts are mounted and have become interchangeable, the technician must use the information from the provisional prostheses. One such transfer of information is the incisal guide table (Fig 37). This is fabricated by placing acrylic resin (GC America, Alsip, IL, USA) within the table that houses the pin. When the acrylic resin is in the doughy stage, the upper member of the articulator with the provisional cast is moved against the opposing cast in all directions to replicate the guidance. This movement creates a trough through the acrylic resin. After the acrylic resin

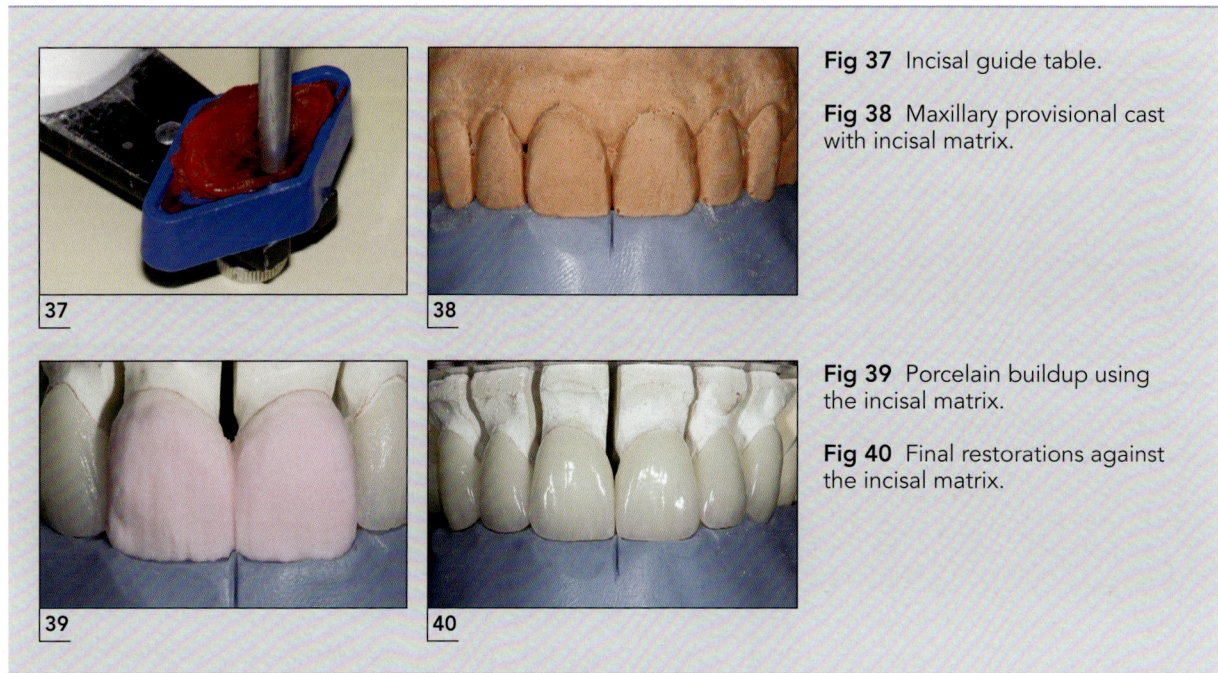

Fig 37 Incisal guide table.

Fig 38 Maxillary provisional cast with incisal matrix.

Fig 39 Porcelain buildup using the incisal matrix.

Fig 40 Final restorations against the incisal matrix.

hardens, the trough will guide the lingual contours of the restorations on the preparation cast to match the provisional cast.

The next transfer of critical information in the laboratory is the fabrication of matrices. The main matrices used in the laboratory are the facial matrix, the lingual matrix, and the incisal matrix. The first two allow verification or reduction of either the waxup or framework, as well as comparison of the final prosthesis to the provisional prosthesis from a facial and lingual contour perspective. This saves time because the technician does not have to remake the waxup. Because the provisional prosthesis is the pattern for the final prosthesis, all the esthetic and functional information is present. The next step is to open the pin by 1 mm and fabricate a matrix against the incisal edges and cusp tips of the maxillary provisional cast (Fig 38). When the provisional cast is replaced with the preparation cast, the laboratory technician knows exactly how much material to add incisally in the frame to support the ceramics and for the final length of the ceramics. This matrix can be used to fabricate the ideal porcelain buildup. If the technician knows how much shrinkage will result, the pin can be opened by that amount, and after the first bake, the incisal edge will be nearly in the perfect position (Figs 39 and 40). The final prostheses should fit intimately to the incisal matrix.

CONCLUSION

It is evident that the transfer of information throughout the rehabilitation process is critical. Although it may take a bit more time in the diagnostic phase of treatment, accurate means of transferring information throughout the rehabilitation process is paramount to predictability. In severe wear cases where the teeth are too short and need to be lengthened, the incisal plane guide is an indispensable tool. By transferring the critical esthetic determinants to the articulator, the process of waxing becomes easier and more predictable. If the patient needs crown lengthening, all the information necessary for esthetic success is already incorporated in the provisional prosthesis because the critical esthetic determinants were used for fabrication. Once the provisional prosthesis is idealized and the correct occlusal relationships are taken to allow cross-mounting the casts, fabrica-

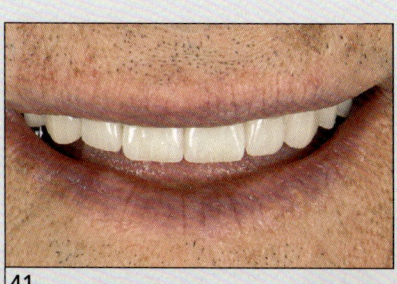

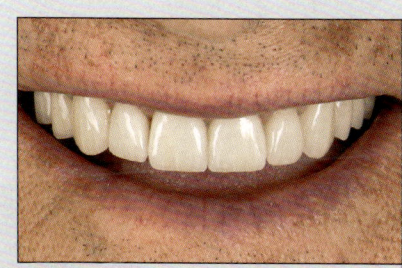

Fig 41 Final incisal edge at rest.

Fig 42 Final smile. Note the level maxillary occlusal plane.

Fig 43 Final intraoral frontal view. Note the level maxillary and mandibular occlusal planes.

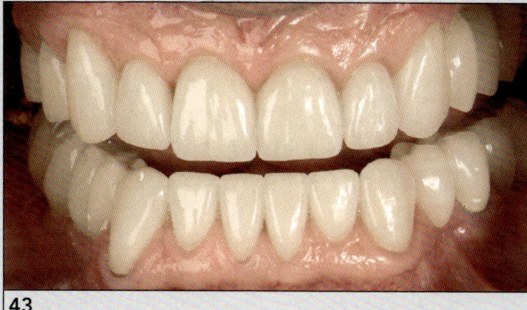

tion of the incisal guide table and matrices from these casts will guide the laboratory technician to ensure esthetic and functional predictability in the final restorations (Figs 41 to 43).

ACKNOWLEDGMENTS

A special thanks to Drs John Kois and Dean Kois for the use of their diagrams and research findings. Also, a special thanks to Harald Heindle (Aesthetic Dental Creations, Mill Creek, Washington) for the beautiful ceramic work.

REFERENCES

1. Frush F, Fisher R. How dentogenics interprets the sex factor. J Prosthet Dent 1956;6:160–172.

2. Frush F, Fisher R. How dentogenics interprets the personality factor. J Prosthet Dent 1956;6:441–449.

3. Frush F, Fisher R. The Age Factor in Dentogenics. J Prosthet Dent 1957;7:5–13.

4. Frush F, Fisher R. The dynesthetic interpretation of the dentogenic concept. J Prosthet Dent 1965;8:558–581.

5. Lombardi RE. The principles of visual perception and their clinical application to denture esthetics. J Prosthet Dent 1973;29:358–382.

6. Lombardi RE. A method for the classification of errors in dental esthetics. J Prosthet Dent 1974;32:501–513.

7. Tjan AH, Miller GD, The JG. Some esthetic factors in a smile. J Prosthet Dent 1984;51:24–28.

8. Vig RG, Brundo GC. The kinetics of anterior tooth display. J Prosthet Dent 1978;39:502–504.

9. Rufenacht CR. Fundamentals of Esthetics. Chicago: Quintessence, 1990:67–134.

10. Chiche GJ, Pinault A. Esthetics of Anterior Fixed Prosthodontics. Chicago: Quintessence, 1994:13–32.

11. Arnett GW, Bergman RT. Facial keys to orthodontic diagnosis and treatment planning. Part I. Am J Orthod Dentofacial Orthop 1993;103:299–312.

12. Phillips K, Morgan R. The acrylic occlusal plane guide: A tool for esthetic occlusal reconstruction. Compend Contin Educ Dent 2001;22;302–306.

13. Kokich VO Jr, Kiyak HA, Shapiro PA. Comparing the perception of dentists and lay people to altered dental esthetics. J Esthet Dent 1999;11:311–324.

14. Kois JC, Kois D. Simplified facebow rationale and technique. In press.

15. Bonwill WGA. The scientific articulation of the human teeth as founded on geometrical, mathematical, and mechanical laws. Dent Items of Interest 1899:617–643.

16. Weinberg LA. An evaluation of basic articulators and their concepts. Part I: Basic concepts. J Prosthet Dent 1963;13:622–644.

17. Weinberg LA. An evaluation of basic articulators and their concepts. Part II: Arbitrary, positional, semiadjustable articulators. J Prosthet Dent 1963;13:645–663.

18. Monson GS. Occlusion as applied to crown and bridge work. JADA 1920;7:399–413.

ZIRCONIUM OXIDE CAD/CAM-GENERATED RESTORATIONS: AN ESSENTIAL OPTION IN CONTEMPORARY RESTORATIVE DENTISTRY

Ricardo Mitrani, DDS, MSD[1]

Roberto Duran, DDS[2]

Eduardo Nicolayevsky, DDS[3]

Joel Lopez, MDT[3]

Two of the most important characteristics of modern restorative dentistry are:

1. The ability to integrate an interdisciplinary treatment plan
2. A full understanding of current restorative materials and technology

[1]Affiliate Assistant Professor, Graduate Prosthodontics, University of Washington, Seattle, Washington, USA; Visiting Professor, Universidad Nacional Autónoma de México; private practice, Mexico City, Mexico.

[2]Director, Nogales Implant Center, Nogales Sonora, Mexico; private practice, Nogales Sonora and Mexico City, Mexico.

[3]Private practice, Mexico City, Mexico.

Correspondence to: Dr Ricardo Mitrani, Paseo de los Laureles #458-302B, Bosques de las Lomas, Mexico City 05120, Mexico. E-mail: ricardomitrani@hotmail.com

The treatment planning phase unquestionably represents the foundation of contemporary dentistry.[1] Whether dealing with the restoration of a single tooth, an implant, or a full-mouth reconstruction, it is through this planning phase that the dental team must set the road map for therapy. While the final outcome may be reached through a variety of pathways, close communication between specialists is essential to choose the ultimate route of treatment.

Indeed, there is no better investment than the time spent during treatment planning. The interdisciplinary team should not overlook even the slightest detail regarding the treatment options.

The starting point for any therapy should be a full understanding of the patient's needs, desires, and complaints. Clinicians should explore the patient's mind before diagnosing his or her mouth, and devote as much time as necessary during the initial consultation to obtain all pertinent information.

A simple rule of thumb in the business world is to listen to the client's requests before offering any products or services. This is certainly applicable to the clinician-patient relationship. There are a few common roadblocks to proper communication: *(1)* the patient and clinician may speak different languages, *(2)* the clinician may not truly listen to the patient, and *(3)* the clinician may overwhelm the patient with medical terminology. However, it seems reasonable to state that in the majority of cases, patients are simply looking for a long-lasting, esthetic restoration.

Thus, the clinician begins the quest to find the best restorative material, which historically has been a challenging task. There is a broad range of restorative materials from which to choose.

Selection criteria are based fundamentally on the following:

1. Strength
2. Fit
3. Biocompatibility
4. Esthetics

High-strength aluminum oxide crowns have been recommended with increasing frequency, especially for anterior restorations, since they satisfy all of these requirements. Further, the successful clinical performance of this material has been documented longitudinally. Conversely, with the advent of CAD/CAM-generated zirconium oxide crowns, the possibility of using these materials for both single and multiple units in the posterior is now a clinical reality.[2–5]

One interesting advantage of these restorations is that they minimize the potential for crack propagation. This is because the tetragonal crystal configuration of partially stabilized zirconium oxide is transformed to the monoclinic phase when occlusal load is applied. The monoclinic crystals are about 3% to 5% larger than the tetragonal crystals. This volume increase seals the microscopic cracks.[6]

CASE PRESENTATIONS

Case 1

A 50-year-old female presented with a maxillary first premolar fractured slightly above the free gingival margin (Figs 1 and 2).

The tooth had previously undergone root canal therapy with a cast post and core and an ill-fitting ceramometal restoration that was frequently decementing.

The patient was presented with three treatment options:

1. Saving the tooth, which would entail the following steps: *(1)* endodontic retreatment, *(2)* placement of a post and core, *(3)* crown lengthening surgery to gain adequate ferrule, and *(4)* fabrication of a new crown.
2. Extraction and fabrication of a three-unit fixed partial denture; however, this would mean preparing perfectly sound adjacent teeth.
3. Extraction and implant placement, along with fabrication of an implant-supported single tooth restoration.

After carefully analyzing and discussing with the patient the advantages and disadvantages of each option, it was decided, based on predictability and longevity, to remove the tooth and place an implant immediately at the time of extraction. A 4.3 × 13-mm implant was placed (Nobel Replace, Nobel Biocare, Göteborg, Sweden) (Fig 3).

A flipper-type removable provisional restoration was delivered, and 3 months were allotted to ensure osseointegration.

The restorative therapy consisted initially of making an implant-level impression using the open-tray technique (Fig 4) and polyvinyl siloxane (Virtual, Ivoclar Vivadent, Schaan, Liechtenstein) and fabricating a screw-retained provisional restoration made from a plastic temporary abutment (Nobel Biocare) and a light-cured composite material (Adoro, Ivoclar Vivadent) to adequately groom the gingival tissue (Figs 5 to 7).[7]

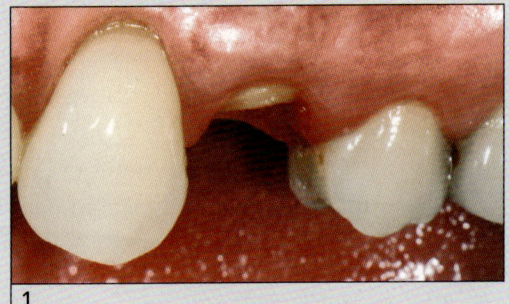

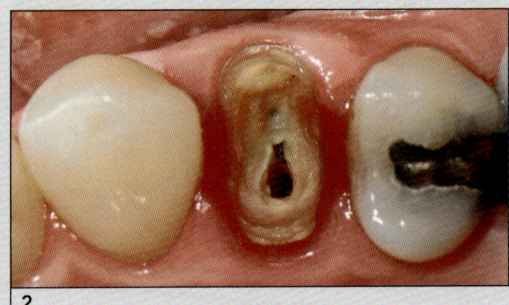

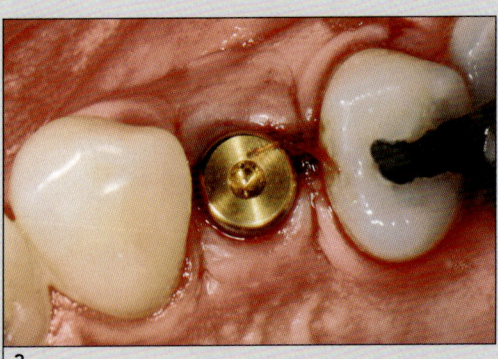

Fig 1 Preoperative view of the maxillary left first premolar fractured just above the free gingival margin.

Fig 2 Occlusal view of the maxillary left first premolar, depicting the extent of the fracture.

Fig 3 After implant placement, a healing abutment was secured.

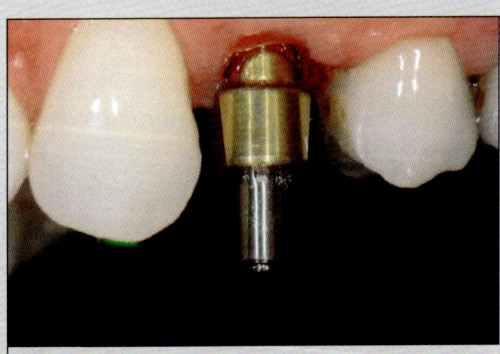

Fig 4 An open-tray impression coping was secured.

Fig 5 Screw-retained provisional restoration.

Fig 6 Insertion of the provisional restoration.

Fig 7 Buccal view of the screw-retained provisional restoration.

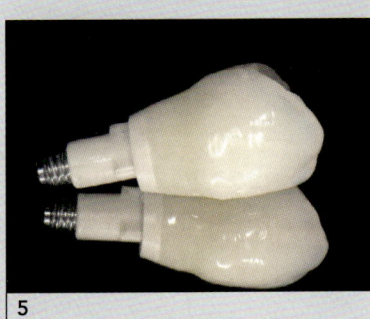

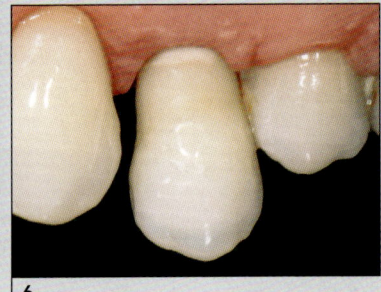

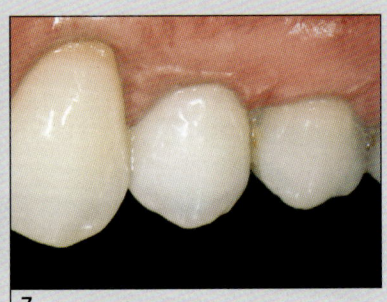

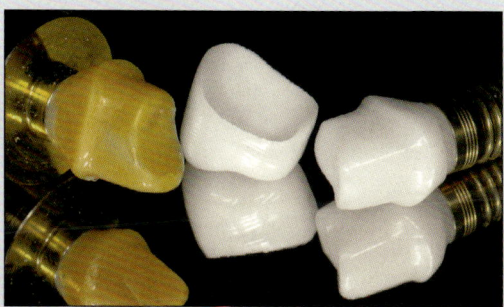

Fig 8 Waxed-up prototype abutment and zirconium oxide abutment and crown.

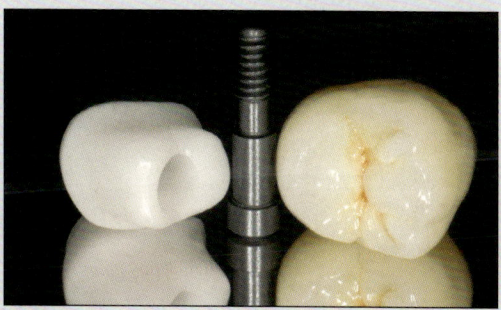

Fig 9 Zirconium oxide abutment, abutment screw, and ceramic crown.

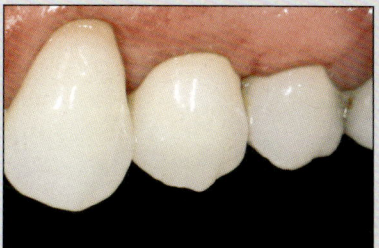

Fig 10 Buccal aspect of the definitive restoration.

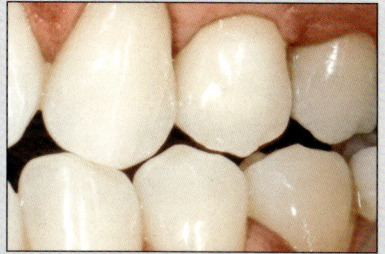

Fig 11 Occlusal scheme depicting the canine rise.

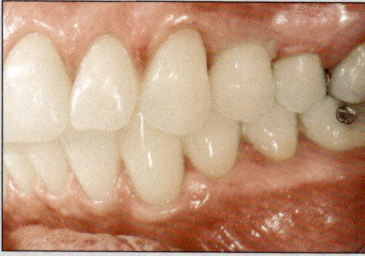

Fig 12 Buccal aspect of the restoration in occlusion.

Next, the definitive restoration, which consisted of a customized zirconium oxide abutment and a zirconium oxide ceramic crown, was fabricated.

The abutment was waxed, and using a touch probe and computer software to allow remote fabrication (Procera System, Nobel Biocare), a zirconium oxide abutment and coping were obtained (Fig 8), followed by the ceramic application of the veneering porcelain (Fig 9).

The insertion of the restoration consisted of the following:

- Securing the abutment and confirming the fit using a radiograph
- Torquing the screw to 35 Ncm
- Sequential torquing to avoid the embedment relaxation effect
- Obliterating the screw access hole
- Cementing the crown using resin-modified glass-ionomer cement

A light centric contact was obtained and verified using shimstock, and a canine rise was verified (Figs 10 to 12).

Case 2

A 48-year-old female presented with the complaint that her teeth barely showed when she smiled, which made her look older. Further, she had old restorations that she wanted to be replaced.

The patient's concern was valid, since the incisal edges were almost invisible in repose. This is usually seen only in elderly patients.[8]

After a thorough clinical and radiographic evaluation, the patient showed the following dental problems (Figs 13 to 18):

1. Missing teeth
2. Defective restorations
3. Uneven gingival margins
4. Short clinical crowns

The treatment plan for the patient consisted of a maxillary full-arch reconstruction. In the mandible, it was decided to replace the ill-fitting pre-existing four-unit fixed partial denture in the mandibular left quadrant, and to replace the

CASE 2 (Figs 13 to 53)

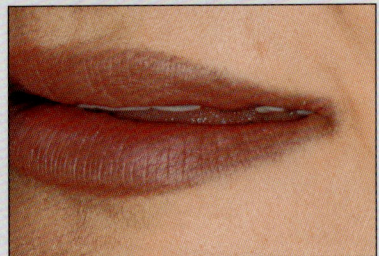

Fig 13 Preoperative condition. Minimal tooth display in repose is evident.

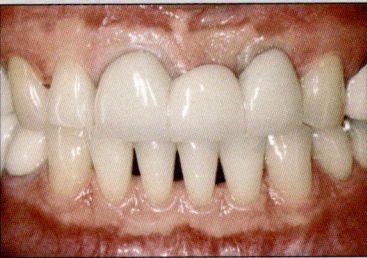

Fig 14 Intraoral frontal view of the preoperative condition.

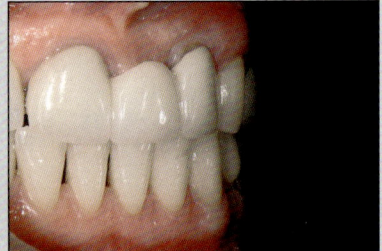

Fig 15 Lateral view of the preoperative condition.

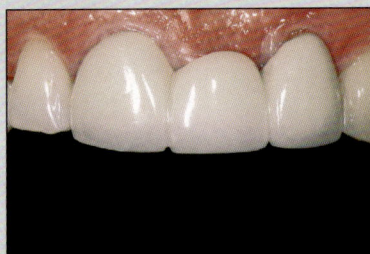

Fig 16 The maxillary anterior sextant, showing uneven gingival margins.

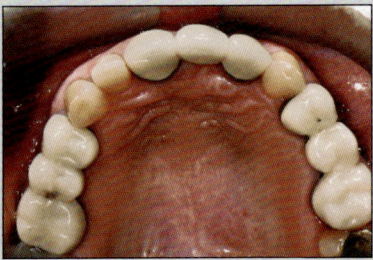

Fig 17 Occlusal view of the maxillary arch, showing multiple metal-ceramic restorations.

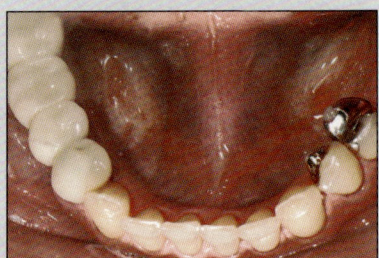

Fig 18 Occlusal view of the mandibular arch.

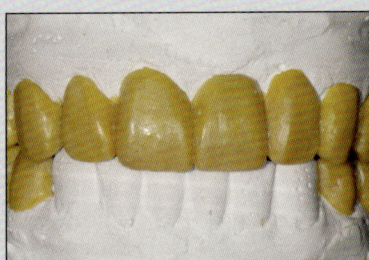

Fig 19 Diagnostic waxup on mounted casts in a semiadjustable articulator.

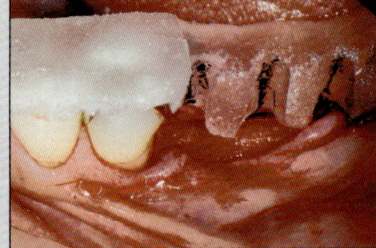

Fig 20 Surgical template in place for the surgical insertion of the implants.

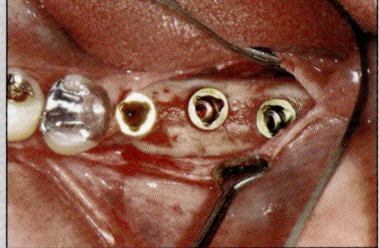

Fig 21 Occlusal view of the implant placement.

mandibular right posterior dentition using osseointegrated implants.

Once the diagnostic casts were mounted in a semiadjustable articulator using a facebow transfer and a centric relation record, a diagnostic waxup was elaborated, lengthening the incisal edges of the anterior teeth and modifying the interincisal angle (anterior guidance) (Fig 19).

For the mandibular right quadrant, the missing teeth were waxed up and a surgical template was fabricated to assist the precise placement of three osseointegrated implants in four aspects (mesiodistal, buccolingual, apicocoronal, and angulation) (Fig 20).

Three 4.3 × 13-mm implants (Nobel Replace, Nobel Biocare) were placed and left submerged for 2 months to ensure integration (Fig 21).

Fig 22 Frontal view of the maxillary preparations.

Fig 23 Occlusal view of the full-arch provisional restoration.

Fig 24 Frontal view of the provisional restoration.

Fig 25 Frontal view of the provisional restoration in occlusion.

Fig 26 A more esthetically pleasing tooth display during repose was achieved.

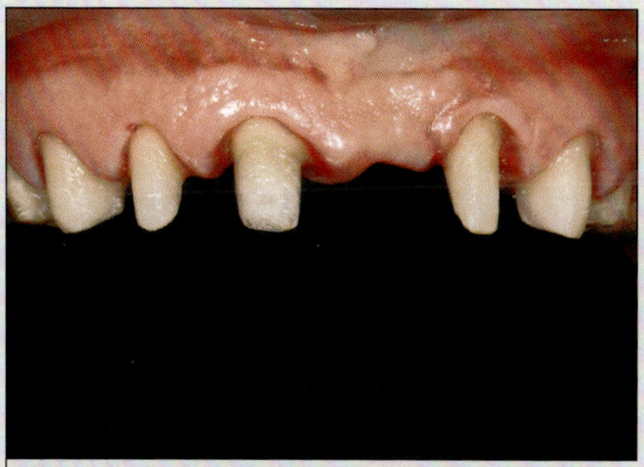

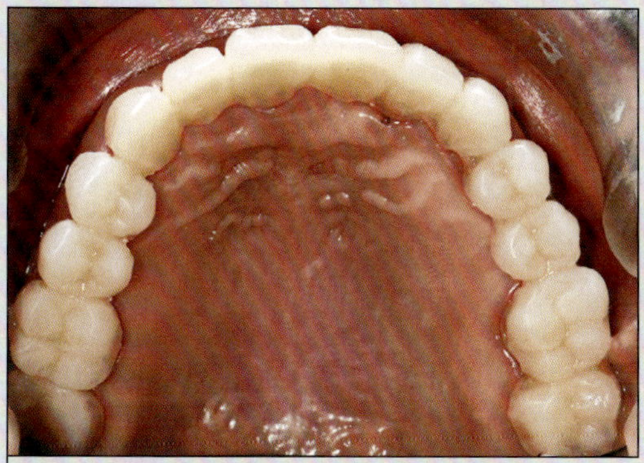

Meanwhile, maxillary full-arch preparations were performed (Fig 22) using reduction guides previously fabricated from the diagnostic waxup, and an acrylic resin shell was relined with autopolymerizing acrylic resin using copious irrigation and a vertical motion to avoid locking in the provisional restoration.[9,10]

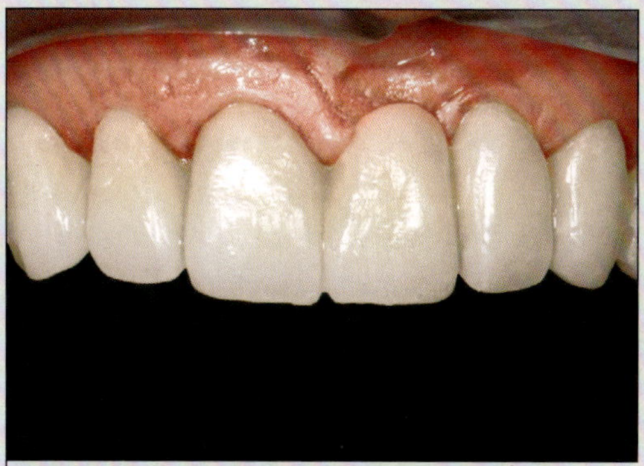

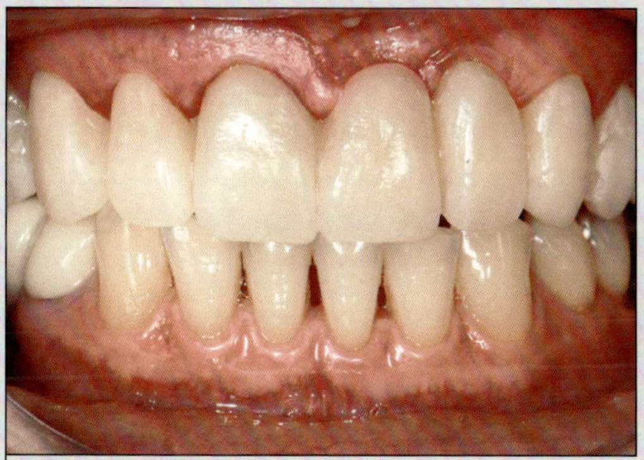

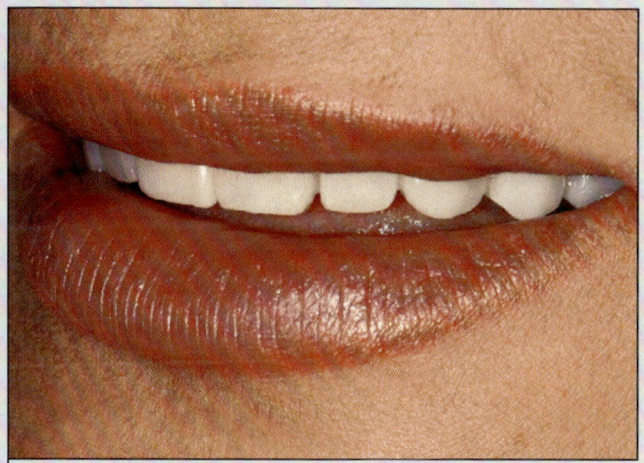

Once the acrylic resin had fully polymerized, the provisional restoration was then trimmed, polished, and cemented (Figs 23 to 26).

Enhancement of the pontic site was scheduled for a subsequent appointment, and in the meantime, a ridge lap configuration was used.

For the maxillary arch, custom trays were fabricated and impressions were taken using the dual-cord technique and polyvinyl siloxane impression material (Fig 27). For the mandible, implant-level impressions were taken using closed-tray impression copings (Nobel Biocare), because the implants (especially the most distal implant) were

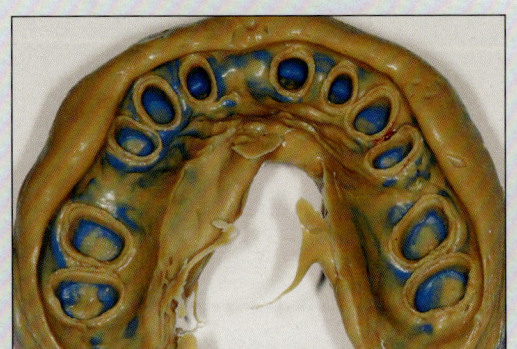

Fig 27 Maxillary arch impression using polyvinyl siloxane material.

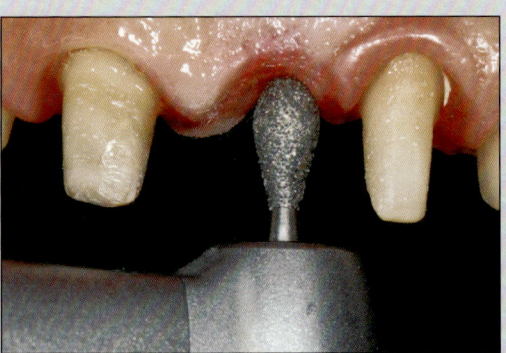

Fig 28 The pontic site was prepared using a coarse diamond bur.

too far back and could not be adequately manipulated.

Once the impressions were poured, alginate impressions of the provisional restorations were taken. A facebow transfer along with the maxillomandibular records, which comprised the provisional against the preparations and preparations against preparations, were obtained by sectioning the maxillary provisional and leaving only the anterior three-unit fixed partial denture, to hold the vertical dimension and ensure an accurate centric relation record.

Cross-mounting the casts of the provisional allowed the technician to obtain valuable information regarding length, midline, and incisal-occlusal plane orientation.

Using the contours of the provisional restorations facilitated the design of the implant abutments as well as the framework configuration.

The dies were obtained, and a Procera Forte unit (Nobel Biocare) was used to scan the preparations where fixed partial dentures were planned. A Piccolo scanner (Nobel Biocare) was used to scan the implant abutments and the single-tooth copings, which were then sent to the laboratory.

While the laboratory procedures were performed, enhancement of the pontic site was carried out. This procedure consisted of grinding the undersurface of the pontic of the provisional and adding contour with autopolymerizing acrylic resin to obtain a highly polished ovate shape.

The provisional was placed back into the mouth, and the patient was asked to bite on a cotton roll. A blanching response was evident as a result of the manipulation of tissue in the area.

After 5 minutes, the provisional was removed and the tissue was dimpled using a football-shaped coarse diamond bur (Fig 28), thus creating space for the full seating of the provisional. The provisional was cemented and the site was left undisturbed for proper healing.

Once the zirconium oxide abutments, copings, and frameworks were received from production (Figs 29 to 32), they were tried in. During this appointment, the soft tissue topography of the pontic area was also transferred to the laboratory.[11,12] Starting with the maxillary anterior framework, the provisional restoration was removed (Fig 33), followed by the immediate seating of the framework, and cold-cured autopolymerizing acrylic resin was used to accurately copy the groomed soft tissue topography (Fig 34). The rest of the maxillary copings and frameworks were tried in (Fig 35).

In the mandible, the zirconium oxide abutments were secured (Fig 36), and a radiograph was taken to ensure they were fully seated. The frameworks were tried in (Fig 37), and a polyvinyl siloxane pickup impression was made. Because there was no reason to remove the abutments, they were sequentially torqued at 35 Ncm, and a provisional restoration was relined.

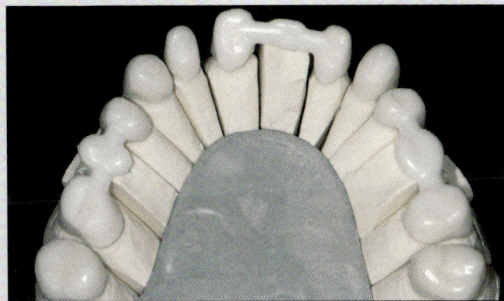

Fig 29 Occlusal view of the maxillary arch zirconium oxide copings and frameworks.

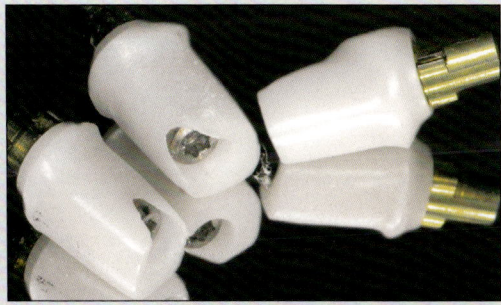

Fig 30 CAD/CAM-generated Procera zirconium oxide abutments.

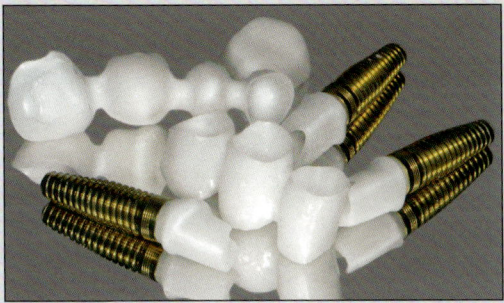

Fig 31 Mandibular copings and zirconium oxide frameworks.

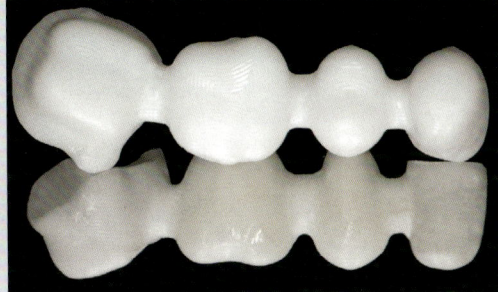

Fig 32 Closeup view of the Procera four-unit zirconium oxide fixed partial denture framework.

Fig 33 Removal of the provisional restoration.

Fig 34 Insertion of the anterior framework; the pontic site was picked up using acrylic resin.

Fig 35 Occlusal view of the framework and copings try-in.

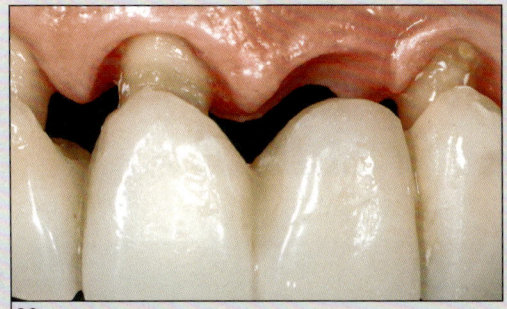

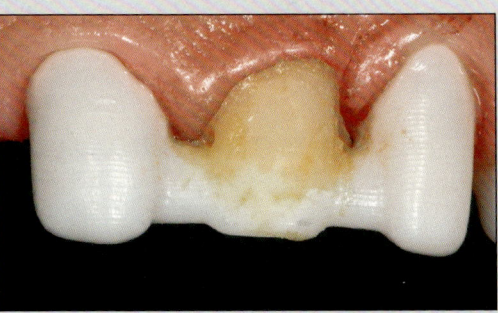

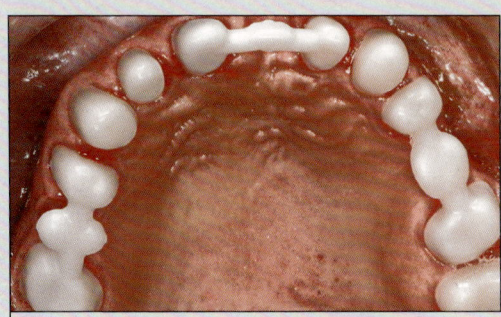

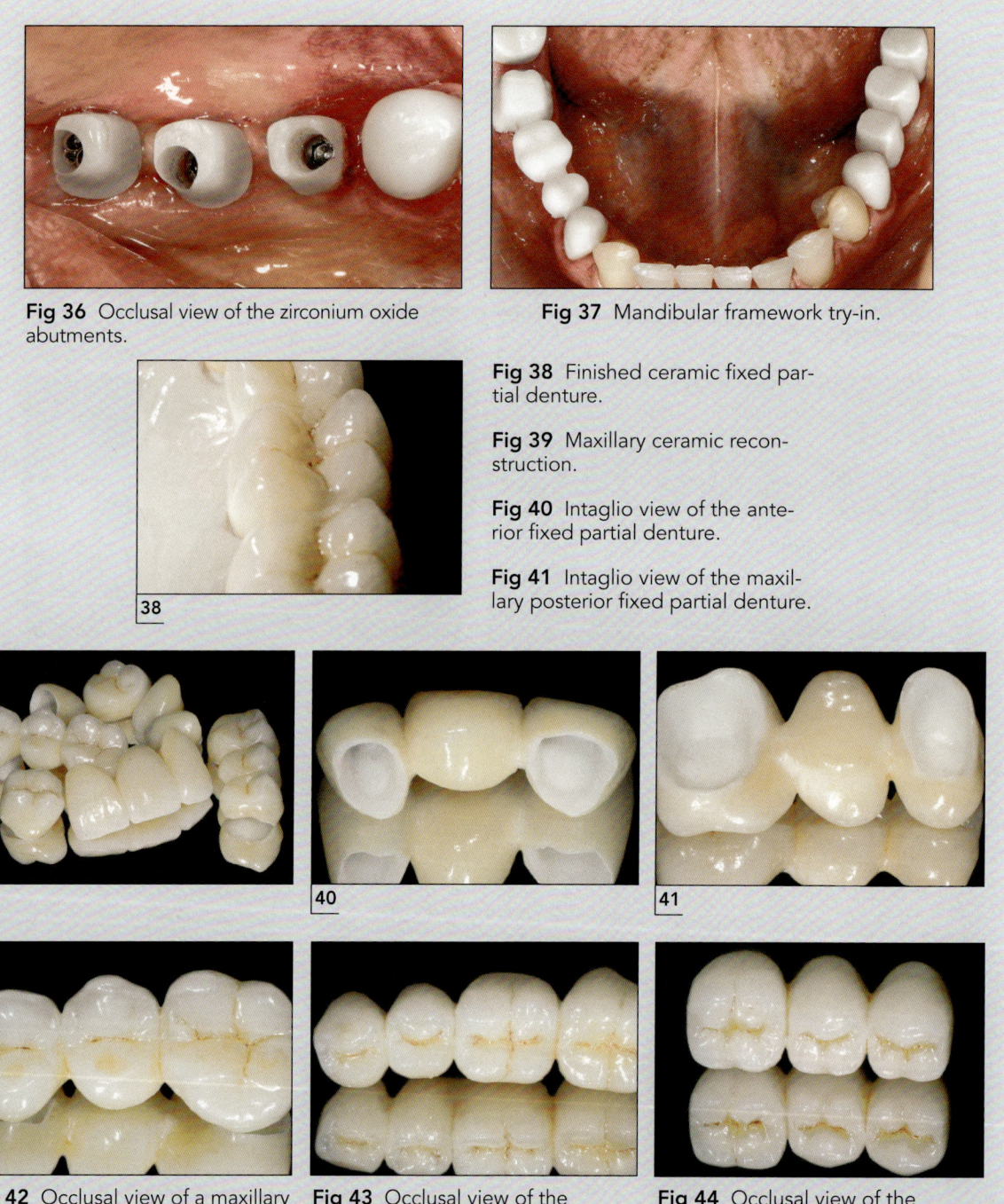

Fig 36 Occlusal view of the zirconium oxide abutments.

Fig 37 Mandibular framework try-in.

Fig 38 Finished ceramic fixed partial denture.

Fig 39 Maxillary ceramic reconstruction.

Fig 40 Intaglio view of the anterior fixed partial denture.

Fig 41 Intaglio view of the maxillary posterior fixed partial denture.

Fig 42 Occlusal view of a maxillary posterior fixed partial denture.

Fig 43 Occlusal view of the mandibular tooth-supported four-unit Procera fixed partial denture.

Fig 44 Occlusal view of the mandibular implant-supported fixed partial denture.

The ceramic layering of both arches was then completed (Figs 38 to 44). The zirconium oxide–based restoration was tried in (Fig 45) and then cemented using resin-modified glass-ionomer cement following conventional protocols (Figs 46 to 53).[13,14]

A mutually protected occlusal scheme was obtained. The patient was given a night guard and scheduled for a 6-month recall.

Fig 45 Insertion of the three-unit maxillary anterior fixed partial denture.

Fig 46 Cemented three-unit maxillary anterior fixed partial denture.

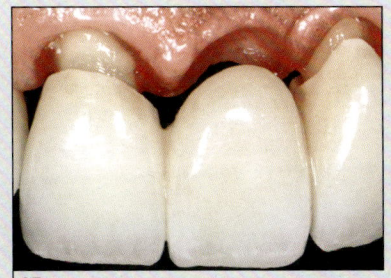

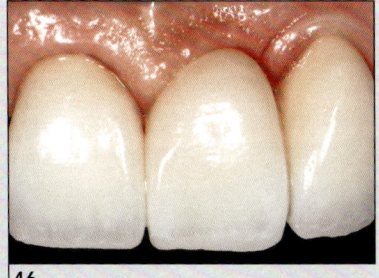

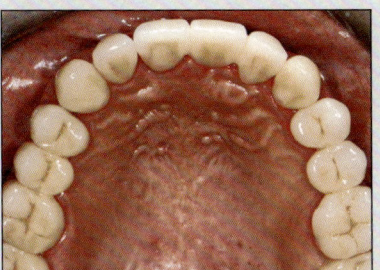

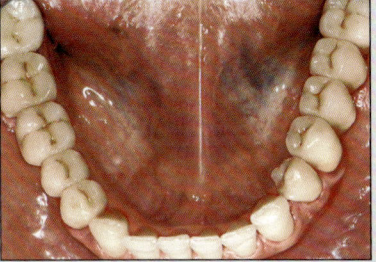

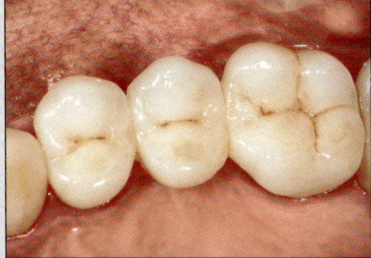

Fig 47 Occlusal view of the maxillary ceramic reconstruction.

Fig 48 Occlusal view of the mandibular ceramic reconstruction.

Fig 49 Closeup view of the maxillary posterior tooth-supported ceramic fixed partial denture.

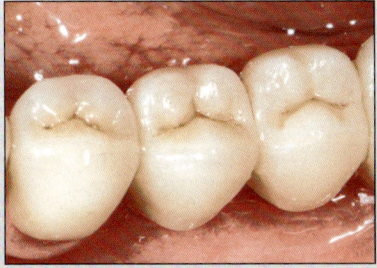

Fig 50 Closeup view of the mandibular posterior implant-supported ceramic fixed partial denture.

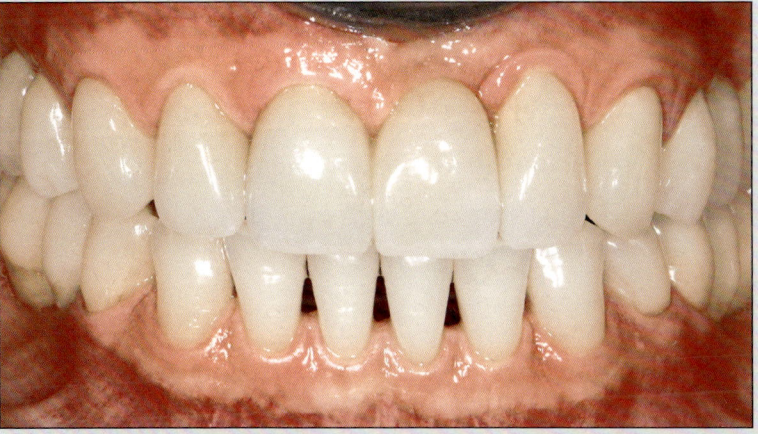

Fig 51 Frontal view of the ceramic reconstruction.

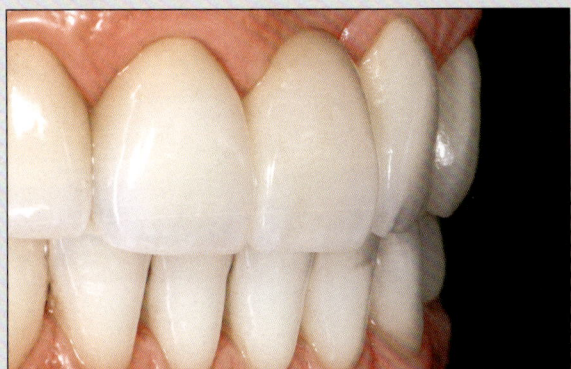

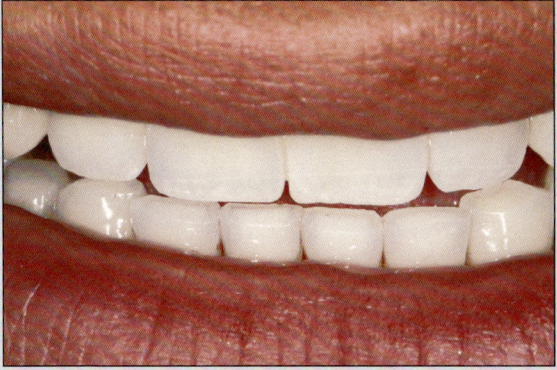

Fig 52 Lateral view of the ceramic reconstruction.

Fig 53 Extraoral view of the ceramic reconstruction.

CONCLUSION

Implementing CAD/CAM-generated zirconium oxide restorations for single-tooth restorations, implant therapy, and full-mouth rehabilitations has become a common practice in contemporary restorative dentistry.

The esthetic possibilities and increased fracture resistance have made zirconium oxide one of today's top contenders in the search for the optimal restorative material.

ACKNOWLEDGMENT

The authors would like to thank Dr Norberto Ruiz for scanning the frameworks in Case 2.

REFERENCES

1. Mitrani R, Kois JC. Restorative dentistry using a multidisciplinary approach. Compend Contin Educ Dent 2000;21:316–318, 320, 322–323.

2. Andersson M, Razzoog ME, Odén A, Hegenbarth EA, Lang BR. Procera: A new way to achieve an all-ceramic crown. Quintessence Int 1998;29:285–296.

3. Odman P, Andersson M, Procera All-ceram crowns followed for 5 to 10.5 years: A prospective clinical study. Int J Prosthodont 2001;14:504–509.

4. Sadan A, BLatz MB, Lang B. Clinical considerations for densely sintered alumina and zirconia restorations: Part 1. Int J Periodontics Restorative Dent 2005;25:213–219.

5. Sadan A, BLatz MB, Lang B. Clinical considerations for densely sintered alumina and zirconia restorations: Part 2. Int J Periodontics Restorative Dent 2005;25:343–349.

6. McLaren EA, White SN. Glass-infiltrated zirconia/alumina-base ceramic for crowns and fixed partial dentures. Pract Periodontics Aesthet Dent 1999;11:985–994.

7. Phillips K, Kois JC. Aesthetic peri-implant site development. The restorative connection. Dent Clin North Am 1998;42:57–70.

8. Vig RG, Brundo GC. The kinetics of anterior tooth display. J Prosthet Dent 1978;39:502–504.

9. Yuodelis RA, Faucher R. Provisional restorations: An integrated approach to periodontics and restorative dentistry. Dent Clin North Am 1980;24:285–303.

10. Rieder CE. Use of provisional restorations to develop and achieve esthetic expectations. Int J Periodontics Restorative Dent 1989;9:122–139.

11. Mitrani R, Rubenstein JE, Kois JC, Phillips KM. Alternative uses of a visible light-polymerized material. J Prosthet Dent 2001;86:107–110.

12. Gamborena I, Blatz M. A clinical guide to predictable esthetics with zirconium oxide ceramic restorations. Quintessence Dent Technol 2006;29:11–23.

13. Blatz MB, Sadan A, Martin J, Lang B. In vitro evaluation of shear bond strengths of resin to densely-sintered high-purity zirconium-oxide after long-term storage and thermal cycling. J Prosthet Dent 2004;91:356–362.

14. Palacios RP, Johnson GH, Phillips KM, Raigrodski AJ. Retention of zirconium oxide ceramic crowns with three types of cement. J Prosthet Dent 2006;96:104–114.

REPRODUCING OPALESCENT AND COUNTER-OPALESCENT EFFECTS WITH DIRECT RESIN COMPOSITES

Luis Guilherme Sensi, DDS, MS, PhD[1]

Fabiano de Oliveira Araujo, DDS, MS, PhD[2]

Fabiano Carlos Marson, DDS, MS, PhD[2]

Sylvio Monteiro, Jr, DDS, MS, MSD, PhD[3]

The goal of esthetic and restorative dentistry is to replace lost or damaged structures with artificial materials that possess biological, physical, and functional properties similar to natural teeth.[1] In recent years, numerous resin composite systems have been developed with a multitude of shades, translucencies, opacities, and effects, which in conjunction with innovative placement techniques, makes it possible to fabricate restorations that faithfully emulate the polychromatic variations and optical characteristics of natural teeth.[2–16] However, to achieve a direct resin composite restoration with a truly natural appearance, a comprehensive knowledge and understanding of the optical characteristics of natural teeth and resin composites, proper selection and application of current restorative systems, and rigorous training are imperative.[2,11,16] The optical characteristics present in natural teeth are determined by the interaction between light and the dentin, enamel, and underlying pulp, and include the varying degrees of translucency and opacity of enamel and dentin, fluorescence, and opalescence.[2,7,9,10,17,18]

When a ray of light reaches the surface enamel of an intact natural tooth, several events occur: some of the light is reflected, some is transmitted, and some penetrates the enamel and is absorbed and spread within the tooth structure.[17] The light that penetrates the enamel and reaches the dentin is also reflected backward, and thus reflects the color of the dentin.[2] The final perceived color of a tooth depends on the thickness and translucency characteristics of the overlaying

[1]Assistant Professor, Department of Endodontics, Prosthodontics, and Operative Dentistry, University of Maryland Dental School, Baltimore, Maryland, USA.

[2]Graduate student, Operative Dentistry, Federal University of Santa Catarina, Florianópolis, Santa Catarina, Brazil.

[3]Professor, Department of Operative Dentistry, Federal University of Santa Catarina, Florianópolis, Santa Catarina, Brazil.

Correspondence to: Dr Luis Sensi, University of Maryland Dental School, 650 West Baltimore Street, Baltimore, Maryland 21201, USA. E-mail: lsensi@umaryland.edu

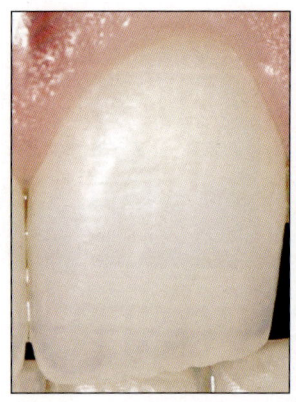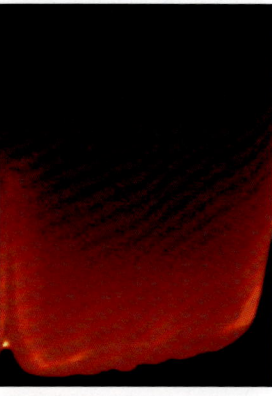

Figs 1a and 1b **(a)** Under reflected light, the natural tooth presents a bluish appearance at the incisal third. **(b)** Under transmitted light, an orange appearance is observed.

enamel, as well as how the underlying dentin influences the enamel appearance. On the cervical third, the enamel is very thin (approximately 0.3 mm), and therefore it is easier to observe the dentin shade underneath. On the middle third, the enamel is approximately 1.0 mm thick, and increased light scattering is observed. However, it is on the incisal third where infinite kinds of characteristics can be seen, with varying degrees of opacities and translucencies. The enamel thickness in this area can vary from 0.9 to 1.2 mm, and this region may present a totally translucent area, because little or no underlying dentin may be present and the facial and lingual enamel may be in direct contact.[4,17] These characteristics can result in the creation of opalescence and counter-opalescence, which are clinically relevant effects that must be identified and understood before they can be recreated.

OPALESCENCE

Opalescence is a phenomenon that causes the enamel of natural teeth, some resin composites, and some types of porcelain to change color as a result of the type of lighting (reflected or transmitted) and angle of view.[2] The opalescent effect occurs when the light that reaches the enamel is ab-

sorbed and refracted within microcrystals and colloidal inclusions. The space between the enamel rods causes this light to be scattered.[17] This results in the reflection of shorter wavelengths (ie, blue) and the transmission of longer wavelengths (ie, orange) under direct illumination. This means that the bluish translucency visible on the incisal third is a result of opalescence.[2,4,17–19] In fact, the enamel in this region is actually colorless.[17]

However, under transmitted, indirect illumination (ie, if light is positioned on the lingual aspect), the opalescent effect occurs in the opposite way. The short, blue wavelengths are transmitted, while the longer, orange wavelengths are reflected.[2,4,17–19] Thus, natural teeth, under reflected light, frequently show bluish areas in the region of the incisal third, while under transmitted light, they show a reddish-orange appearance (Figs 1a and 1b). However, the opalescent effect is not limited to the incisal third; it occurs in the whole enamel structure. It is simply more evident on the incisal third, because the enamel thickness is greater and there is little to no underlying dentin. The opalescent effects of enamel brighten the tooth and provide optical depth and vitality.[18] Opalescence affects the hue, luminosity, and chroma of objects without influencing their translucency.

Arguably, however, the most important function of the opalescence of natural tooth enamel is that it produces counter-opalescence.[2]

COUNTER-OPALESCENCE

Counter-opalescence results from light penetration of an opalescent material and its reflection within the material itself. This effect causes orange and pinkish-orange hues in the incisal edges of the dentin mamelons of natural teeth (Fig 2). The tips of the mamelons do not present visible orange or pink colors; the appearance is simply an optical event. The light penetrating from the facial side passes through the enamel and reaches the palatal or lingual side. Part of

Fig 2 Counter-opalescence may cause orange and pinkish-orange hues in the incisal edges of the dentin mamelons of natural teeth, and an orange appearance in the opaque incisal halo.

Figs 3a and 3b **(a)** The opaque incisal halo. **(b)** When the tongue is placed on the palatal surface, a remarkable reduction in the opaque incisal halo occurs because the reflection index of the enamel becomes smaller than that of the saliva, thus increasing its translucency.

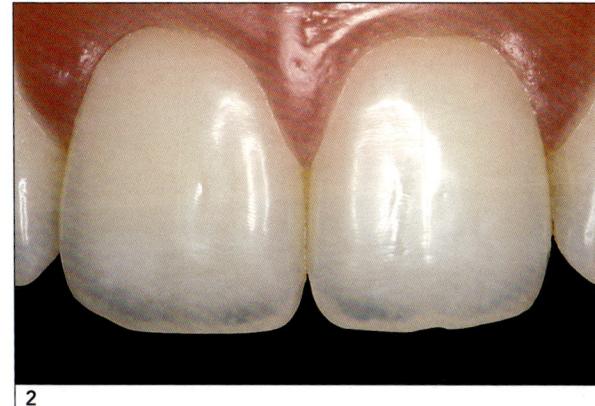

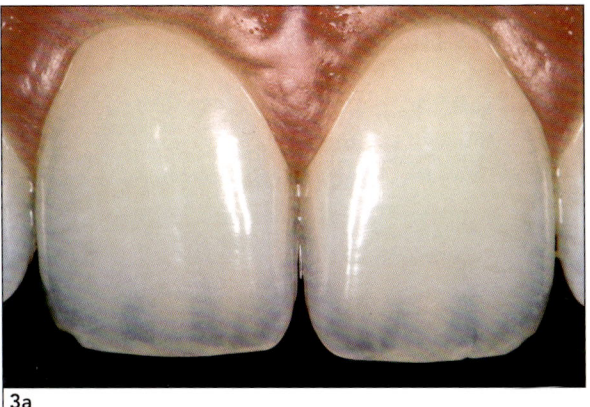

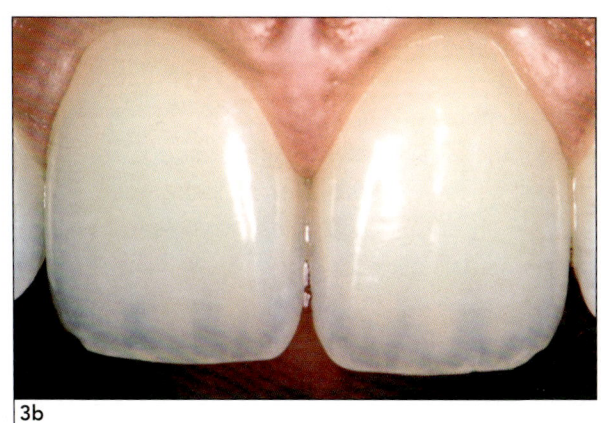

this light is reflected and returns to the facial side as an orange shade.[2]

Although dental enamel is a translucent tissue, the incisal edges of some anterior teeth may present an opaque halo that generally shows an orange color. This may also occur on small portions of the proximal surfaces and is related to the total reflection of the light in these regions, because the light emission and light reflection angles coincide as a result of the inclination of the lingual surface.[2,17] This phenomenon can be observed when the tongue is placed on the palatal or lingual side of a tooth. The orange appearance is reduced as a result of a change in the reflection index of the dental enamel, which becomes smaller in relation to that of saliva, thus increasing its translucency (Figs 3a and 3b).

Both opalescence and counter-opalescence are important factors in the final color buildup of resin composite restorations. For that reason, the use of opalescent materials is recommended for enamel

layers in which creating a natural appearance is a treatment goal.

OPALESCENT RESIN COMPOSITES

Resin composites used for enamel reproduction can be divided into generic enamels (pearled, value enamel), intense white enamels (opaque), or opalescent enamels. The resin composites designated as opalescent enamels have very high translucency and varying hues, such as blue, orange, gray, yellow, or violet (Figs 4a and 4b). These resin composites are also known as incisal or translucent resin composites and are generally identified by their characteristics, for example: I (incisal), T (transparent), ST (super transparent), SL (super light), TB (transparent with blue pigment), and TG (transparent with gray pigment).[2]

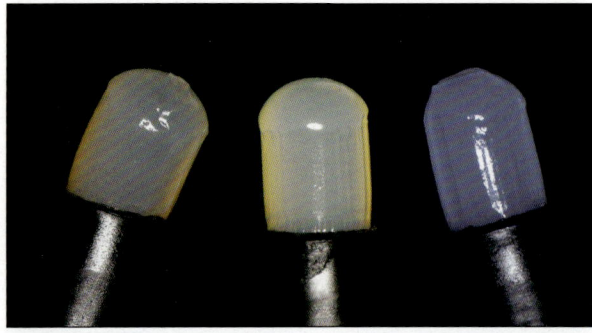 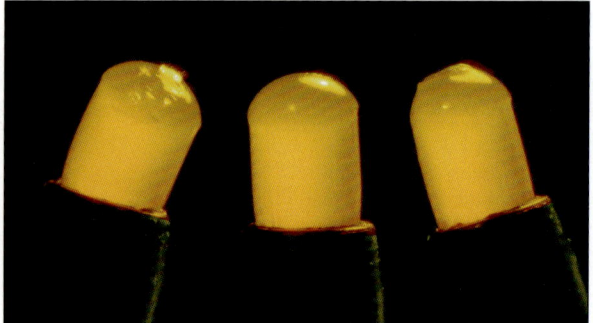

Figs 4a and 4b An example of resin composites that present opalescence: **(a)** under reflected light; **(b)** under transmitted light.

Using opalescent resin composites only in the incisal third is a common mistake. In fact, these resin composites are indicated for the reproduction of incisal and internal proximal opalescence, as well as for the last layer of facial enamel, to provide an appearance of optical depth. Opalescent materials allow changes to hue and chroma and increase the luminosity of the restorations without changing the translucency.[2]

The opalescence of some available resin composites was recently determined with a color-measuring spectrophotometer.[20] A few of the resin composites displayed opalescence, and this effect varied according to the material and shade. The opalescence of resin composites is influenced by the difference in the refractive indices between the resin matrix and filler. To show opalescence, the resin matrix of the material must be translucent. If the resin matrix is opaque, the scattered light from fillers will not be visible.[20] However, not every translucent resin composite will show true opalescence. The majority of translucent resin composites used for enamel provide a pseudo-opalescent effect that is clinically satisfactory for reproducing the incisal characteristics, especially in young patients.[5,7–9] In a laboratory study, the opalescent properties of resin composites did not change after accelerated aging, suggesting stability of this effect in the long-term.[21]

The key to reproducing opalescence is extensive observation of the characteristics of the adjacent dentition, the selection of appropriate resin composites, and the placement of these resin composites in the proper locations.

CASE PRESENTATION

A 15-year-old female model presented with a small incisal fracture on the discolored maxillary left central incisor. The fracture was caused by a ground-level traumatic injury and was followed by endodontic treatment (Figs 5 and 6). Because the traumatic injury led to initial root resorption, no internal bleaching could be performed; therefore, a veneer was indicated. Due to the young age of the patient, a direct resin composite veneer presented a more conservative option compared to a ceramic veneer. Further, since all teeth presented with a yellowish hue, an in-office external bleaching procedure was conducted with a 35% hydrogen peroxide gel (Whiteness HP Maxx, FGM, Joinville, SC, Brazil) (Fig 7a). The bleaching procedure reduced the amount of sound tooth structure to be prepared on the left central incisor, since the initial discoloration was reduced (Fig 7b). When observing the optical characteristics present on the right central incisor, a remarkable bluish incisal area outlined by an opaque halo was noted (Fig 8). When indirect white lighting was used, the orange opalescent effect was visible only on the right central incisor (Fig 9).

A diagnostic waxup served as a reference to produce two silicone putty matrices, one to facilitate development of an accurate incisal edge contour and the other to guide veneer preparation (Figs 10a and 10b). The teeth were cleaned with pumice and shade selection was performed before field isolation to prevent improper color matching caused by tooth dehydration. Shade selection was

CASE PRESENTATION

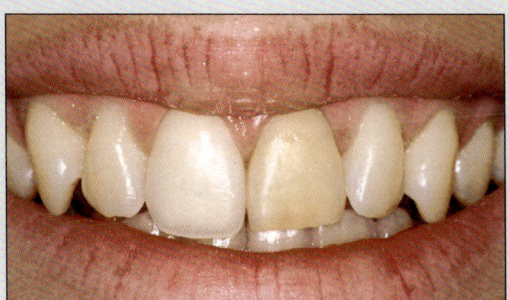

Fig 5 Frontal view of the patient's smile.

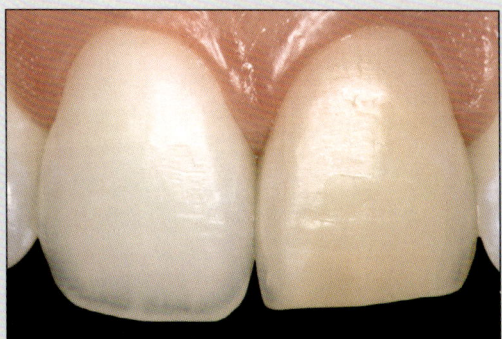

Fig 6 The central incisors. Note the translucency on the incisal third of the right central and the discoloration of the left central.

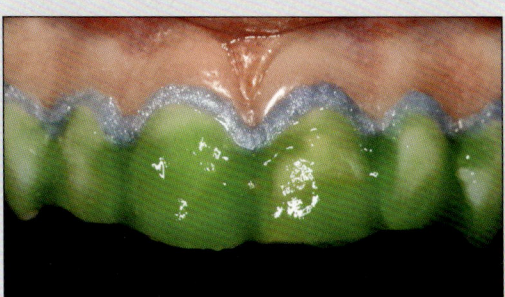

Fig 7a An in-office bleaching procedure was performed with a 35% hydrogen peroxide gel (Whiteness HP Maxx, FGM).

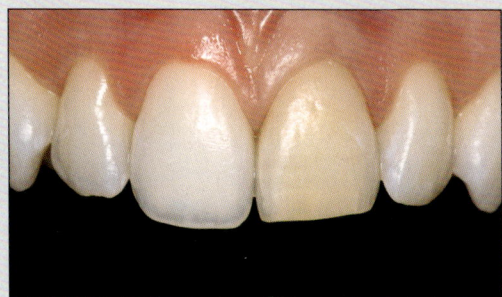

Fig 7b The anterior teeth 7 days after bleaching.

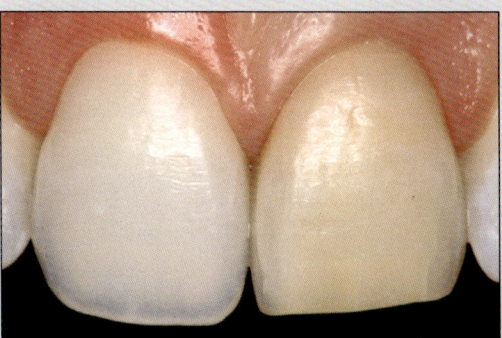

Fig 8 Under direct illumination, the right central incisor showed a remarkable bluish incisal area outlined by an opaque halo.

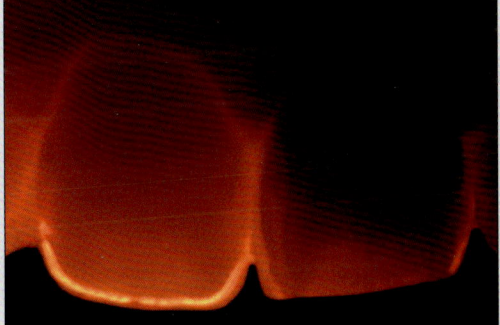

Fig 9 Under indirect lighting, the incisal opalescent effect could only be observed on the right central incisor.

initially accomplished with a digital spectrophotometer (VITA Easyshade, Vident, Brea, CA, USA) (Fig 11) and confirmed after the positioning and light curing of small increments of the selected resin composites over the adjacent tooth structure.

This is a crucial step, as the shade of microhybrid resin composites will change after polymerization, becoming darker and more translucent.[2,22] The veneer preparation was completed, and the amount of tooth reduction was kept to a minimum (Fig 12).

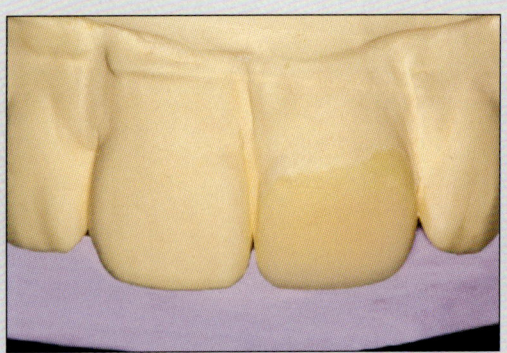
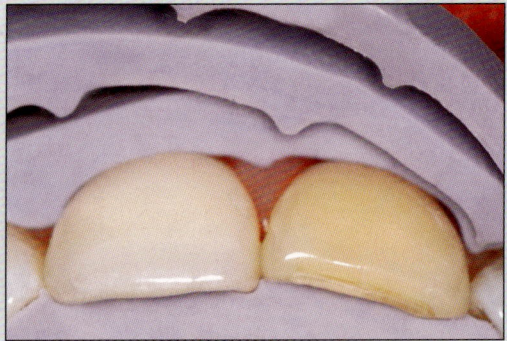

Figs 10a and 10b Silicone putty matrix used to facilitate the development of the incisal edge contour **(a)** and guide the veneer preparation **(b)**.

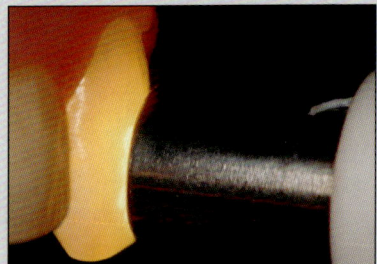

Fig 11 A spectrophotometer was used for the shade selection (VITA Easyshade, Vident).

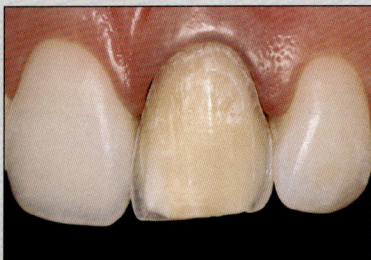

Fig 12 The completed veneer preparation.

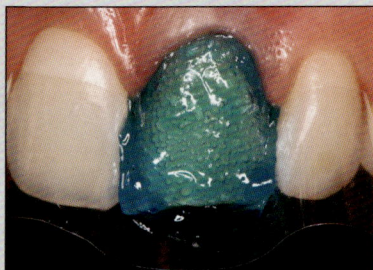

Fig 13 Following field isolation, a 37% phosphoric acid gel (Total Etch, Ivoclar Vivadent) was applied for 15 seconds.

Field isolation was accomplished with a lip and cheek retractor and retraction cord. A 37% phosphoric acid (Total Etch, Ivoclar Vivadent, Schaan, Liechtenstein) was applied to the enamel and dentin for 15 seconds (Fig 13), rinsed with an air-water spray for 15 seconds, and dried slightly with a mild air stream to prevent dentin dehydration. A one-bottle adhesive system (Excite, Ivoclar Vivadent) was applied according to the manufacturer's instructions and light cured for 10 seconds (Fig 14). The initial layer of a hybrid resin composite (White Effect, 4 Seasons, Ivoclar Vivadent) was positioned to mask the underlying discoloration and match the value of the adjacent teeth (Fig 15). The same resin composite was positioned on the silicone matrix with a spatula and smoothed with a sable brush (no. 4, National Keystone, Cherry Hill, NJ, USA) (Fig 16). The silicone matrix was positioned and the resin composite was carefully internally adapted to the tooth structure (Fig 17). This layer

was initially light cured for 20 seconds with the silicone matrix in position, and completed through the palatal surface for another 20 seconds after removal of the silicone matrix. This thin layer reproduced the incisal opaque halo effect and allowed for the reproduction of the bluish incisal area (Fig 18). A hybrid resin composite (Blue Effect, 4 Seasons, Ivoclar Vivadent) was layered to reproduce the opalescent area. A blue tint (Kolor + Plus, Kerr, Orange, CA, USA) was applied to accentuate the bluish appearance (Fig 19). The artificial enamel was created in two resin composite layers to impart a more lifelike depth of color. After application of a thin artificial internal enamel layer (High Value, 4 Seasons, Ivoclar Vivadent), the artificial facial enamel layer was recreated with a Trans Clear hybrid resin composite (4 Seasons, Ivoclar Vivadent), applied and contoured with a long-bladed instrument (IPCL, Cosmedent, Chicago, IL, USA), and smoothed with an artist brush (no. 4 National Key-

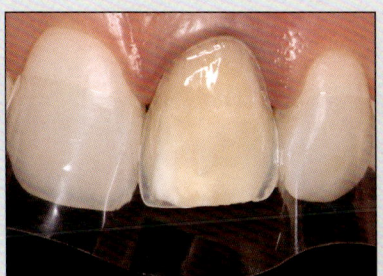

Fig 14 The acid gel was rinsed with an air/water spray and the tooth surface was gently air-dried. A one-bottle adhesive system (Excite, Ivoclar Vivadent) was applied to the etched surface.

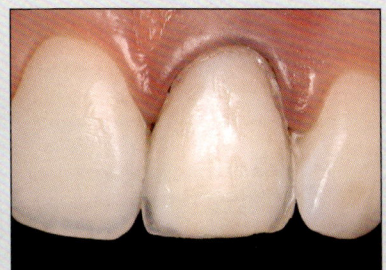

Fig 15 An initial layer of a White Effect hybrid resin composite (4 Seasons, Ivoclar Vivadent) was placed to mask the underlying discoloration and match the value (luminosity) of the adjacent teeth.

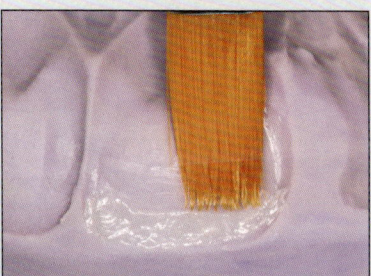

Fig 16 The White Effect hybrid resin composite was placed on the silicone matrix with a spatula and smoothed with a sable brush (no. 4, National Keystone).

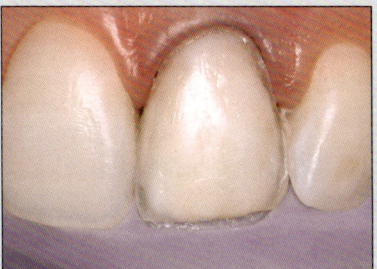

Fig 17 The silicone matrix was positioned and the resin composite was internally adapted to the tooth structure.

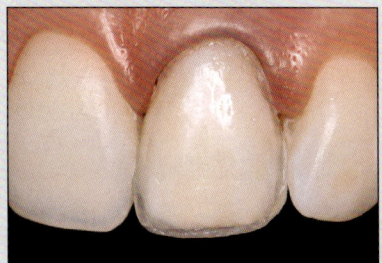

Fig 18 After light curing, it was observed that the opaque incisal halo effect had been recreated, thus allowing for the reproduction of the bluish incisal area.

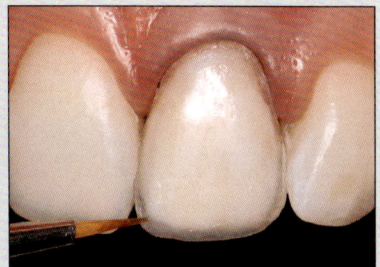

Fig 19 A blue tint (Kolor + Plus, Kerr) was applied to accentuate the bluish appearance of the incisal third.

stone). The restoration was light cured through an oxygen inhibitor gel for 1 minute from the facial and palatal sides.

Figure 20 shows the completed restoration prior to the finishing and polishing procedures. Major excesses were removed, the occlusion was checked and adjusted, and the patient was dismissed. In a subsequent appointment, the surface texture, anatomic morphology, and luster were defined.

It is important to spend enough time on the finishing and polishing procedures, since this is when the morphology and texture are recreated. Sometimes, in fact, more time is spent on finishing and polishing than on layering. A finishing and polishing protocol will now be presented; however, it should be noted that specific procedures will vary according to each case.

The interproximal contour was established with finishing strips of varying abrasiveness (Epitex, GC America, Alsip, IL, USA) (Figs 21a to 21c). The incisal angles and facial and proximal surfaces were finished with an extra-fine aluminum oxide disk (Flexi-Discs, Cosmedent) (Fig 22). A tapered diamond bur was used to recreate the flat areas on the contralateral incisor (Fig 23). The reflectance areas were outlined with colored graffiti, with a green line marking the ideal positioning and a red line marking the current positioning. A long tapered extra-fine diamond bur was used to adjust the positioning of the reflectance area (Figure 24) by making both lines (green and red) overlap (Figure 25). Small depression areas on the contralateral incisor were outlined with gray graffiti and reproduced with a short tapered extra-fine diamond bur (Figs 26 and 27). These areas were polished

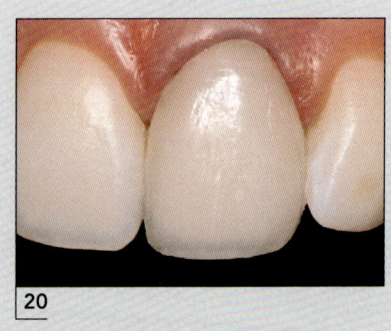

20

Fig 20 The completed restoration prior to the finishing and polishing procedures.

Figs 21a to 21c The interproximal contour was established with finishing strips of varying abrasiveness (Epitex, GC America).

Fig 22 The incisal angles and buccal and proximal surfaces were finished with an extra-fine aluminum oxide disk (Flexi-Discs, Cosmedent).

Fig 23 The flat areas present on the contralateral incisor were recreated with a tapered diamond bur.

Fig 24 A long tapered extra-fine diamond bur was used to adjust the positioning of the reflectance areas.

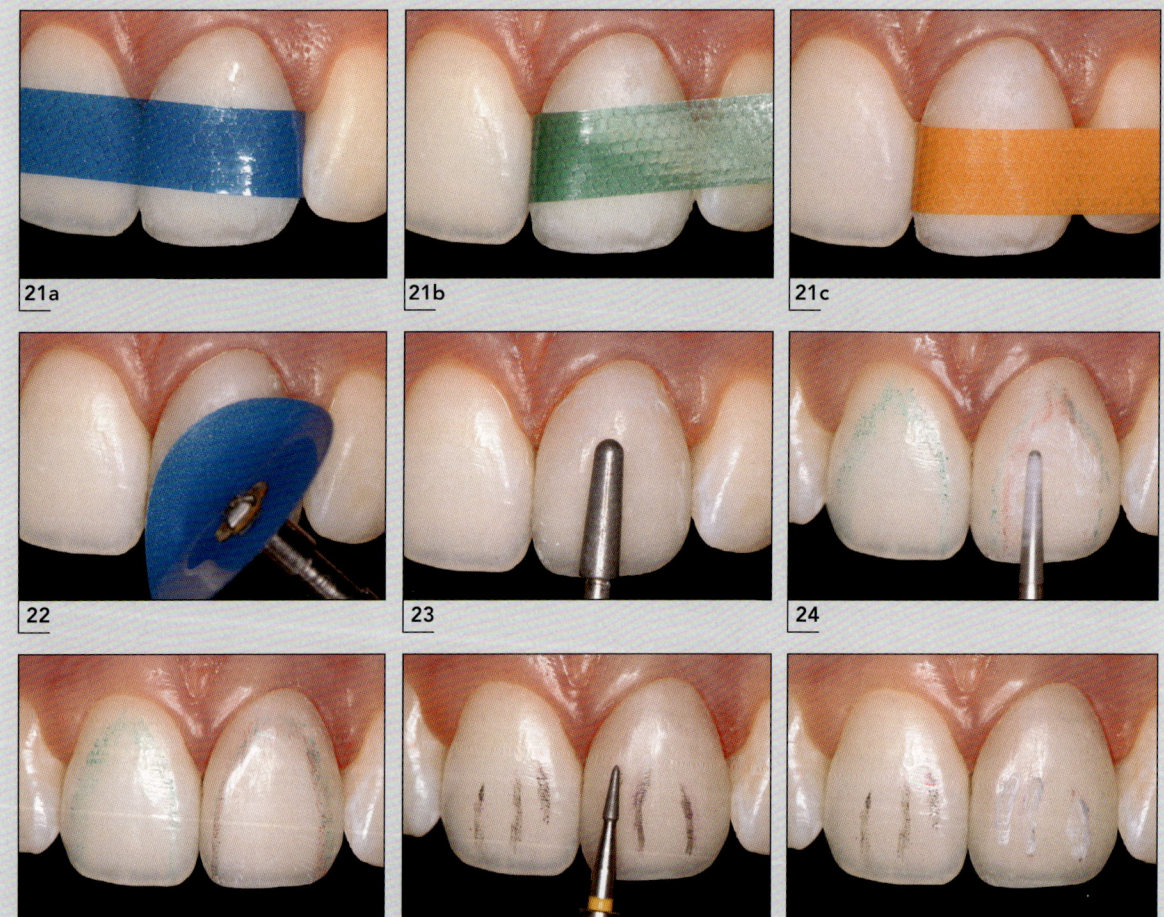

21a

21b

21c

22

23

24

Fig 25 When both lines (green and red) overlapped, the reflectance areas were considered adjusted.

Fig 26 A short tapered extra-fine diamond bur was used to reproduce the depression areas.

Fig 27 The completed depression areas before polishing.

with a silicone rubber point (Flexi-Point, Cosmedent) to eliminate undesired accentuated characterization (Fig 28). The surface texture was recreated with a straight-edge diamond bur (Fig 29), which was used to produce horizontal lines from the cervical to the incisal third (Fig 30). A buff wheel (Flexi-Buff, Cosmedent) was used with a polishing paste (Enamelize, Cosmedent) to create light reflectance and a high luster while maintaining the established texture and surface morphol-

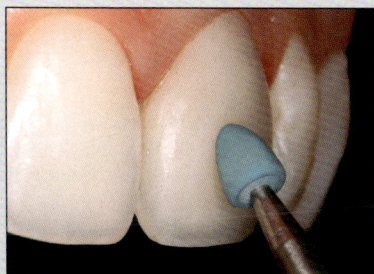

Fig 28 The depression areas were polished with a silicone rubber point (Flexi-Point, Cosmedent) to eliminate undesired accentuated characterization.

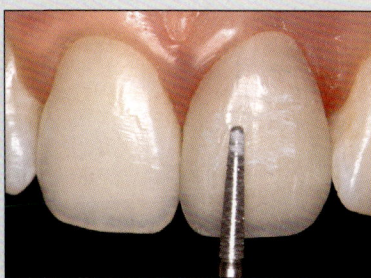

Fig 29 To recreate the surface texture, an extra-fine straight-edge diamond bur was used to produce horizontal lines from the cervical to the incisal third.

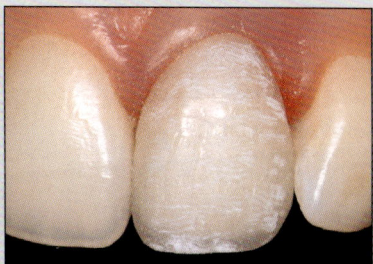

Fig 30 The established horizontal lines prior to polishing.

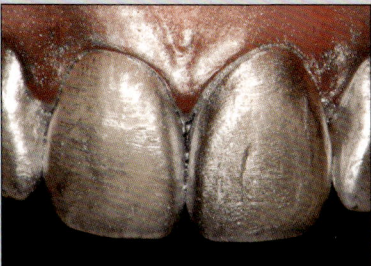

Fig 31 Silver powder was used to highlight the morphology of the teeth and check the final texture.

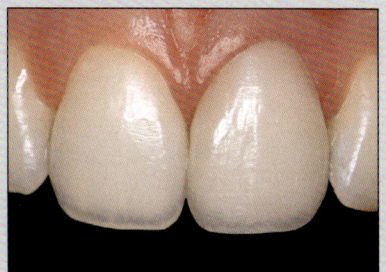

Fig 32 The finished and polished restoration. Note the blue opalescent effect achieved on the left maxillary incisor (compare with Fig 8).

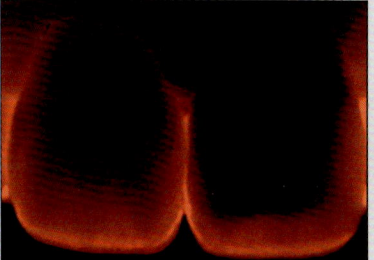

Fig 33 With indirect lighting, the transmission of the orange opalescent effect was observed on both central incisors (compare with Fig 9).

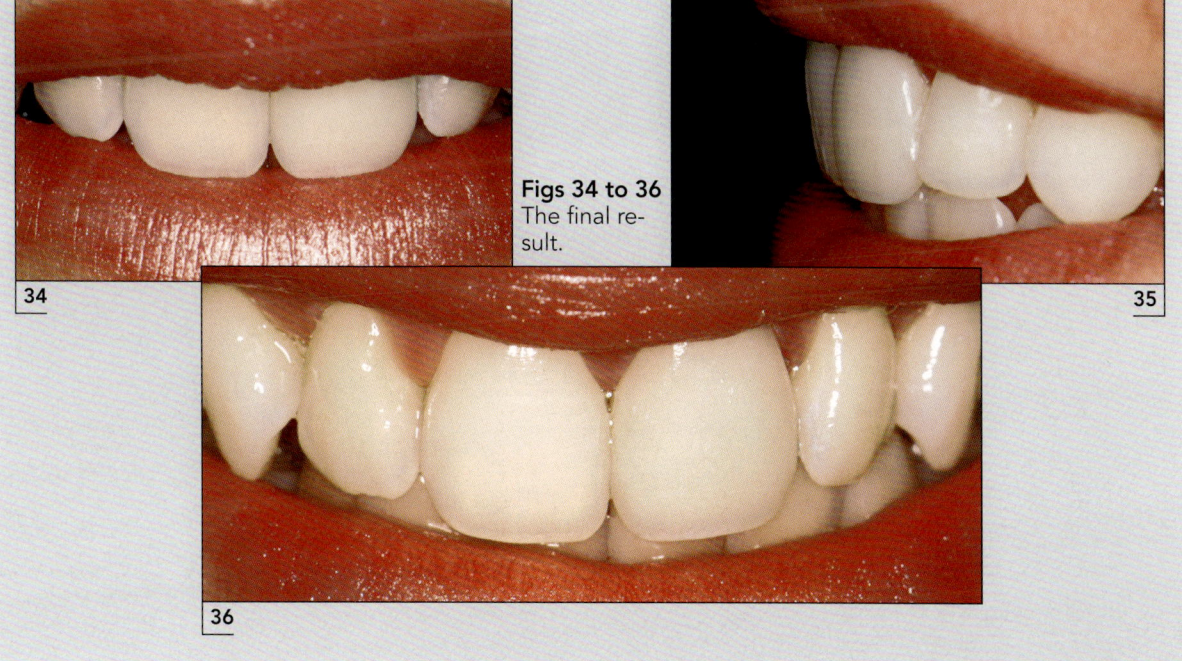

Figs 34 to 36 The final result.

ogy. Silver powder was used to highlight the morphology of the teeth and check the final texture (Fig 31). Figure 32 shows the polished restoration.

The teeth were again indirectly illuminated to observe the opalescence (Fig 33). The final result is shown in Figs 34 to 36.

CONCLUSION

Opalescence is an important optical property of natural teeth, and its careful reproduction is necessary when highly esthetic restorations are desired. Knowledge of all available opalescent resin composites and an understanding of their placement are imperative for the achievement of satisfactory results.

REFERENCES

1. Chu SJ, Ahmad I. Light dynamic properties of a synthetic, low-fusing, quartz glass-ceramic material. Pract Proced Aesthet Dent 2003;15:49–56.

2. Baratieri LN, Araujo EM Jr, Monteiro S Jr. Composite Restorations in Anterior Teeth: Fundamentals and Possibilities. Chicago: Quintessence, 2005.

3. Sensi LG, Marson FC, Roesner, TH, Baratieri LN, Monteiro S Jr. Fluorescence of composite resins: Clinical considerations. Quintessence Dent Technol 2006;29:43–53.

4. Buda M. Form and color reproduction for composite resin reconstruction of anterior teeth. Int J Periodontics Restorative Dent 1994;14:34–47.

5. Dietschi D. Free-hand composite resin restorations: A key to anterior aesthetics. Pract Periodontics Aesthet Dent 1995;7:15–25.

6. Fahl N Jr, Denehy GE, Jackson RD. Protocol for predictable restoration of anterior teeth with composite resins. Pract Periodontics Aesthet Dent 1995;7:13–21.

7. Magne P, Holz J. Stratification of composite restorations: Systematic and durable replication of natural esthetics. Pract Periodontics Aesthet Dent 1996;8:61–68.

8. Dietschi D. Layering concepts in anterior composite restorations. J Adhes Dent 2001;3:71–80.

9. Vanini L. Light and color in anterior composite restorations. Pract Periodontics Aesthet Dent 1996;8:673–682.

10. Dietschi D. Free-hand bonding in the esthetic treatment of anterior teeth: Creating the illusion. J Esthet Dent 1997;9:156–164.

11. de Araujo Junior EM, Baratieri LN, Monteiro Junior S, Vieira LC, de Andrada MA. Direct adhesive restoration of anterior teeth. Part 1. Fundamentals of excellence. Pract Proced Aesthet Dent 2003;15:233–240.

12. de Araujo Junior EM, Baratieri LN, Monteiro Junior S, Vieira LC, de Andrada MA. Direct adhesive restoration of anterior teeth: Part 2. Clinical protocol. Pract Proced Aesthet Dent 2003;15:351–357.

13. de Araujo Junior EM, Baratieri LN, Monteiro Junior S, Vieira LC, de Andrada MA. Direct adhesive restoration of anterior teeth: Part 3. Procedural considerations. Pract Proced Aesthet Dent 2003;15:433–437.

14. Jackson RD. Understanding the characteristics of naturally shaded composite resins. Pract Proced Aesthet Dent 2003;15:577–585.

15. Culp L. Replicating natural dentition with composite resin. Pract Proced Aesthet Dent 2004;16:27–30.

16. Terry DA, Leinfelder KF. An integration of composite resin with natural tooth structure: The Class IV restoration. Pract Proced Aesthet Dent 2004;16:235–242.

17. Winter R. Visualizing the natural dentition. J Esthet Dent 1993;5:102–117.

18. Fondriest J. Shade matching in restorative dentistry: The science and strategies. Int J Periodontics Restorative Dent 2003;23:467–479.

19. Primus CM, Chu CC, Shelby JE, Buldrini E, Heckle CE. Opalescence of dental porcelain enamels. Quintessence Int 2002;33:439–449.

20. Lee YK, Lu H, Powers JM. Measurement of opalescence of resin composites. Dent Mater 2005;21:1068–1074.

21. Lee YK, Lu H, Powers JM. Changes in opalescence and fluorescence properties of resin composites after accelerated aging. Dent Mater 2006;22:653–660.

22. Lee YK, Lim BS, Rhee SH, Yang HC, Powers JM. Color and translucency of A2 shade resin composites after curing, polishing, and thermocycling. Oper Dent 2005;30:436–442.

ALL-CERAMIC RESTORATIONS: MATERIAL SELECTION AND OPACITY CONTROL FOR ESTHETICALLY SUPERIOR RESULTS

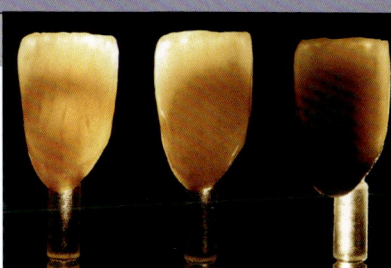

Aki Yoshida, RDT[1]

[1]Private practice, Weston, Massachusetts, USA.

Correspondence to: Mr Aki Yoshida, Gnathos Dental Studio, 56 Colpitts Rd, Weston, MA 02493, USA.
E-mail: akiyoshidainc@verizon.net

In response to increasing patient demands for esthetic dental rehabilitations, more prosthetic restorations are being fabricated using all-ceramic systems, which show superior biocompatibility and similar light characteristics to the natural tooth (Figs 1 and 2).

Further, progress in dental CAD/CAM technology has been so rapid that the marginal fit of copings made via this method show clinically acceptable results[1,2] and are well accepted by clinicians compared to the more complicated indirect process of fabricating cast restorations (Figs 3 to 5). Moreover, the steep rise in the price of precious alloys has provided an added impetus to embrace this technology.

However, from an esthetic standpoint, it is still doubtful whether the best material is being selected for each case (Fig 6). The translucency of all-ceramic crowns is an advantage; however, this translucency is affected by the color of the abutment tooth after cementation (Fig 7).

A minute color difference is less noticeable in multiunit cases, but cannot be ignored in anterior single-unit cases (Figs 8 to 10). It is critical that any crowns made with the selected material exhibit a stable shade under different light sources after cementation.

This article will discuss how to select the most appropriate all-ceramic system for each case.

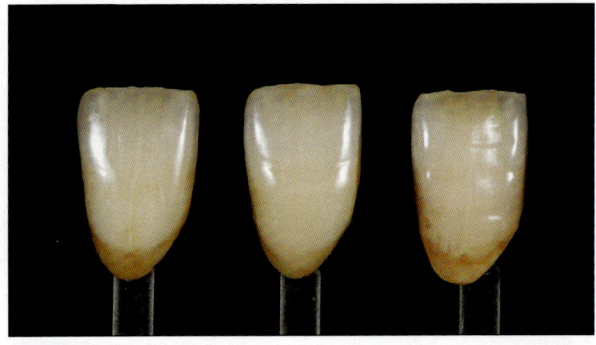
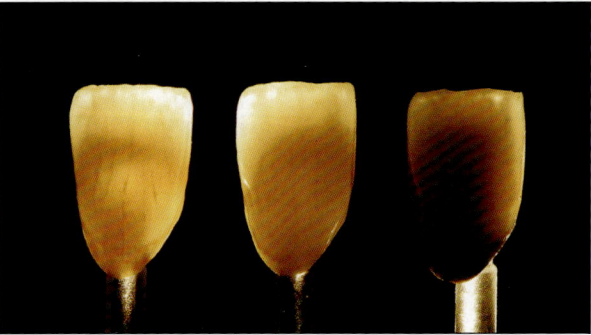

Figs 1 and 2 Three crown systems: Procera *(left)*, zirconia *(middle)*, and metal-ceramic *(right)*. Note that the metal-ceramic crown shows no translucency, which is a significant disadvantage when used for an anterior prosthesis.

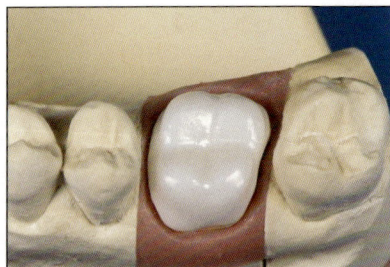

Fig 3 CAD/CAM is an efficient method for fabricating copings.

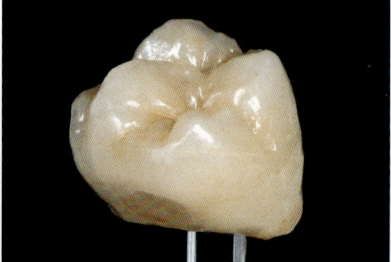

Figs 4 and 5 A zirconia crown made with 100% masking material. It often seems that white zirconia is opaque; however, can you really say that this is opaque?

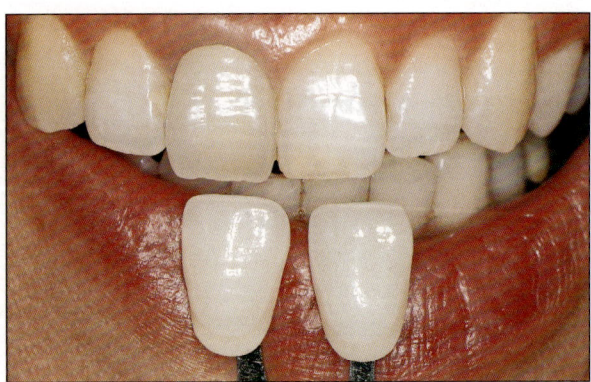

Fig 6 A crown with excellent form, surface detail, and incisal characterization, except for its color disharmony.

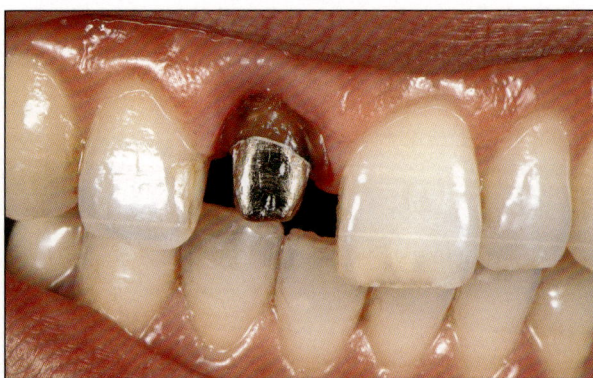

Fig 7 It is impossible to mask the abutment shade without the use of masking materials.

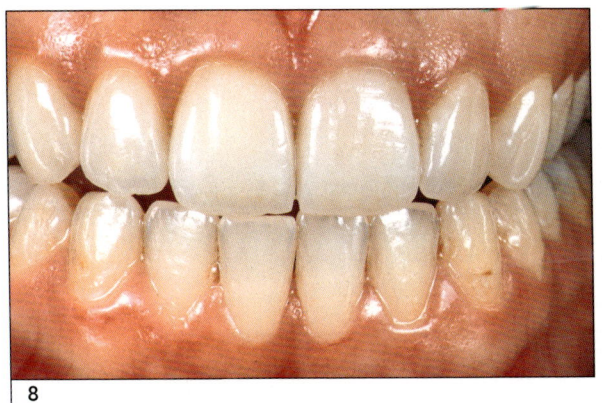

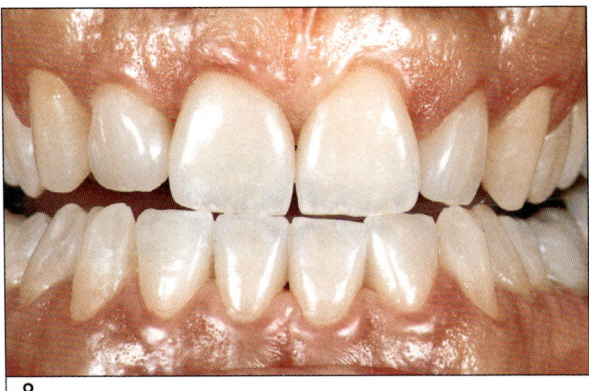

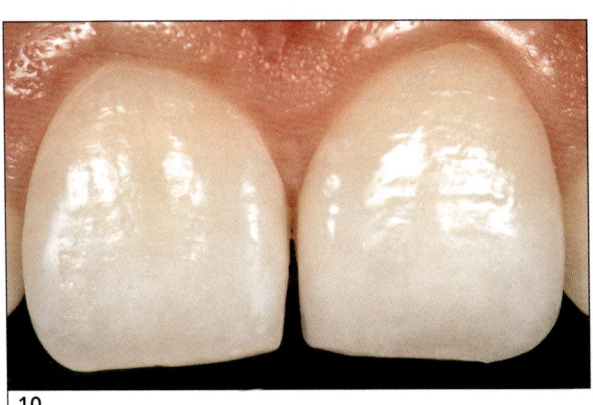

Fig 8 Multiunit prosthesis for six maxillary anterior teeth. In this type of case, the most important goal is to achieve total balance in both the shade and form. Slight differences in shade are usually not visible in multiunit cases.

Fig 9 Maxillary and mandibular all-ceramic four-unit prostheses. Again, slight differences in shade will not be noticeable.

Fig 10 All-ceramic crown for the maxillary left central incisor. Although this is a single-unit case, the color of the final restoration can be estimated since the shade of the abutment tooth is same as that of the final restoration.

TRANSLUCENCY

It is well known that all-ceramic copings are translucent, and so when selecting the proper materials, it is important to know how much translucency each system provides. Therefore, an experiment was carried out to test the translucency of several all-ceramic systems.

First, the author prepared an extracted tooth (Fig 11). After checking for differences in translucency under reflected and transmitted light (Fig 12), the translucency of each coping was measured with the Transmission Densitometer (TD-931, Macbeth, Newburgh, NY, USA) (Fig 13). The results are shown in Table 1.

Interestingly, even the In-Ceram Alumina system (VITA Zahnfabrik, Bad Säckingen, Germany), which is nearly opaque, showed some translucency.[3] It has been established that if opaque porcelain is fired on a metal coping with a gold-colored bonding agent, the gold color will appear orange through the opaque porcelain, which prevents the crown from appearing too dark and helps the color accommodation in the mouth because of the reddish shade.[4]

In this test with this equipment, it was necessary for the opaque metal-ceramic porcelain to be 1 mm thick to achieve perfect opacity. The results suggest that the shade of any all-ceramic system must be checked in the mouth using a try-in paste (Figs 14 and 15).[5]

In Procera (Nobel Biocare, Göteborg, Sweden) and zirconia systems, in which a translucent shade liner is used, the shade may be adjusted before the porcelain buildup, and the translucency of the coping itself is also adjustable (Figs 16 and 17).

It should be noted that while Procera and zirconia are translucent, neither has fluorescence (Figs 18 to 20).[6] Therefore, if the patient has thin gingiva or if the margins are located supragingivally, margin porcelain with fluorescence should be used to achieve better esthetic results (Fig 21).

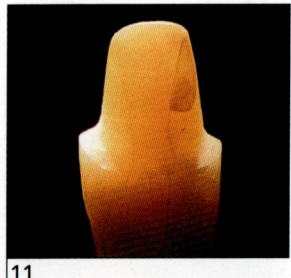

Fig 11 Tooth preparation was carried out on an extracted tooth, and copings were fabricated using five all-ceramic systems.

Fig 12 The study materials under reflected and transmitted light. Note the differences in translucency.

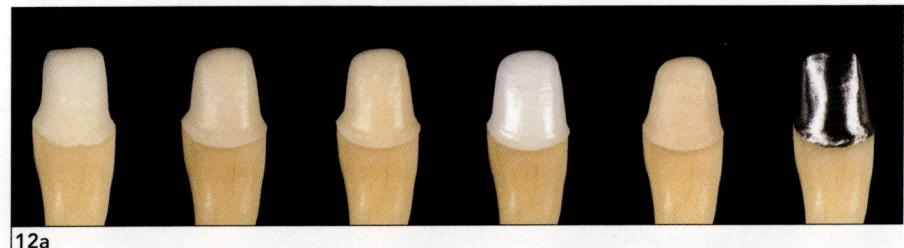

12a

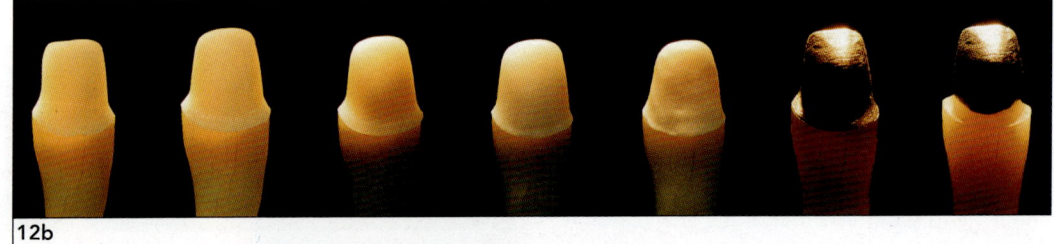

12b

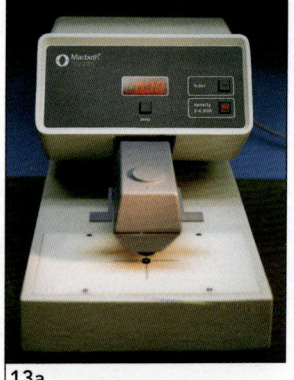

13a

Figs 13a to 13e The Transmission Densitometer (TD-931, Macbeth) **(a)**. Light is transmitted from the base of the device **(b)**. The test specimen is placed at the center of the emission **(c)**. The specimen is covered with black rubber and the transmitted light is measured **(d)**. The top of the device displays the percent of transmitted light **(e)**.

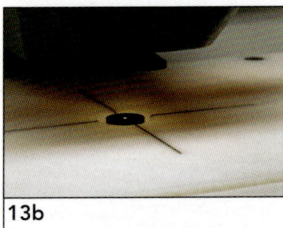

13b

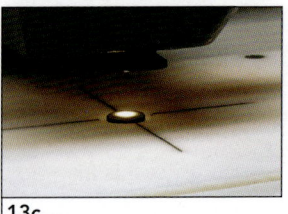

13c

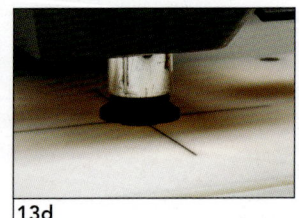

13d

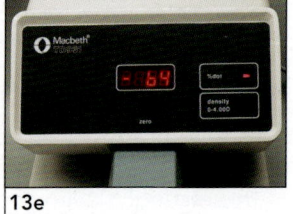

13e

Table 1 Material translucency (% light transmission)

Feldspar	In-Ceram Spinell	Procera	Zirconia	In-Ceram Alumina	Metal
46%	37%	33%	27%	16%	0%

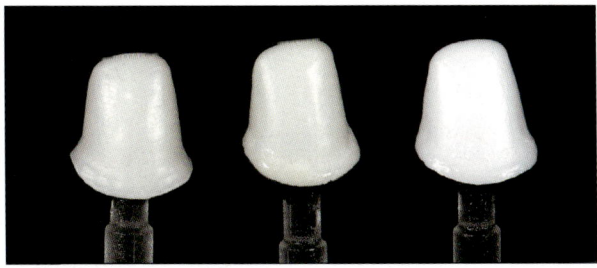

Fig 14 The copings were placed on stumps made from black wax[5]: *(left)* Procera, 0.4 mm thick; *(middle)* Procera, 0.5 mm thick, *(right)* zirconia, 0.5 mm thick. All of the copings appeared opaque.

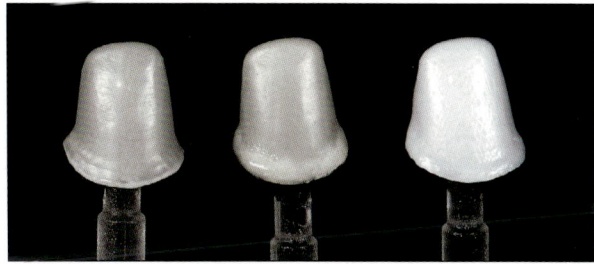

Fig 15 The stain liquid infiltrated the copings.[5] Note how the appearance is affected by the stump shade.

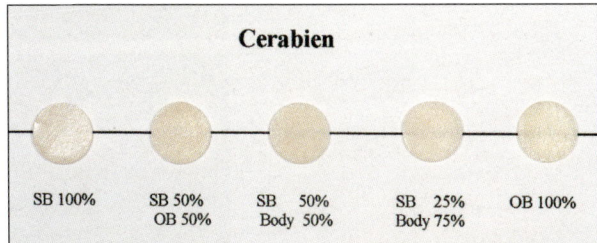

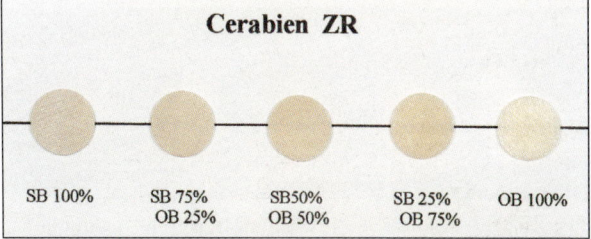

Figs 16 and 17 Shade base for Procera and zirconia copings. Light transmission can be controlled with the use of dentin powder.

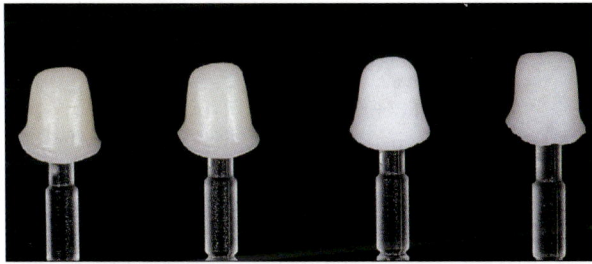

Fig 18 *(left to right)* Procera, 0.4 mm thick; Procera, 0.6 mm thick; zirconia, 0.5 mm thick; Feldspar, 0.4 mm thick.

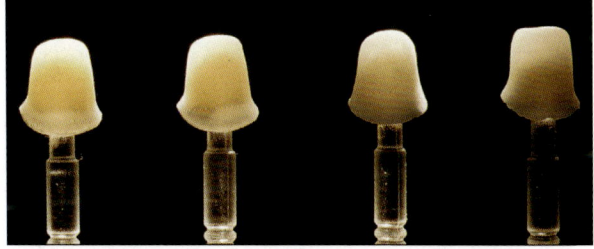

Fig 19 All copings show different degrees of translucency.

Fig 20 Under black light, only feldspar *(far right)* shows fluorescence.

Figs 21a and 21b Step-by-step procedures for the zirconia system using Noritake CZR porcelain. Note the second step from the left, which shows that the margin porcelain is fired on the cervical aspect. Margin porcelain has fluorescence, but zirconia copings do not.

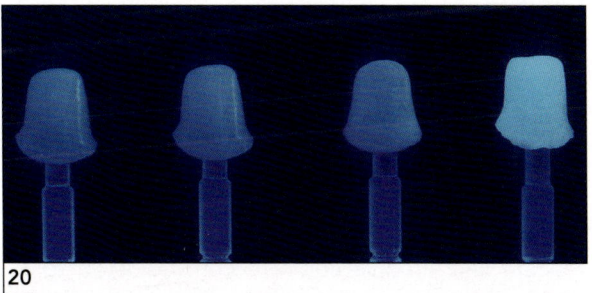

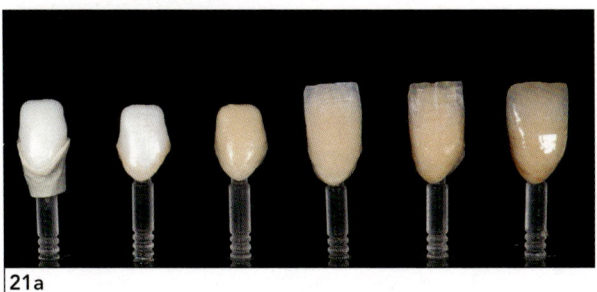

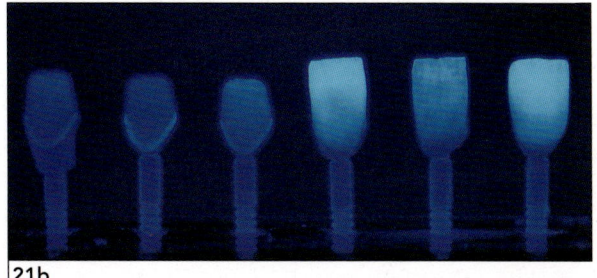

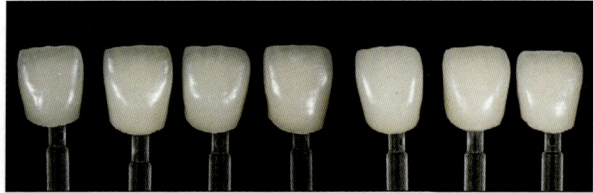

Fig 22 Seven all-ceramic crowns: *(left to right)* Feldspar, In-Ceram Spinell, Procera, Procera with masking, zirconia, zirconia with masking, In-Ceram Alumina.

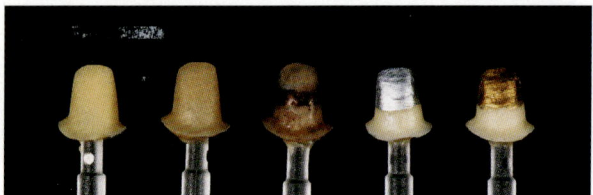

Fig 23 The stumps used to simulate different clinical conditions, *from left:* A3, A4, dark, silver, gold. [5]

SHADE EVALUATION

It should be mentioned that in practice, copings are not used on their own, but are cemented as crowns after porcelain buildup.[7] Therefore, an experiment was performed to evaluate the shade of different all-ceramic systems.

First, seven crowns (Fig 22) were fabricated using the simple three-layer buildup method, where each layer is adjusted to nearly the same thickness. Procera and zirconia crowns were adjusted to have a 0.2-mm-thick masking material. Procera and zirconia copings were adjusted to a thickness of 0.5 mm. The first bake comprised only dentin porcelain, and the thickness after firing was adjusted to 0.7 mm (the thickness of dentin porcelain for a crown with masking material should be 0.5 mm).

Next, the incisal third was covered with enamel porcelain and the entire crown was covered with translucent porcelain. After firing, each crown was adjusted to a thickness of 1.5 mm (including the coping thickness). The shade was A1.

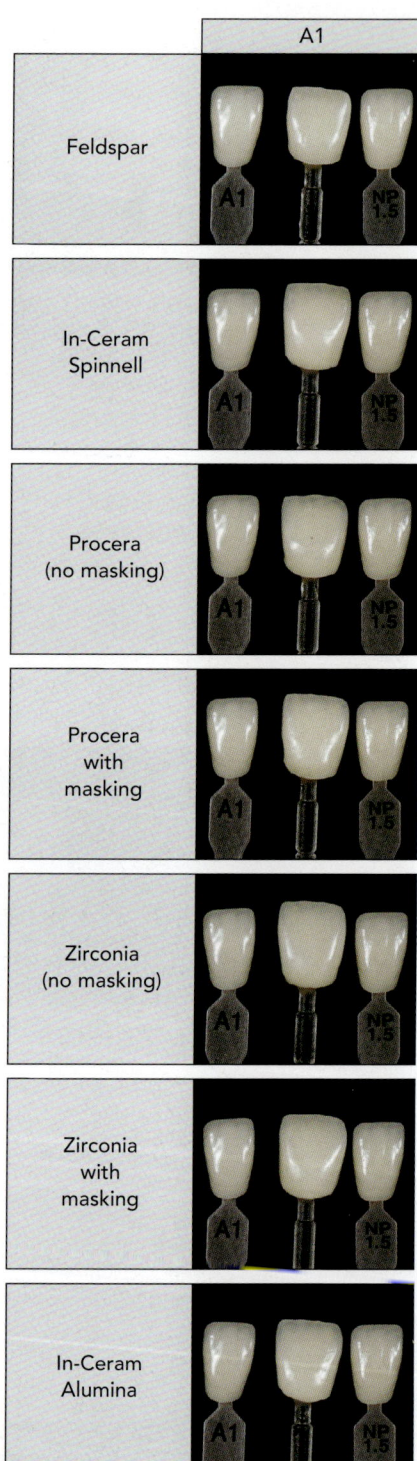

Fig 24 Color evaluation for seven all-ceramic systems with stumps noted.

The seven crowns were placed onto stumps containing a staining liquid to simulate different clinical conditions, and the color change was observed (Fig 23). Photographs were taken

A3	A4	Dark	Silver	Gold

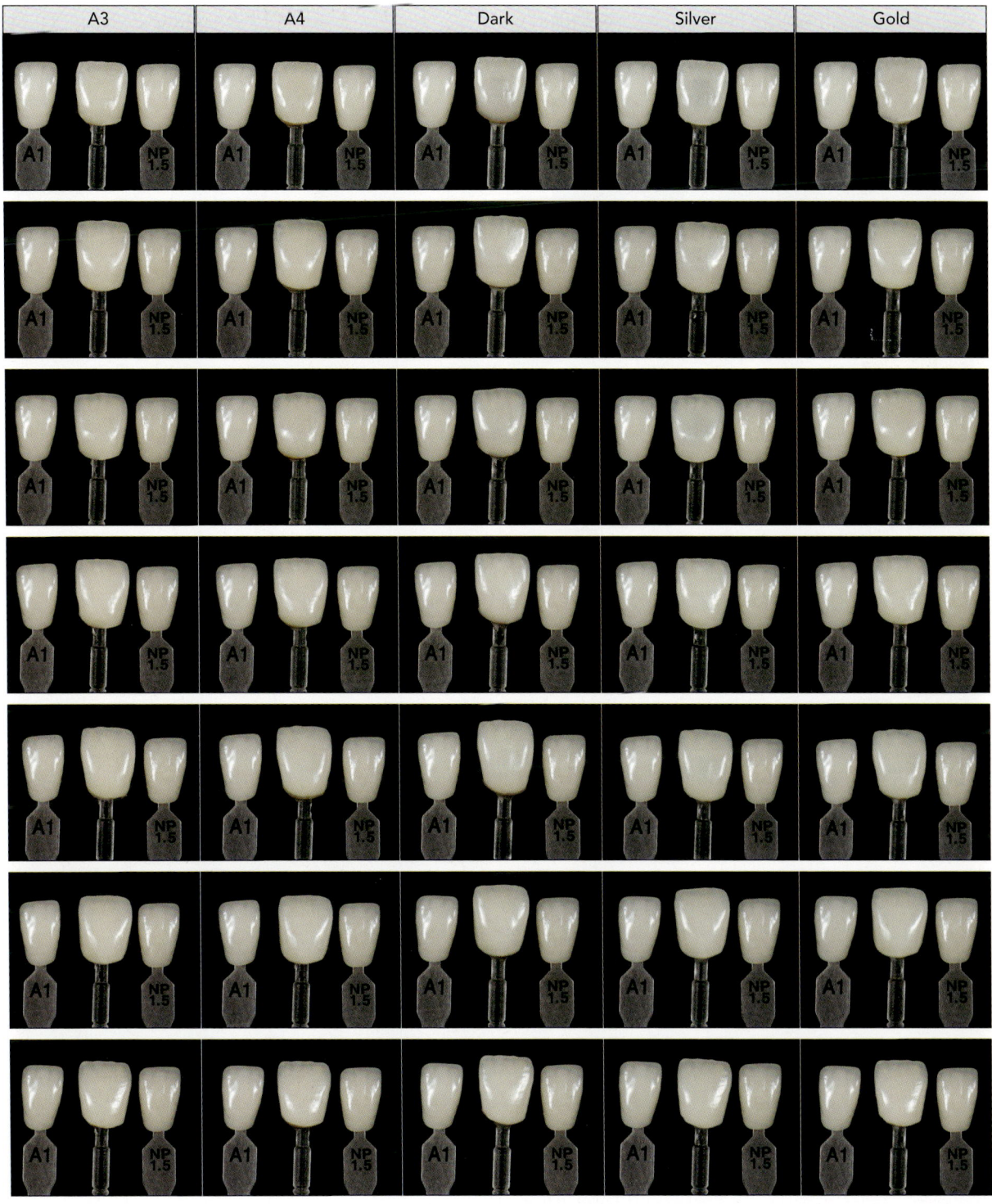

using A1 and NW1.5 (Noritake Shade Guide, Noritake, Aichi, Japan) shade guides (Fig 24). The camera used was a Canon 5D (Canon, Tokyo, Japan) with a custom-set white balance.

The monitor used was a 30-inch LCD (Apple, Cupertino, CA, USA), which was calibrated using the Monaco EZ color system (X-rite, Kentwood, MI, USA).[8,9]

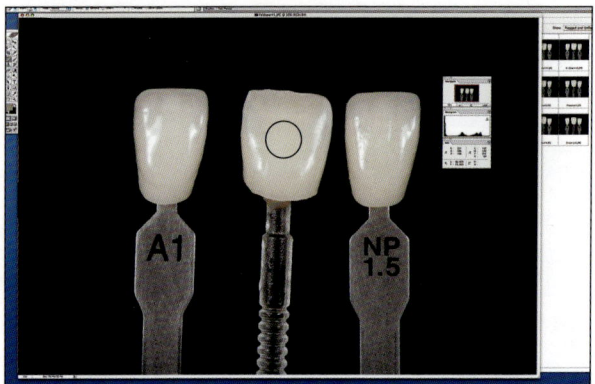

Fig 25a Color measurement with Photoshop (Adobe Systems). The *circle* shows the measurement area between the mesial and distal marginal ridges (which are made visible from the reflection of the flashlight).

	A 1
Feldspar	R 211 G 206 B 186
In-Ceram Spinnell	R 215 G 210 B 188
Procera (no masking)	R 215 G 209 B 193
Procera with masking	R 214 G 208 B 188
Zirconia (no masking)	R 215 G 209 B 187
Zirconia with masking	R 215 G 209 B 191
In-Ceram Alumina	R 215 G 208 B 191

Fig 25b The results of the color measurement. Note the change in number from A1 to Gold.

The RGB numbers of 42 combinations of digital images were measured using Adobe Photoshop (Adobe Systems, San Jose, CA, USA) (Fig 25a), and the results are shown in Fig 25b.

In this experiment, clear stain liquid was used to infiltrate the crowns; however, in clinical situations, opaque cement can be used to control the opacity.[10] The chart may seem too strict, but in reality, any all-ceramic crowns fabricated for patient use will be subject to sunlight, which is more intense and intermittent than the flashlight used in this experiment. Therefore, it is best to use this chart when selecting the proper material.

A 3	A 4	Dark	Silver	Gold
R 204 G 198 B 176	R 199 G 192 B 175	R 186 G 183 B 173	R 186 G 186 B 172	R 198 G 190 B 173
R 213 G 207 B 184	R 205 G 204 B 180	R 198 G 197 B 177	R 19 G 196 B 175	R 203 G 199 B 180
R 211 G 206 B 186	R 206 G 200 B 183	R 202 G 196 B 181	R 196 G 194 B 182	R 204 G 199 B 181
R 213 G 206 B 188	R 209 G 204 B 184	R 204 G 196 B 181	R 204 G 195 B 178	R 207 G 202 B 181
R 213 G 208 B 186	R 210 G 204 B 179	R 207 G 201 B 176	R 206 G 200 B 176	R 209 G 204 B 180
R 215 G 209 B 191	R 214 G 208 B 191	R 209 G 206 B 189	R 207 G 203 B 185	R 213 G 209 B 191
R 214 G 208 B 191	R 214 G 207 B 189	R 213 G 206 B 188	R 213 G 207 B 188	R 214 G 208 B 190

The number of the A1 stump is the standard. Regarding the amount of change, 5 or less is optimal (green boxes), 10 or less is acceptable (yellow boxes), and 11 or more is unacceptable (white boxes).

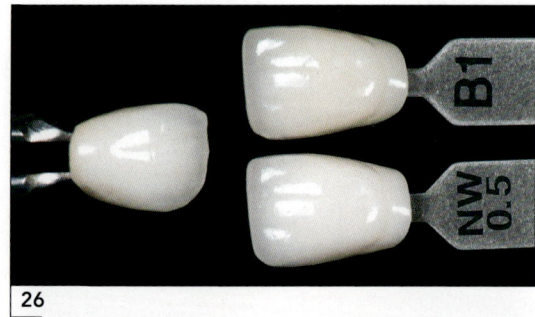

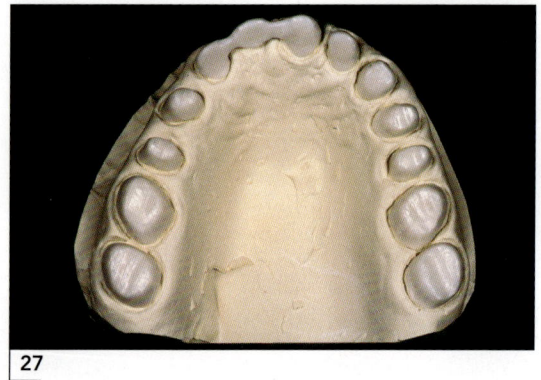

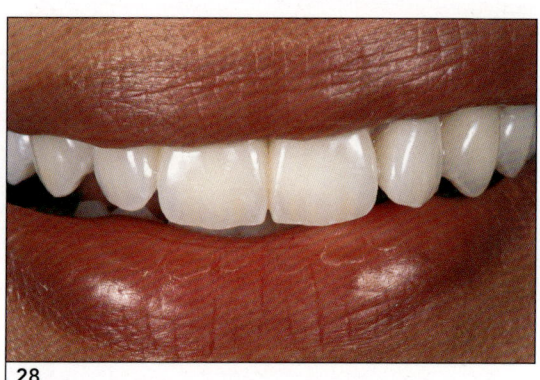

Fig 26 If a bright and translucent appearance is desired, a zirconia coping is recommended.

Figs 27 and 28 Using white zirconia copings, a soft expression was achieved.

OPACITY AND VALUE CONTROL

The value of the restoration depends on the difference in the degree of light transmission from the copings.[11] For example, if a bright and translucent appearance is desired, a zirconia coping is preferable to keep the value high (Fig 26). On the other hand, to express a translucent, low-value shade, a more translucent coping is preferable as long as the background color can be controlled.

In the case shown in Figs 27 and 28, the patient disliked her opaque white crowns and requested a soft translucent bleaching shade. Zirconia was selected as the white coping material. After cementation, the desired color was achieved.

CASE PRESENTATIONS

Case 1

The patient presented with a complaint about the color of the maxillary left central incisor, which had an all-ceramic crown fabricated using a pressure-forming ceramic system. Compared to the natural right central incisor, the translucency was extremely high and the value low. After removal of the crown, the condition of the abutment tooth was observed as a nonvital tooth with slight discoloration (Figs 29 to 33).

The stump shade was A3 to A3.5, and the shade for the final restoration was A1 to A2 with a low value for the incisal third. In this case, a bonding-type material could not be selected because of the condition of the abutment tooth. For the expression of low values, Procera or In-Ceram are advantageous; however, considering the translucency, a Procera coping (with no masking) was judged most appropriate. The tooth showed surface details of low texture and low luster. It is important for the restoration to be in harmony with the surface details of the adjacent teeth.[12]

CASE 1

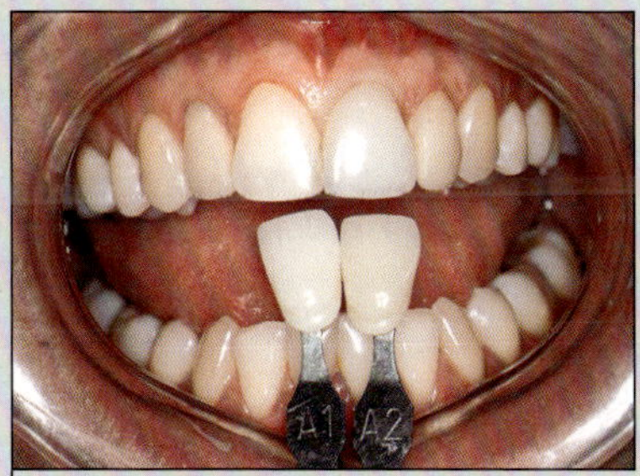

Fig 29 The maxillary left central incisor had a pressure-forming all-ceramic crown.

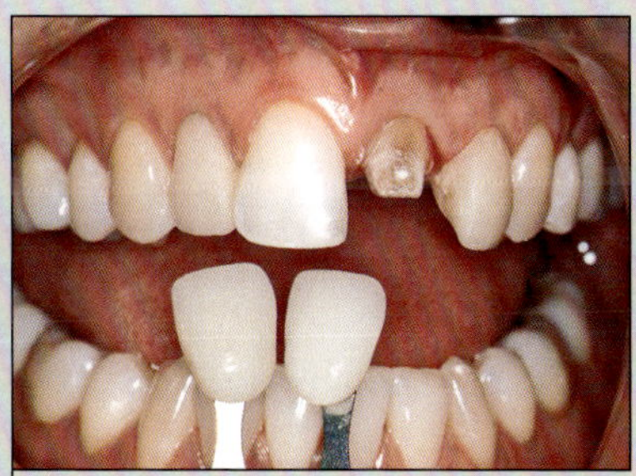

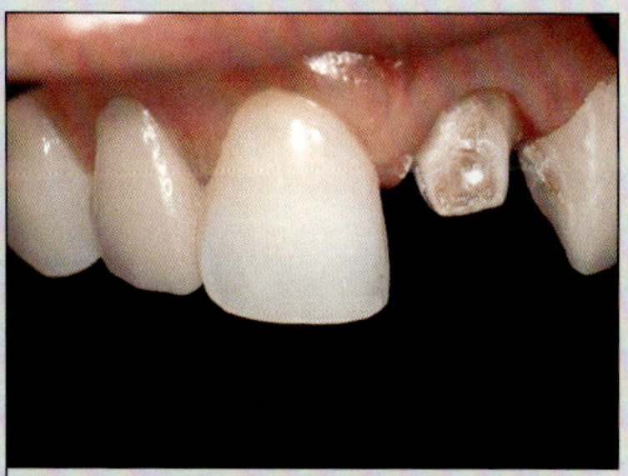

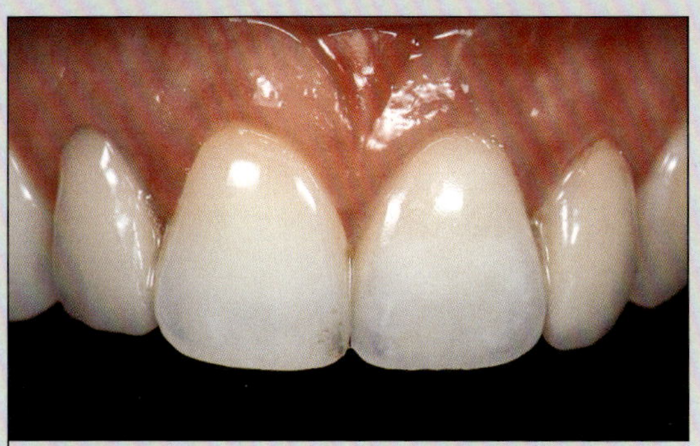

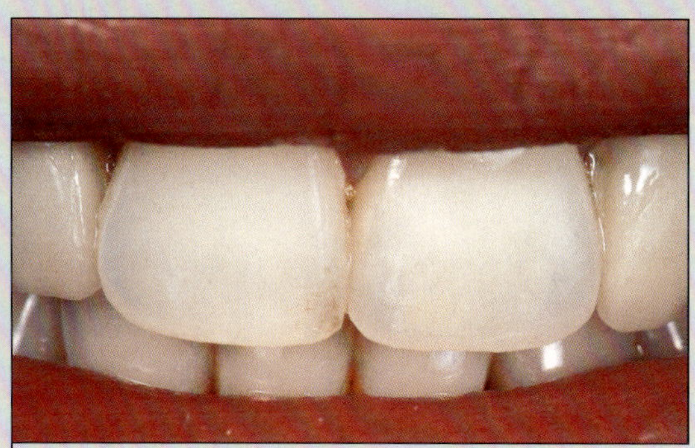

Fig 30 The abutment tooth after removal of the crown.

Fig 31 The dentin of the adjacent tooth showed moderate translucency and value.

Fig 32 Procera crown after cementation. A slight difference in hue at the cervical third was visible; however, it is not obvious because the translucency and value are well matched.

Fig 33 Incisal translucency and value are two of the most important factors when restoring esthetics.

Case 2

A young female patient presented with congenitally missing maxillary lateral incisors. An implant-supported prosthesis was planned. In this case, the crown width needed to be so small that a small-diameter implant was necessary, along with a small custom abutment.

Considering the limited space for the crown, the lateral wall of the custom abutment was created as thin as possible. The abutment was made with cast gold because of its superior strength.

According to the chart, four materials were potentially suitable. When the color of the neighboring teeth was examined, it was observed that they showed low translucency and a high value. Considering the low translucency, the choices were limited to zirconia or In-Ceram Alumina. In this case, a white zirconia coping with a masking material was used to avoid any effects from the gold abutment and to keep the value high (Figs 34 to 40).

CASE 2

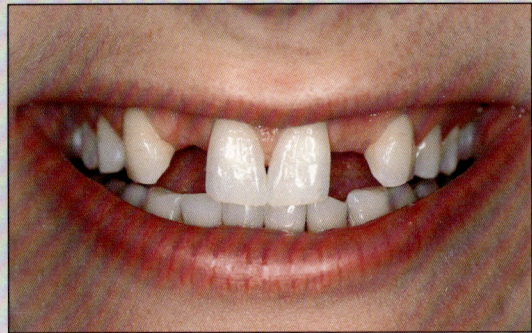

Fig 34a A young female patient presented with congenitally missing maxillary lateral incisors.

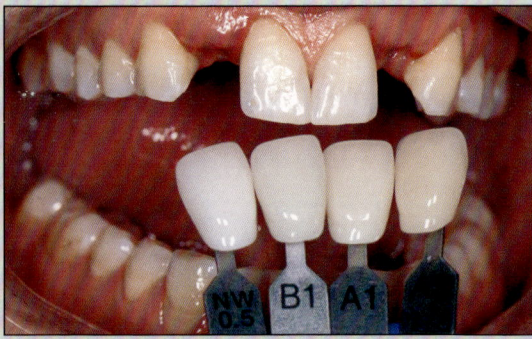

Fig 34b Compared to the shade stub, the crowns of natural teeth were more opaque.

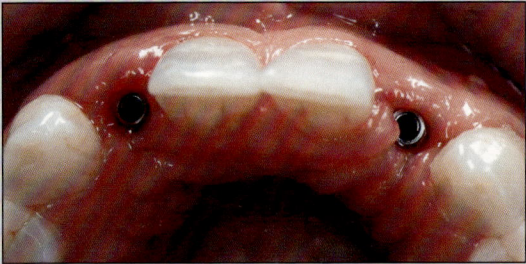

Fig 35 Implants with a diameter of 3.5 mm were inserted.

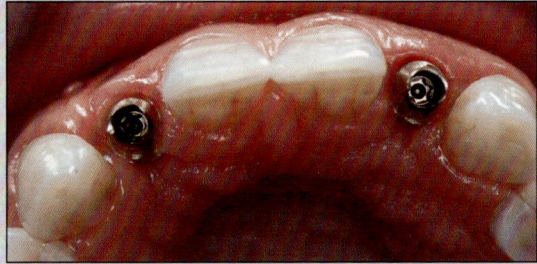

Fig 36 Custom abutments were fabricated using cast gold.

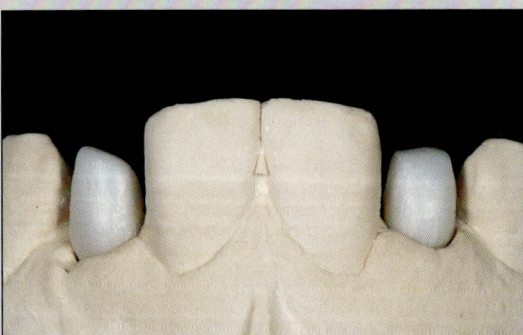

Fig 37 The color of the gold abutment was masked with a high-value white zirconia coping.

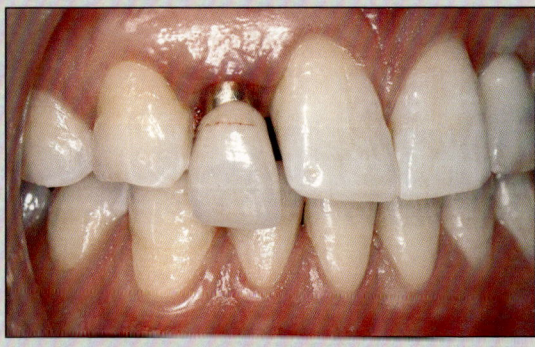

Fig 38 Intraoral try-in. The final shade should be checked using the try-in paste.

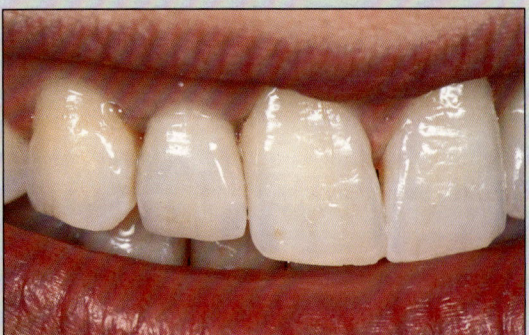

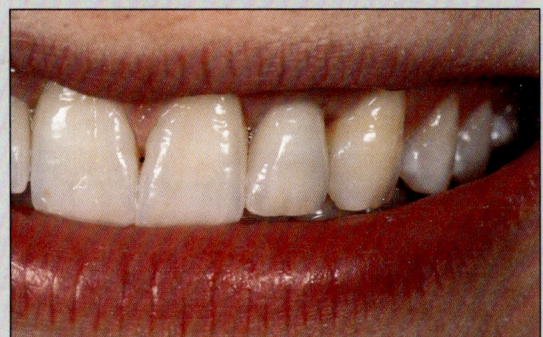

Figs 39 and 40 Right and left lateral views after crown cementation. The value was properly matched with the adjacent teeth.

CASE 3

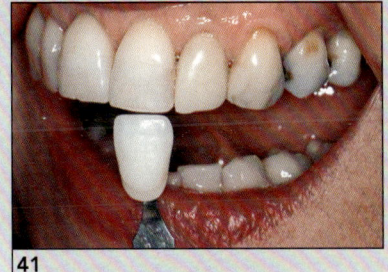

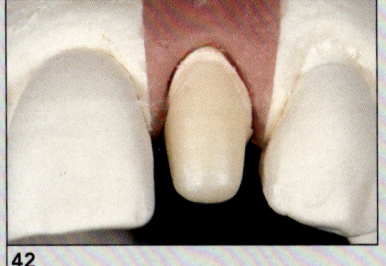

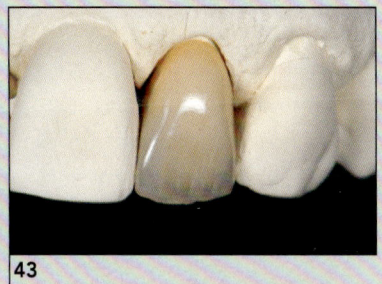

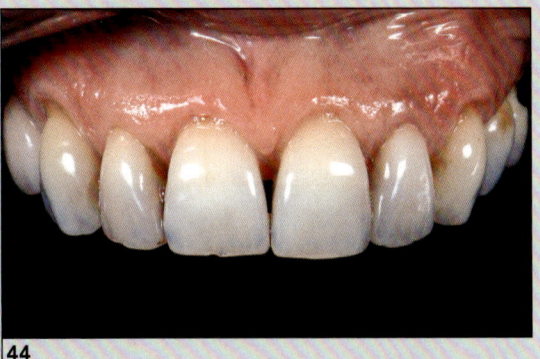

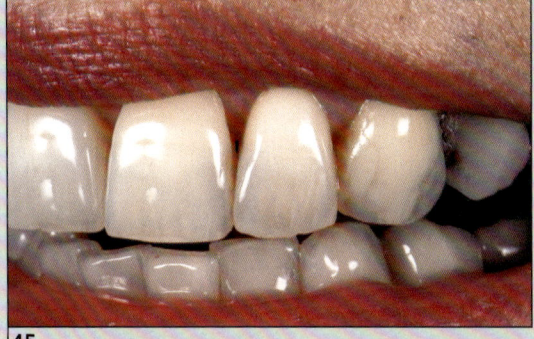

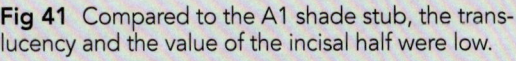

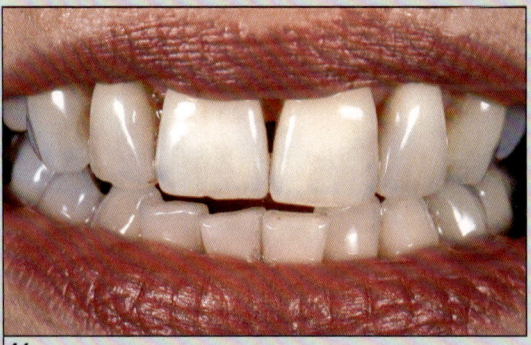

Fig 41 Compared to the A1 shade stub, the translucency and the value of the incisal half were low.

Fig 42 In preparation for a porcelain butt margin, the facial margin of the Procera coping was reduced.

Fig 43 Final restoration on the stone cast.

Fig 44 Final restoration after cementation.

Fig 45 All characterizations were expressed using the internal live stain technique.

Fig 46 Harmony was achieved between the restoration and the natural dentition.

Case 3

The patient presented requesting a single crown at the maxillary left lateral incisor. Because no discoloration of the abutment was visible, it may seem that any material would have been suitable. However, even in cases such as this, it is important to precisely observe the color of the neighboring teeth.

The chroma was A1 to A2. The translucency of the dentin was moderate, and the value of the incisal half was low. Both Procera and zirconia offer moderate translucency; however, Procera was selected because of its low value.

It is important to select a coping material with a different translucency in individual clinical situations to more easily control the value. Internal characterization may be performed with the internal live staining technique (Figs 41 to 46).[13]

CONCLUSION

The chart provided in Fig 25b will not necessarily apply without modification to all clinical cases; rather, it should be used as a basic reference. It is important to remember that different veneering porcelains exhibit different translucencies, and the shade will be affected by the cement and the amount of tooth reduction.

The author recommends that dental technicians modify the chart according to each clinical condition. For better esthetics using all-ceramic crowns, it is important to check every step of the laboratory procedures to avoid frustrating remakes and create successful restorations.

ACKNOWLEDGMENTS

The author would like to thank his good friends Dr Alan Sulikowski and Dr Lloyd L. Miller for the clinical cases presented in this article. The author further thanks Dr Miller for his instruction regarding three-dimensional color and the relationship between translucency and value. This article was translated from Japanese by Dr Takahiro Sato, Roppongi Kasahara Dental Office, Tokyo, Japan.

REFERENCES

1. Coli P, Karlsson S. Precision of a CAD/CAM technique for the production of zirconium dioxide copings. Int J Prothodont 2004;17:577–580.
2. Bindl A, Mormann WH. Marginal and internal fit of all-ceramic CAD/CAM crown-copings on chamfer preparations. J Oral Rehabil 2005;32:441–447.
3. Sieber C. Anterior Porcelain Restorations: Esthetics and Function. Tokyo: Quintessence, 1993:158–160.
4. Herrmann R. Anterior Porcelain Restorations: Esthetics and Function. Tokyo: Quintessence, 1993:67–68.
5. Yamamoto M, Ohata K, Nishimura Y. The possibility of all ceramic restorations. Part 2. What happens at the appearance of "white metal" [in Japanese]. Quintessence Dent Technol 2003;28:32–56.
6. Rutten L, Rutten P. Creating natural esthetics with CAD/CAM. Quintessence Dent Technol 2006;29:24–42.
7. Heffernan MJ, Aquilino SA, Diaz-Arnold AM, Haselton DR, Stanford CM, Vargas MA. Relative translucency of six all-ceramic systems. Part 1: Core and veneer materials. J Prosthet Dent 2002;88:10–15.
8. Saitoh I. Best of digital. Twelve questions about digital cameras: Isamu Saitoh's digital camera course (no. 1 to no. 4) [in Japanese]. Quintessence Dent Technol 2006;31:1–4.
9. Yamamoto M. Looking for the best digital camera for oral photographs—Development of a dental digital camera "eye special" [in Japanese]. Quintessence Dent Technol 2004;29:80–82.
10. Kawahara K, Shima H, Igarashi T. A study on the color of resin cement—The effect of thickness on the color and cutoff performance. J Jpn Prosthodont Soc 2001;45(special issue):112.
11. Benge L, Young R. An alternative technique for value management of densely sintered alumina-based restorations. Quintessence Dent Technol 2001;24:23–27.
12. Sulikowski A, Yoshida A. Surface texture: A systematic approach for accurate and effective communication. Quintessence Dent Technol 2003;26:10–19.
13. Aoshima H. A Collection of Ceramic Works: A Communication Tool for the Dental Office and Laboratory. Chicago: Quintessence, 1992.

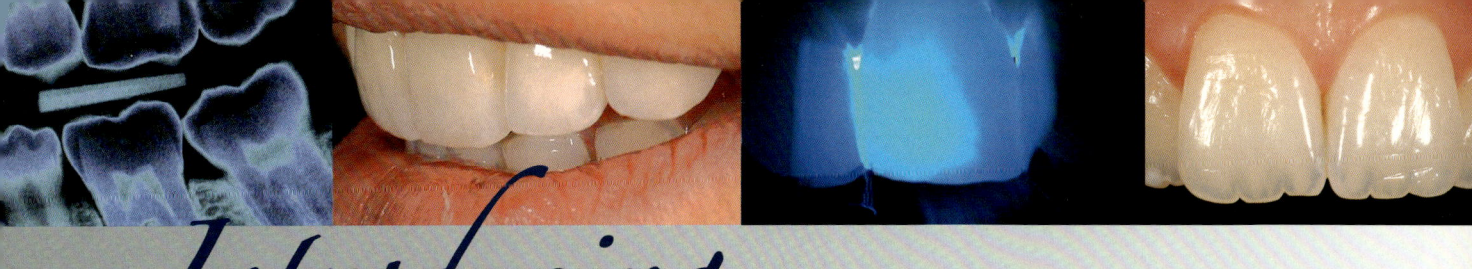

Introducing . . .

Editor-in-Chief
Alessandro Devigus

Associate Editors

Implantology
Ueli Grunder
Nitzan Bichacho

Prosthodontics
Mauro Fradeani
Jörg Strub

Adhesive Dentistry
Didier Dietschi
Roberto Spreafico

Endodontics
Peter Velvart
Oliver Pontius

Orthodontics
Rafi Romano
Vittorio Cacciafesta

Periodontology
Hannes Wachtel
Giano Ricci

Dental Technology
Nicola Pietrobon
Ernst Hegenbarth

Restorative Dentistry
Galip Gürel
Stefano Gracis

Subscription rates (4 issues/year):

Regular rate	$128
Institutional rate	$198
Student rate	$68

To order, contact your nearest
Quintessence office

Quintessence USA
Fax 630.736.3633
E-mail service@quintbook.com
Web www.quintpub.com

Quintessence UK
Fax +44 (0)20 8336 1484
E-mail info@quintpub.co.uk
Web www.quintpub.co.uk

The official publication of
the European Academy of Esthetic Dentistry

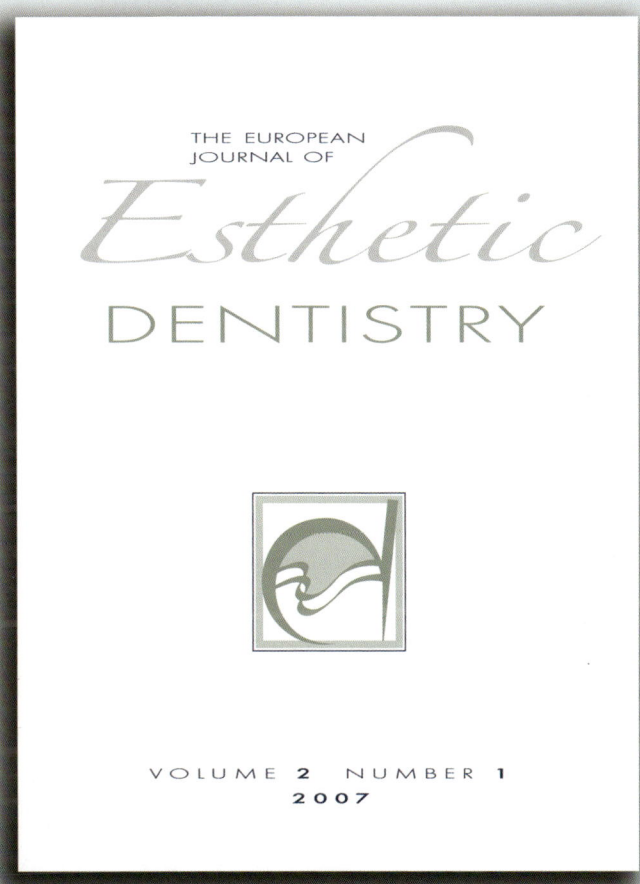

THE EUROPEAN
JOURNAL OF

Esthetic

DENTISTRY

VOLUME **2** NUMBER **1**
2007

The European Journal of Esthetic Dentistry addresses multidisciplinary topics, both clinical and technical, to help you develop and refine your esthetic treatment skills, network with colleagues, and build a successful esthetic dental practice to meet the increasing demands of your patients.

This exceptional journal will enable you to expand your knowledge through case presentations—of failures as well as successes—and treatment-planning sessions from international experts in their fields. Peer-reviewed articles will allow you to explore the latest innovations in methods and materials, and they will inspire and motivate you to maximize your potential. Don't wait—subscribe now and become part of the new and exciting adventure that is Esthetic Dentistry!

SELECTED CASE PRESENTATION

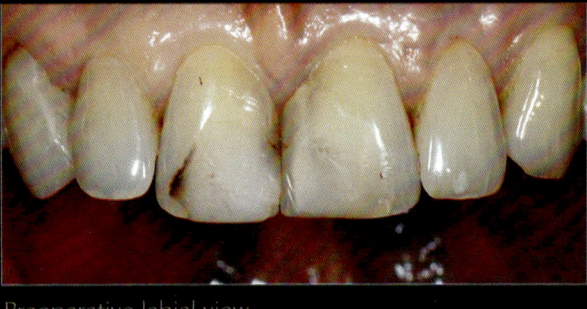

Preoperative labial view.

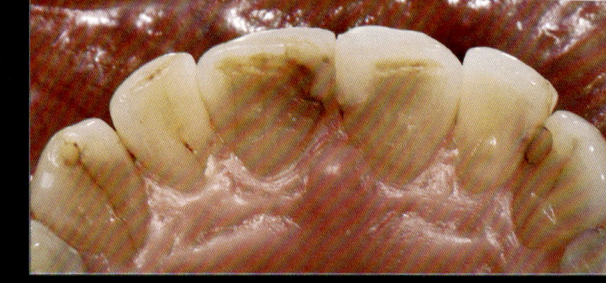

Preoperative lingual view.

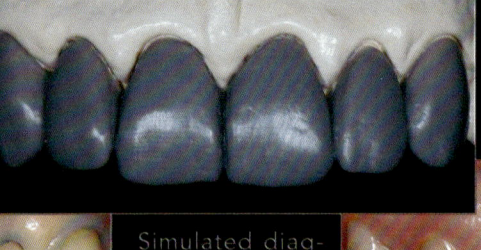

Simulated diagnostic waxup.

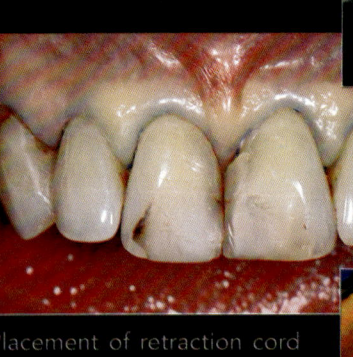

Placement of retraction cord prior to tooth preparation.

Preparations, labial view.

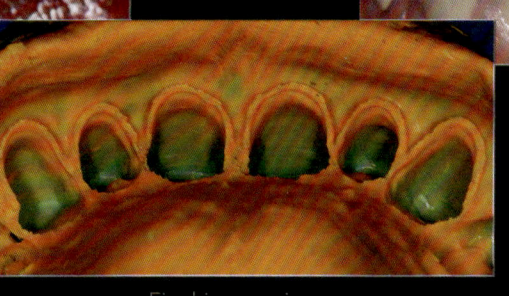

Final impression.

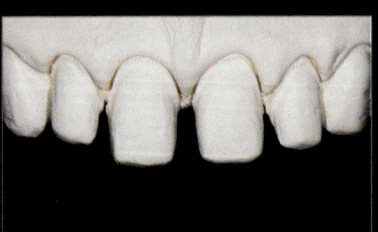

Solid cast.

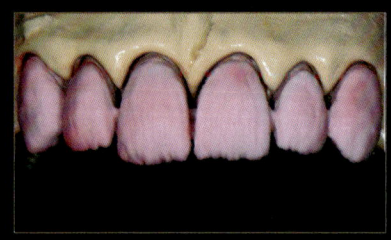

Simulated body buildup.

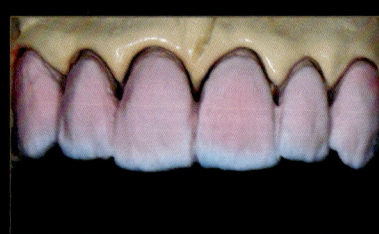

Simulated incisal framing buildup.

Restorative Team

Avishai Sadan, DMD
Professor and Chairman
Department of Comprehensive Care
Case Western Reserve University
School of Dental Medicine
Cleveland, Ohio, USA

Tomikazu Tada, RDT
Master Ceramist and Laboratory Manager
Department of Comprehensive Care
Case Western Reserve University
School of Dental Medicine
Cleveland, Ohio, USA

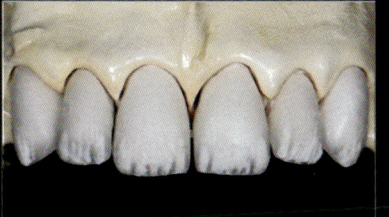
Simulated mamelon buildup.

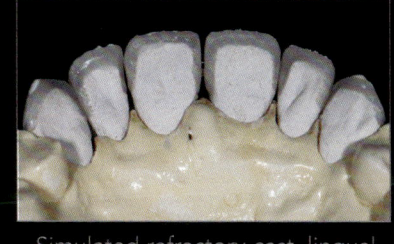
Simulated refractory cast, lingual view.

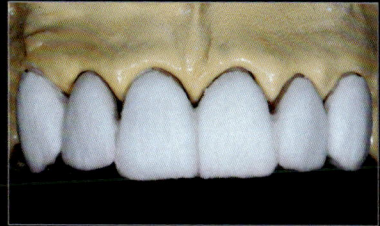
Simulated enamel skin layer buildup.

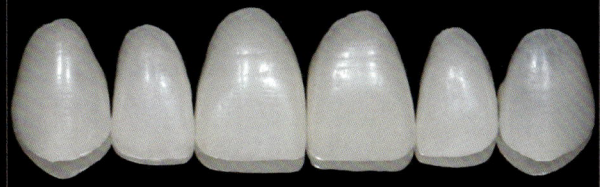
Completed veneers, labial view.

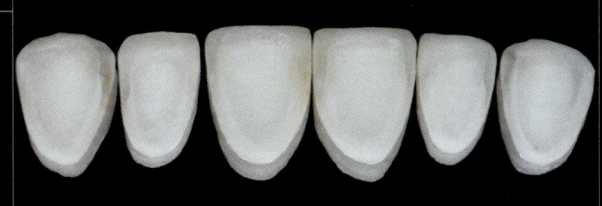
Completed veneers, lingual view.

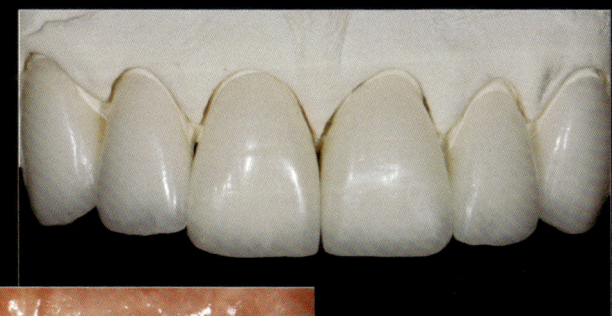
Completed veneers on solid cast.

Postoperative labial views.

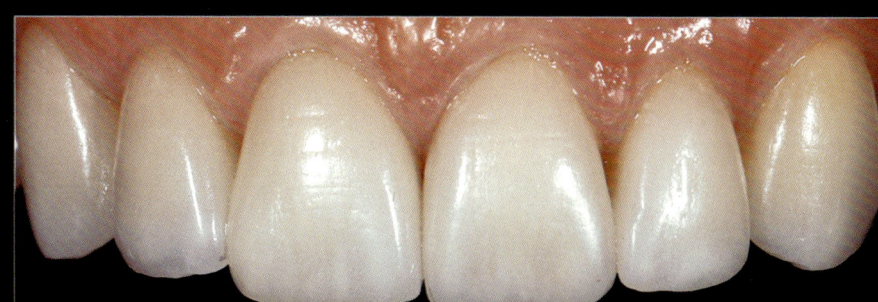

SELECTED CASE PRESENTATIONS

Case 1

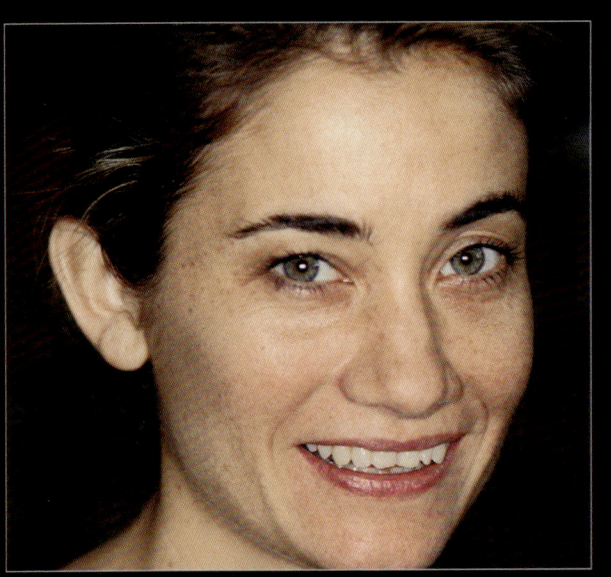

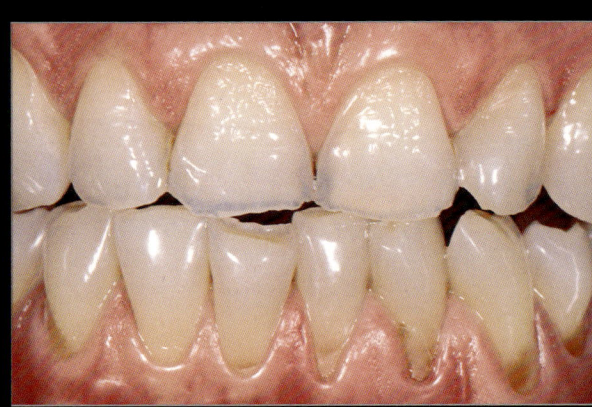

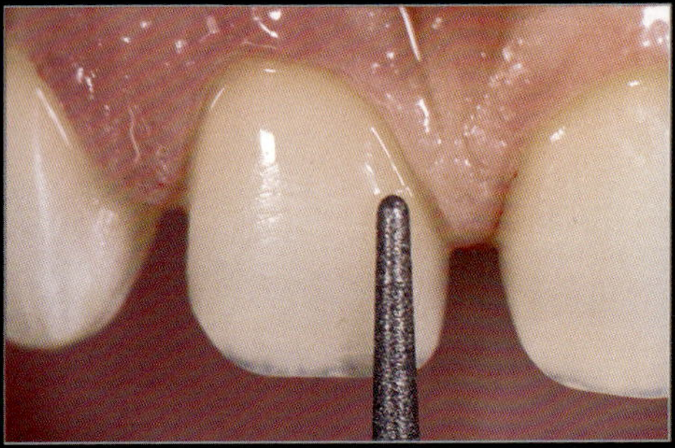

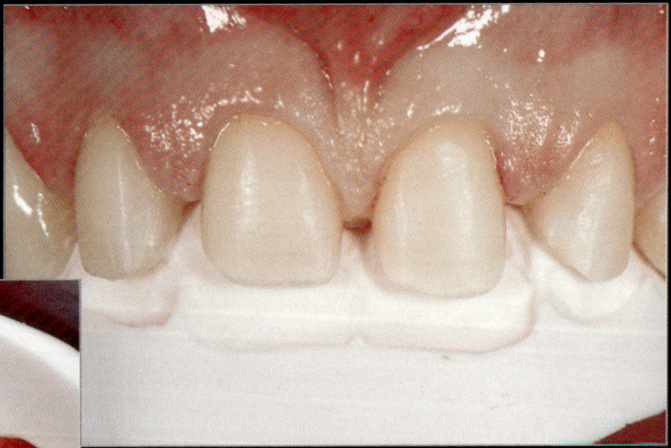

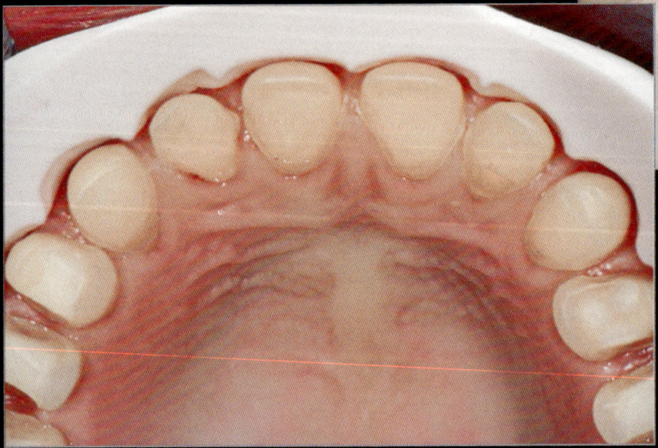

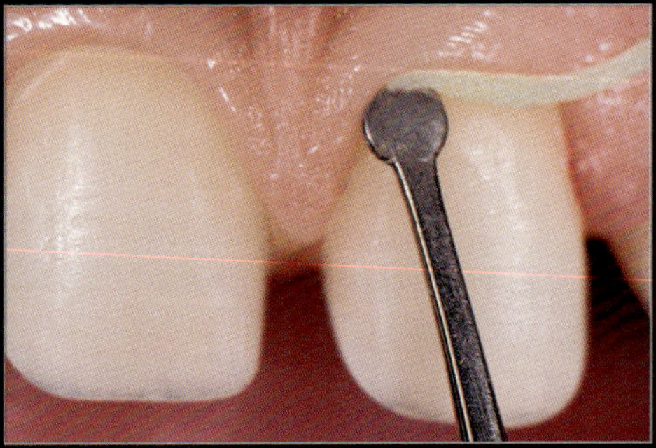

Otto Zuhr, DDS, Dr med dent
Institute for Periodontology and Implantology
Munich, Germany

Uli Schoberer, MDT
Private dental laboratory
Seehausen, Germany

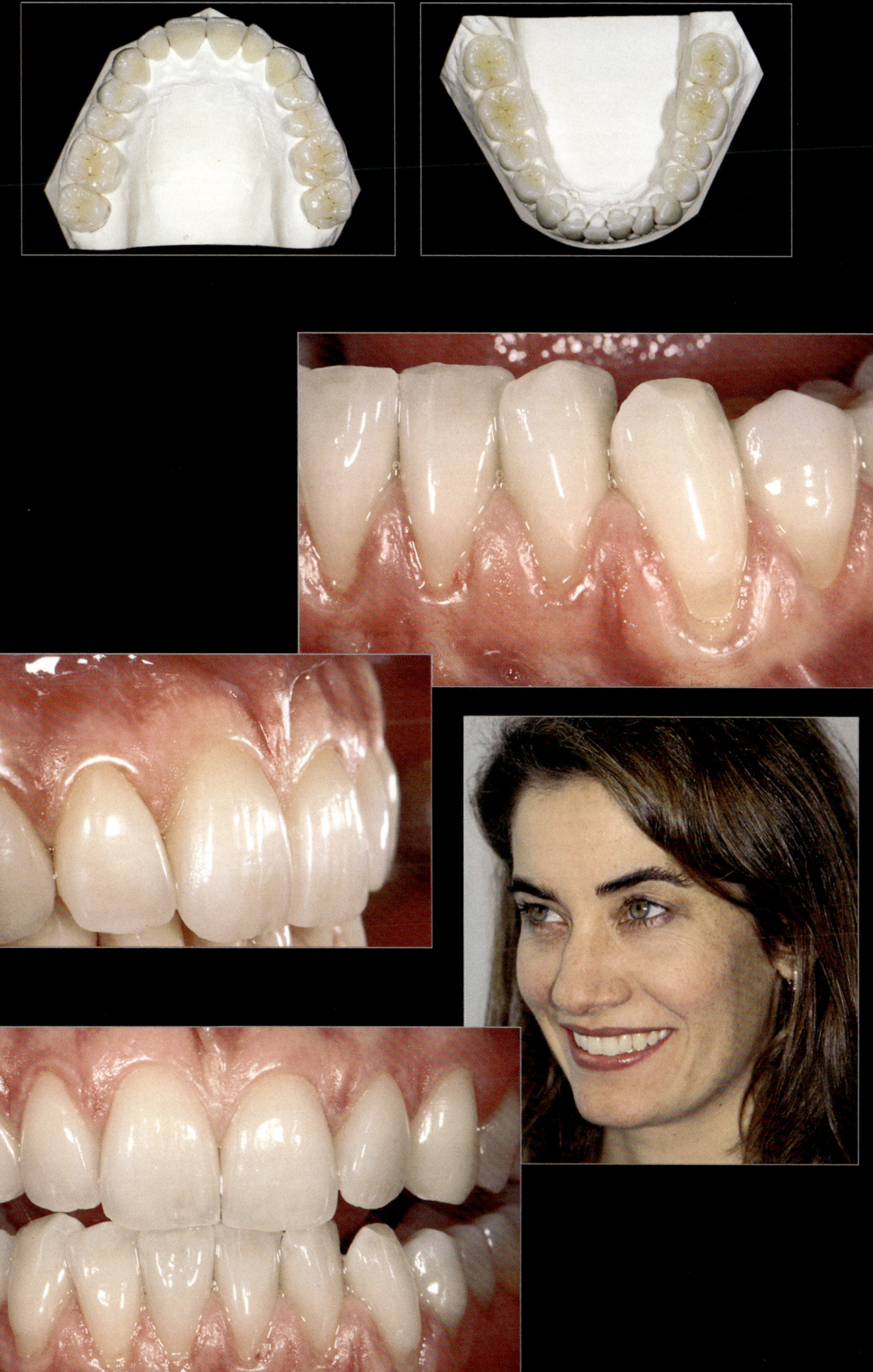

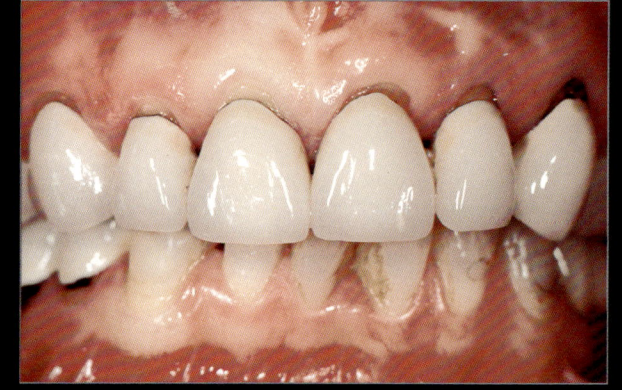

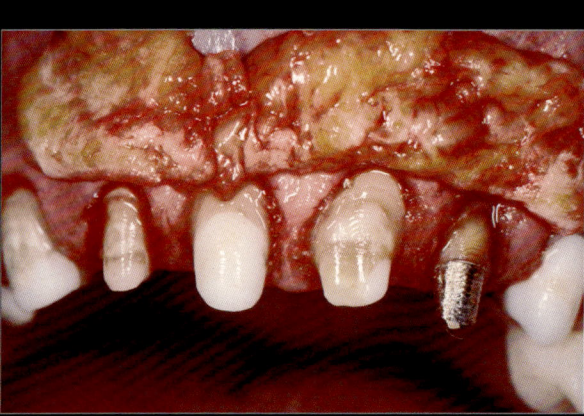
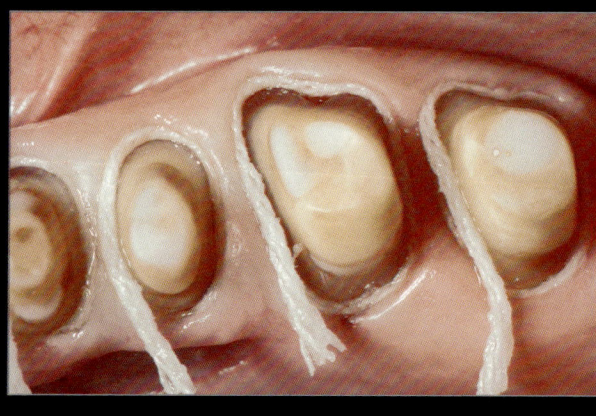

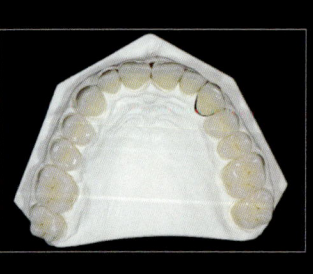
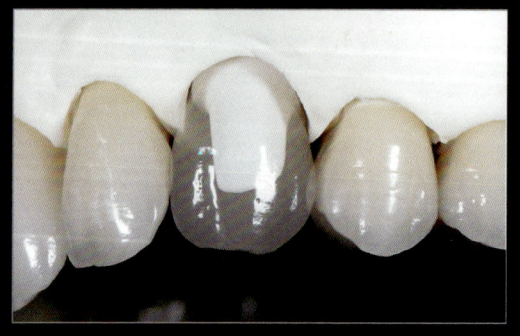
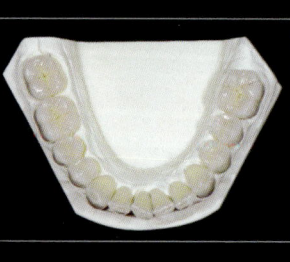

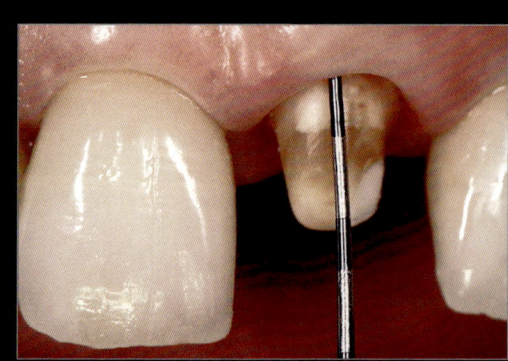
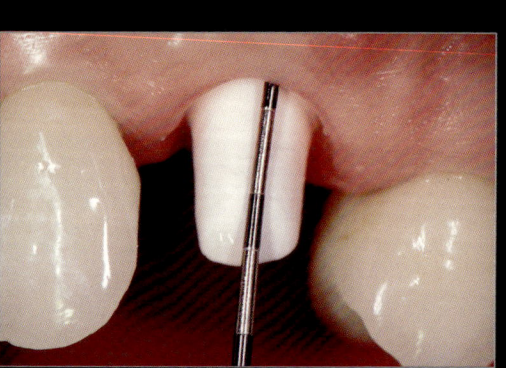

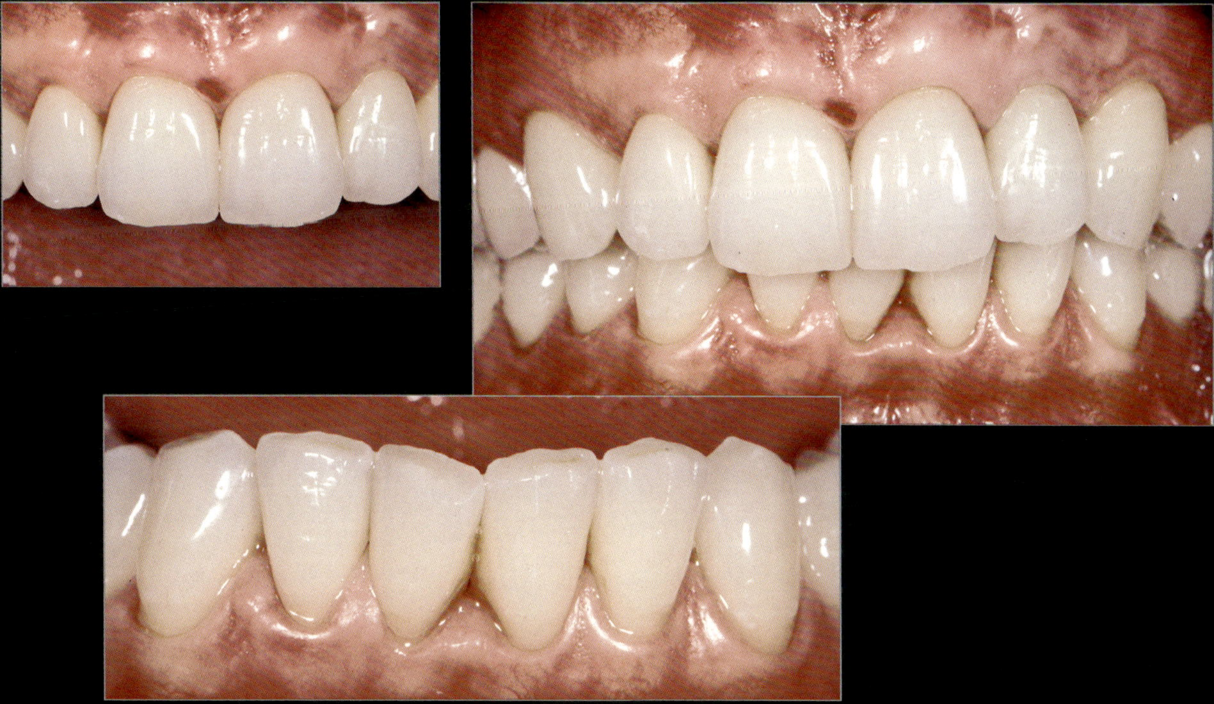

Case 3

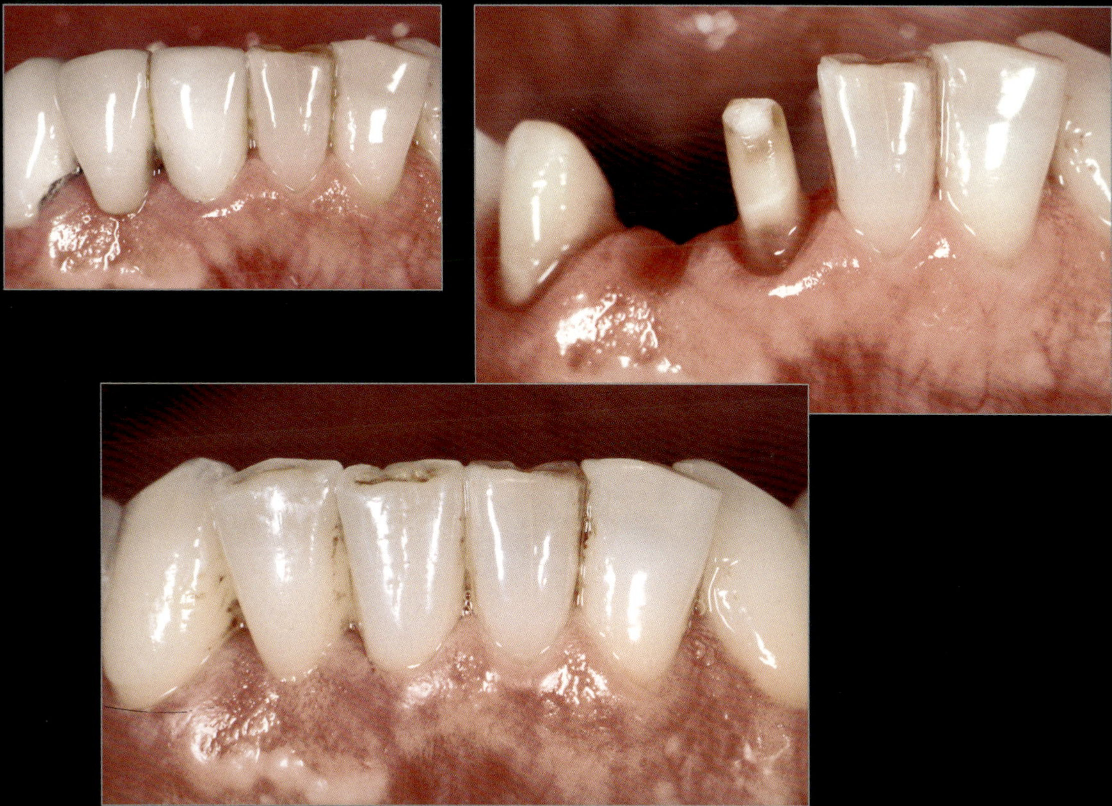

SELECTED CASE PRESENTATIONS

Pontics with Natural-Appearing Emergence Profiles

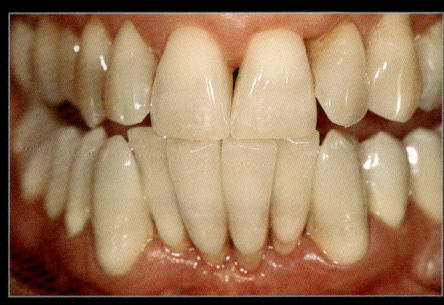

Mandibular eight-tooth fixed partial denture (FPD) with four pontics. The four incisors were extracted due to periodontal disease. A provisional FPD was used to guide the soft tissue healing, and the final prosthesis was inserted 9 months after tooth extractions.

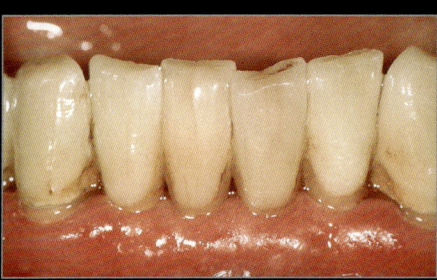

Four mandibular anterior pontics, part of a 12-tooth FPD. Six teeth were extracted and periodontal surgery was performed on the remaining mandibular teeth prior to the insertion of the final prosthesis with supragingival margins.

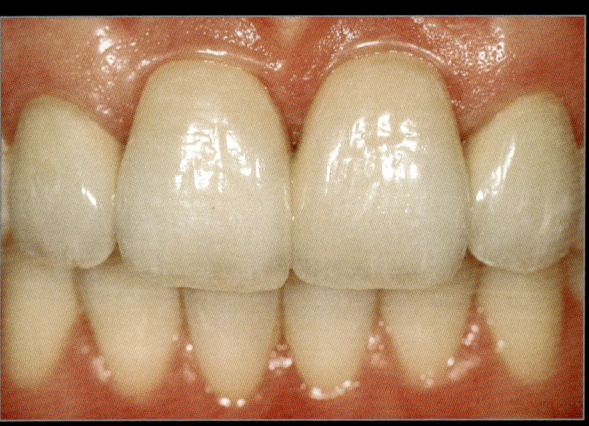

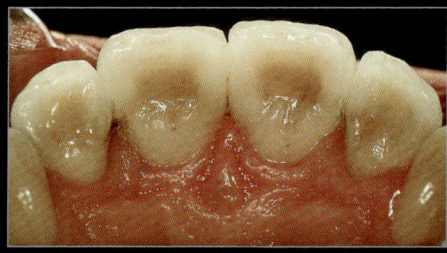

Two-year postinsertion views of a four-tooth FPD with ovate pontics. The maxillary central incisors were extracted post-trauma and a provisional prosthesis was used to guide soft tissue healing and preserve the form of the gingiva and papillae.

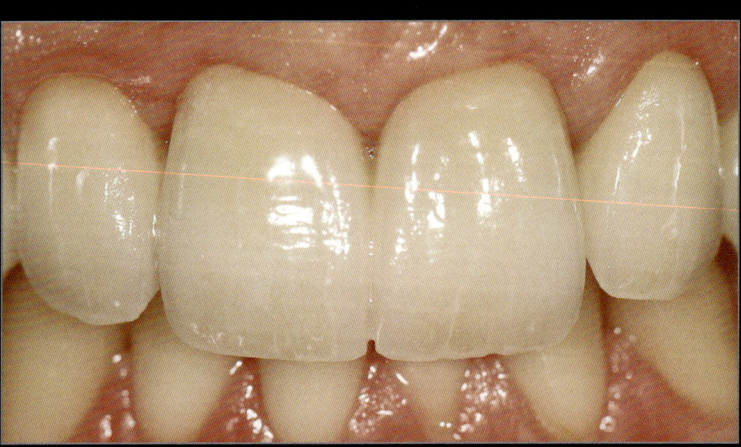

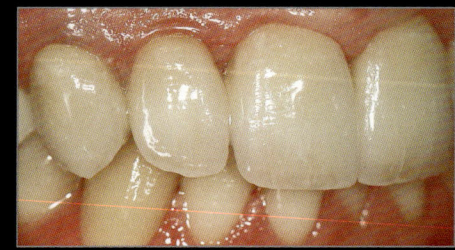

Seven-tooth FPD with pontics for the maxillary right lateral incisor and both central incisors. The teeth were extracted post-trauma and residual ridge–guided healing was accomplished with the provisional restoration.

Clinical and technical procedures by: Robert R. Winter, DDS

Private practice
Newport Beach, California, USA

Clinical Associate Professor, Department of Comprehensive Care
Case Western Reserve University School of Dental Medicine, Cleveland, Ohio, USA

Three-year postinsertion view of a cantilever maxillary lateral incisor pontic with the left canine as an abutment. Connective tissue augmentation was performed to enhance the residual ridge 8 months prior to insertion of the FPD. Ovate pontic design was used to support the gingival tissue and allow for optimal hygiene.

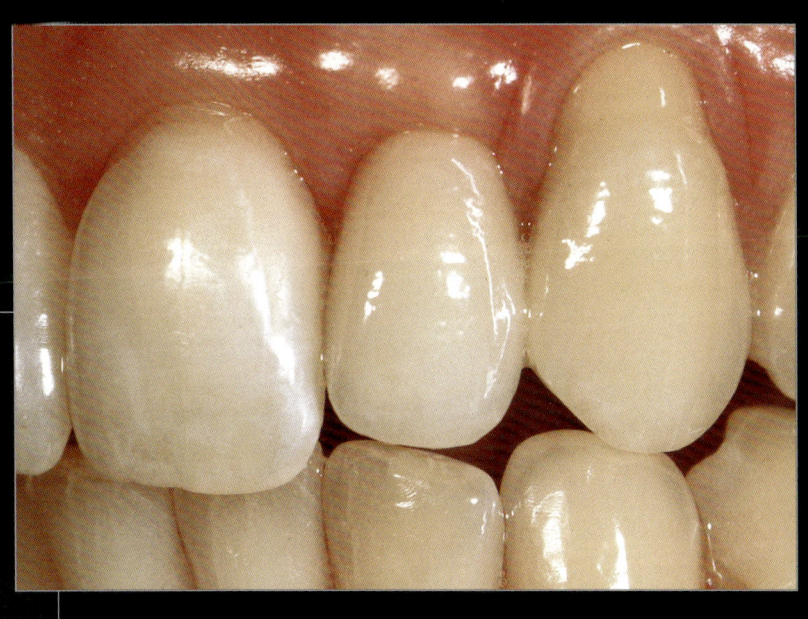

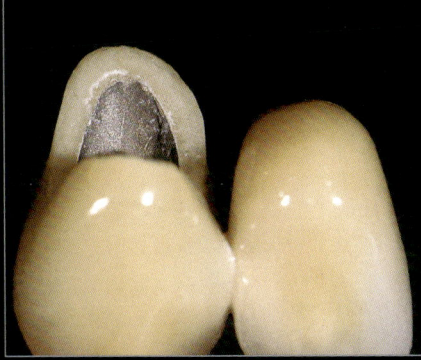

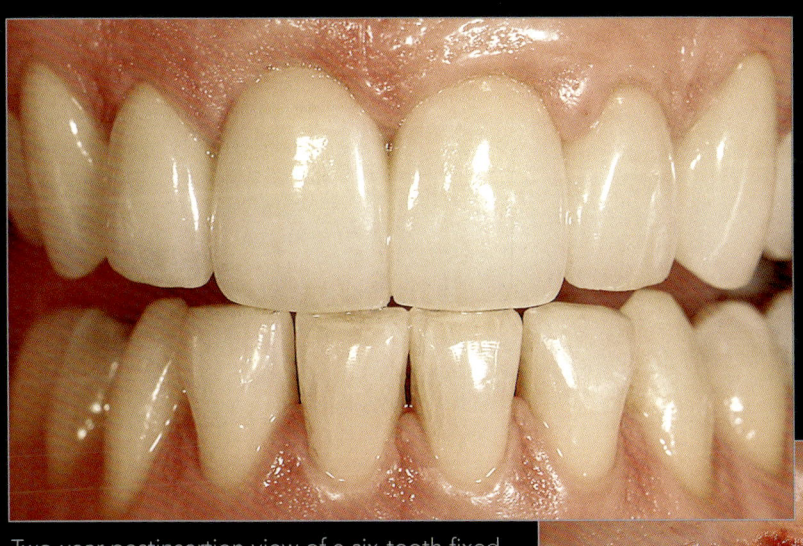

Two-year postinsertion view of a six-tooth fixed partial denture showing healthy, stable gingiva and papillae. The residual ridge was augmented with a connective tissue graft and the provisional restoration guided the healing, forming the ovate pontic sites. At the time of definitive prosthesis insertion, an incision was made 1.5 mm from the facial aspect of the residual ridge at a depth of 3 to 4 mm to allow for slight facial movement of the facial aspect of the ridge, thus positioning the tissue and papilla with ideal pontic forms.

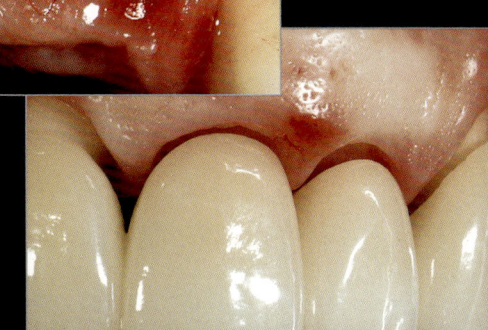

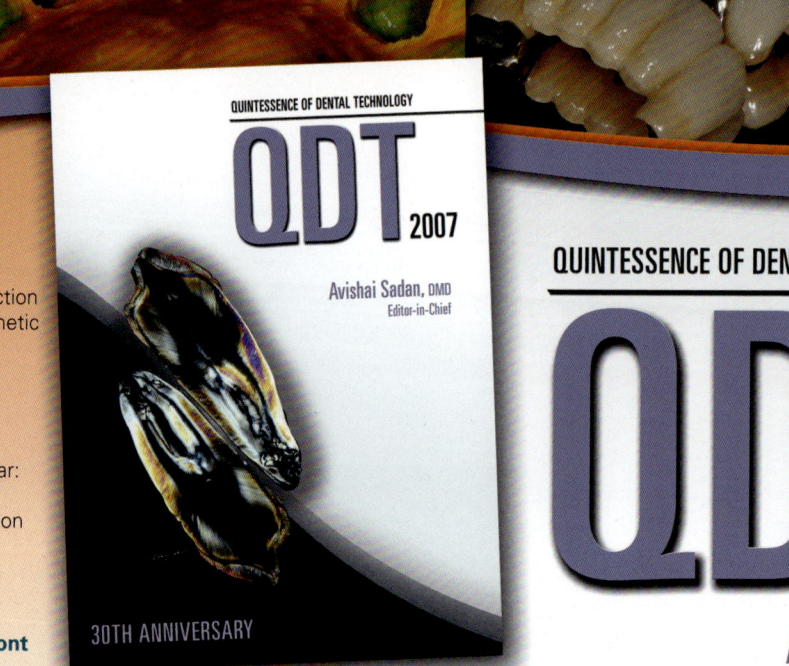

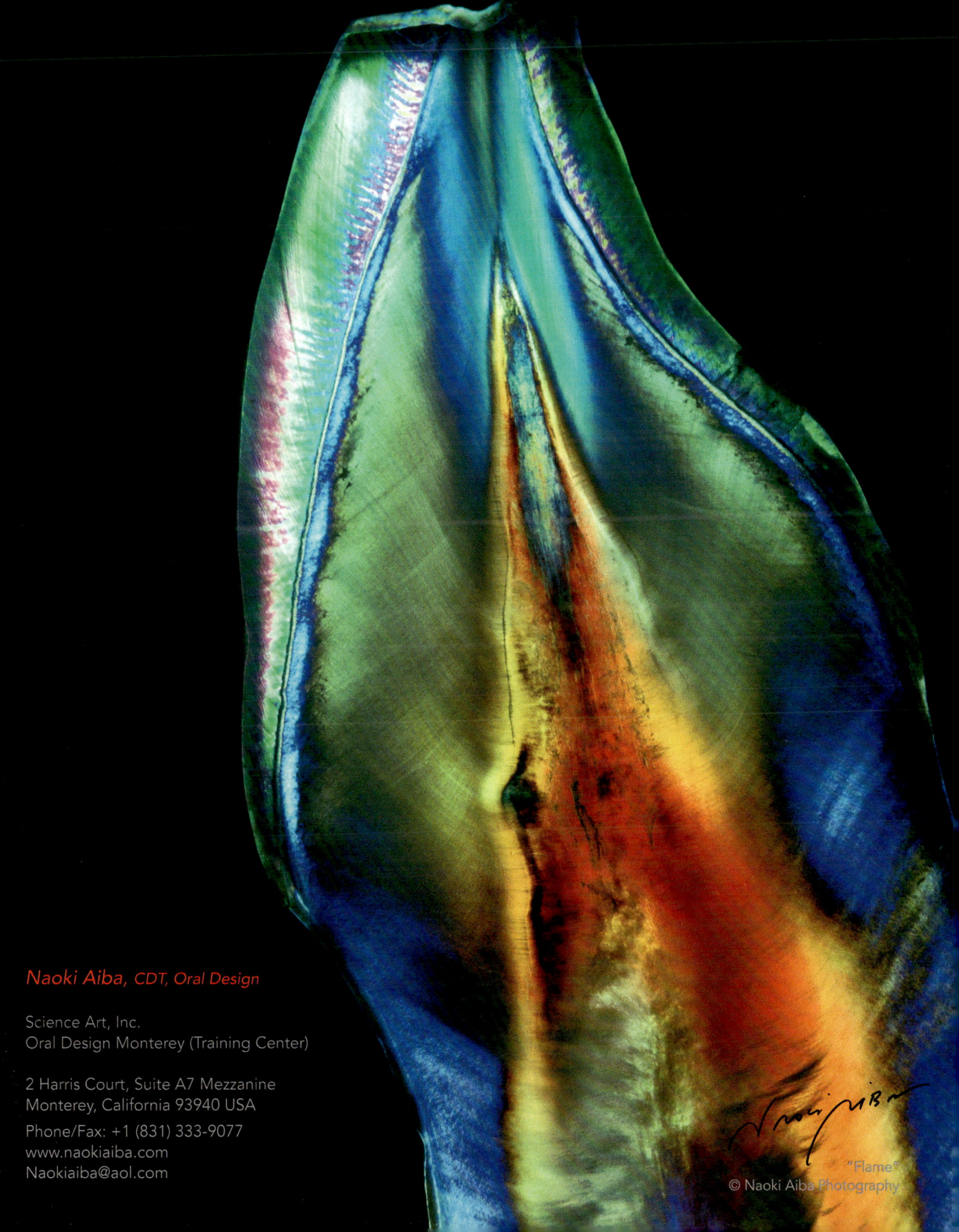

DENTSCAPE
LATERALS

Naoki Aiba, *CDT, Oral Design*

Science Art, Inc.
Oral Design Monterey (Training Center)

2 Harris Court, Suite A7 Mezzanine
Monterey, California 93940 USA

Phone/Fax: +1 (831) 333-9077
www.naokiaiba.com
Naokiaiba@aol.com

"Flame"
© Naoki Aiba Photography

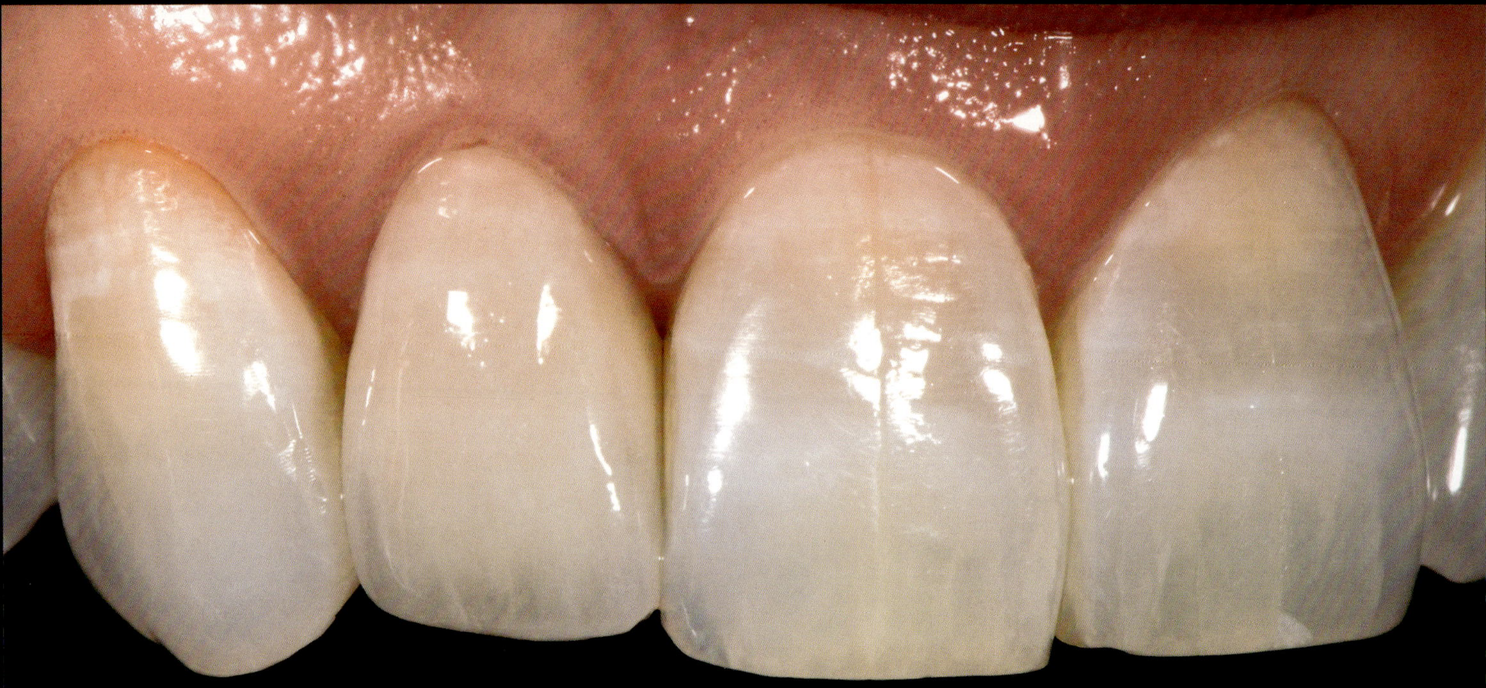

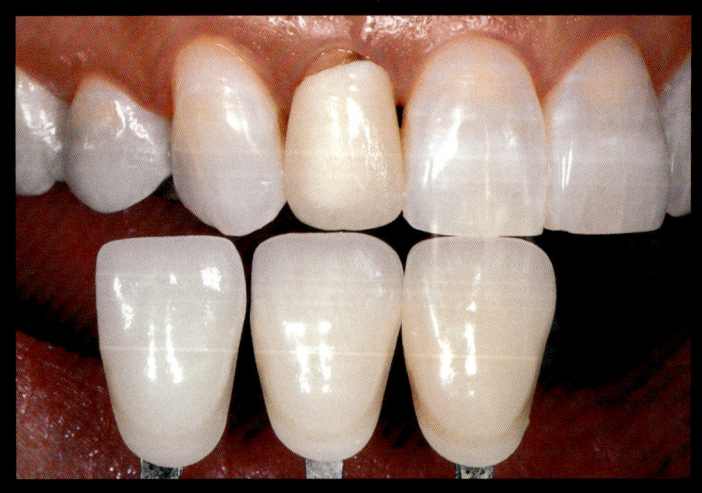

Clinician: Mark J. Bilello, DDS

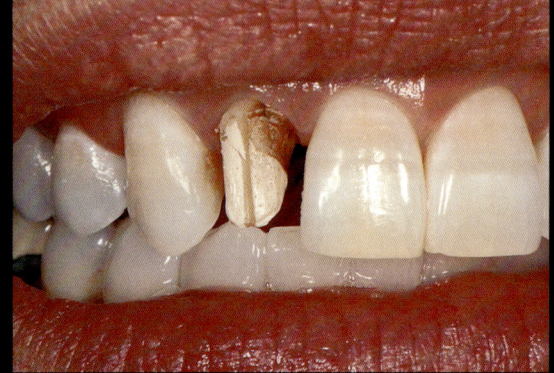

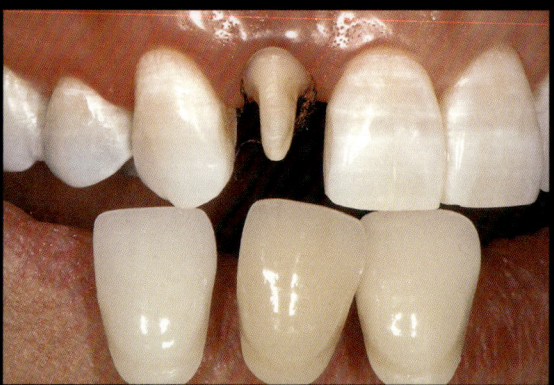

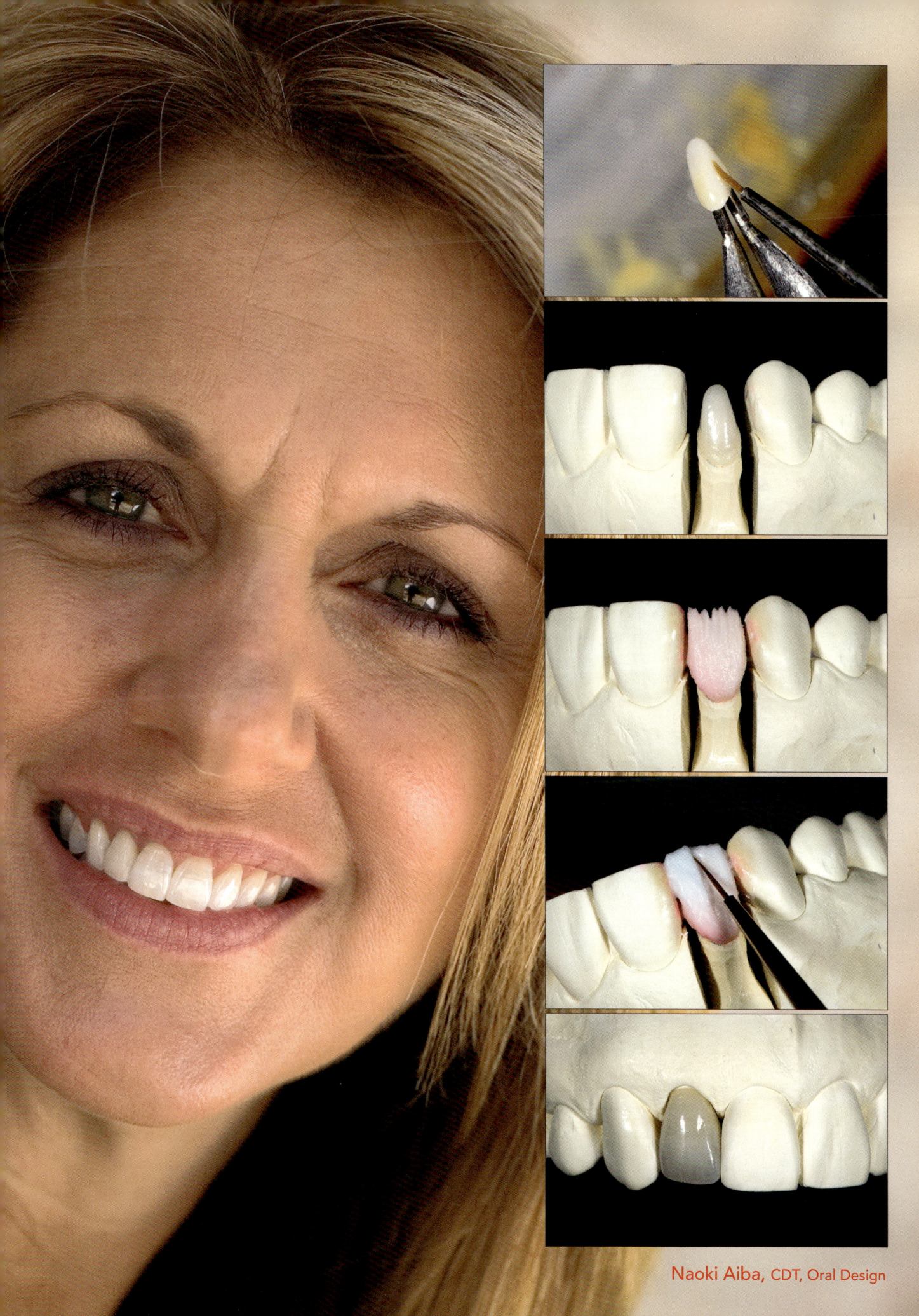

Naoki Aiba, CDT, Oral Design

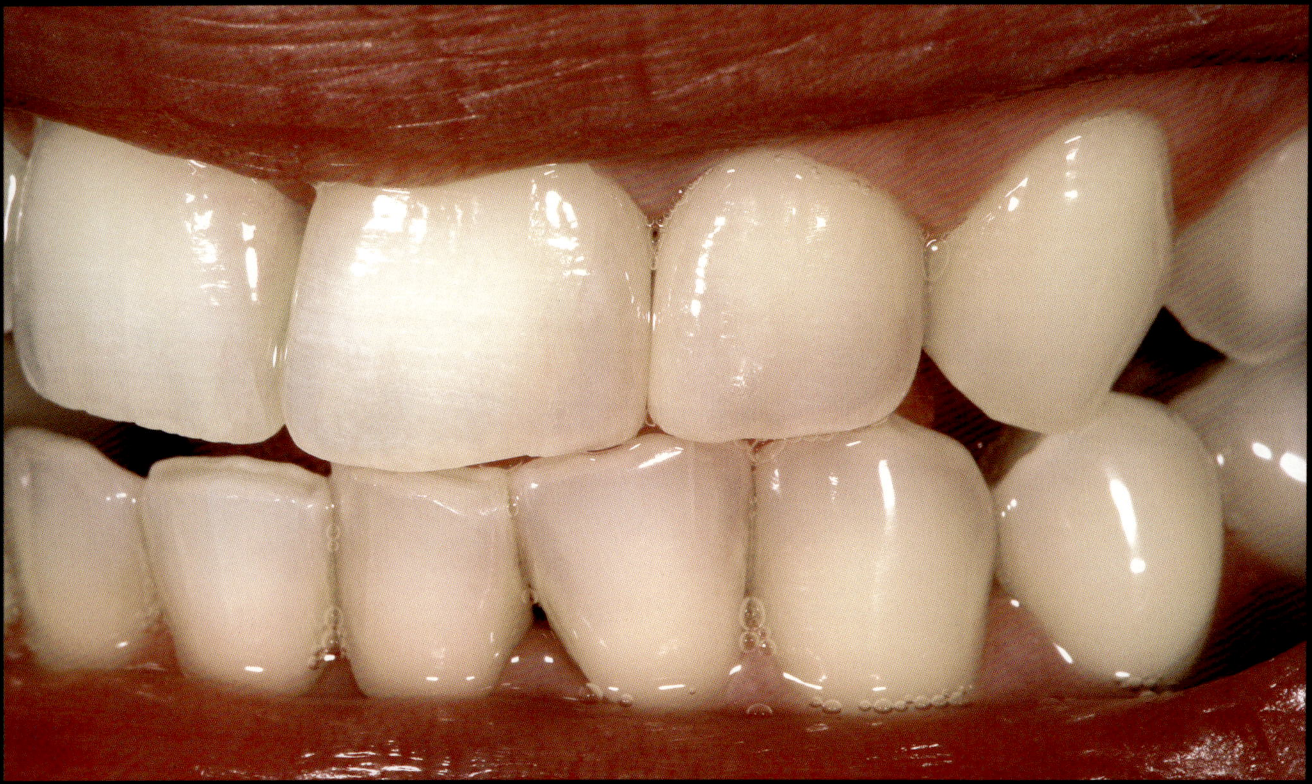

Clinician: Jennifer Wynn, DDS

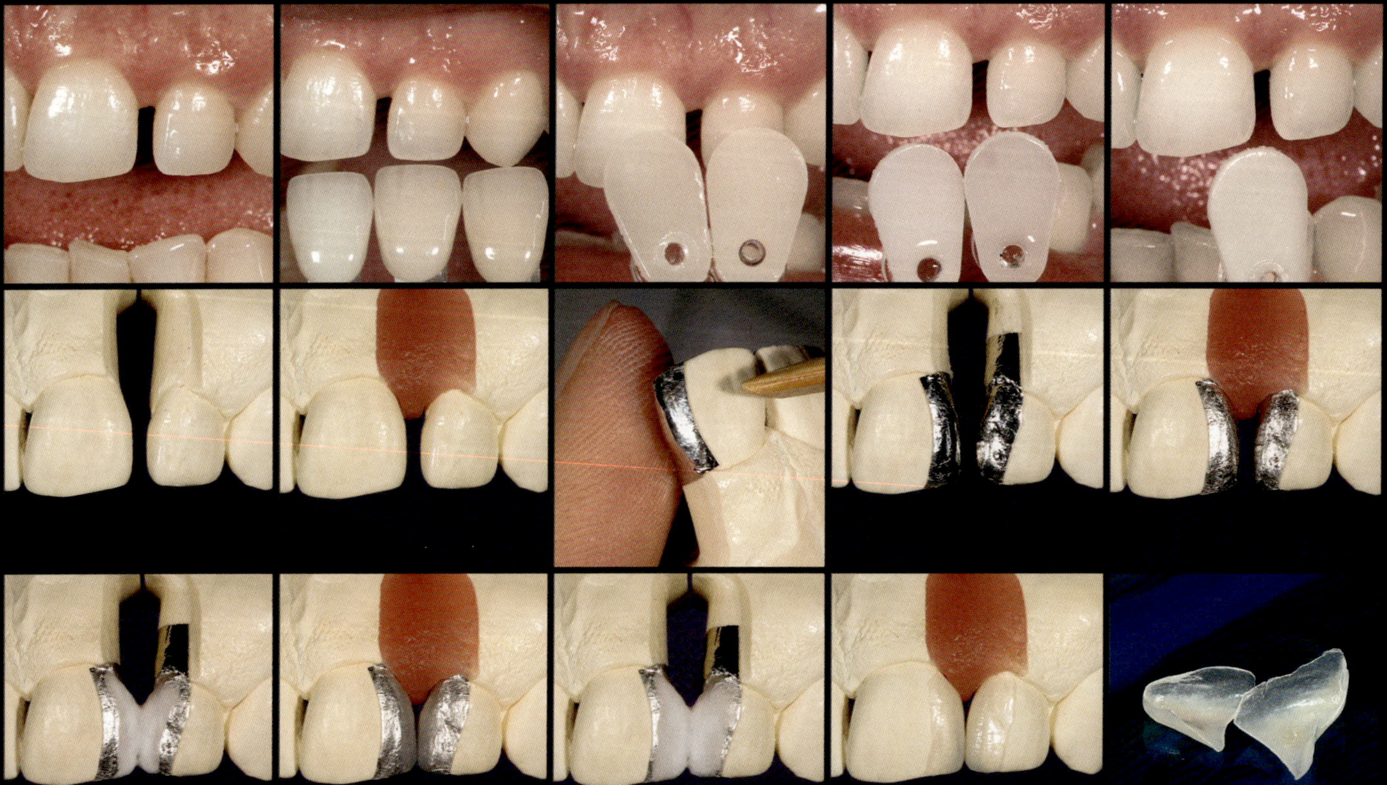

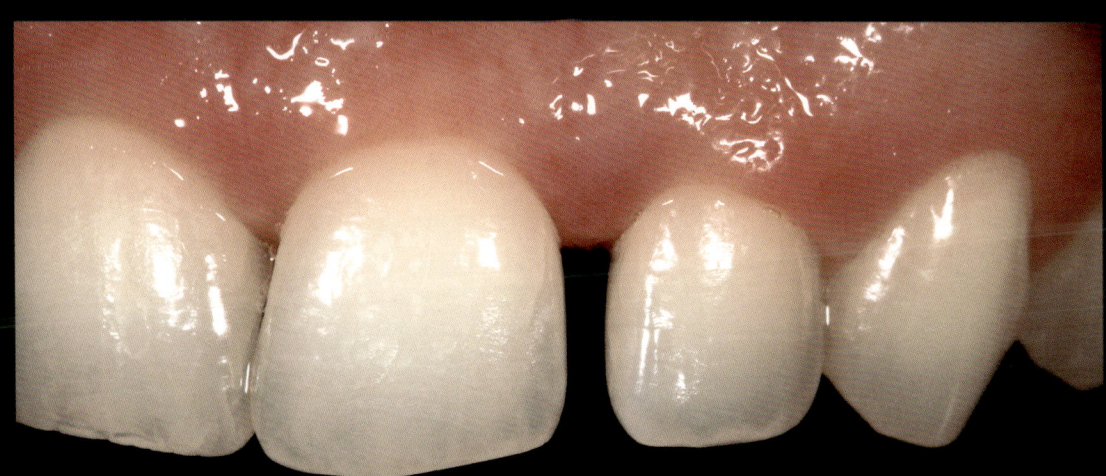

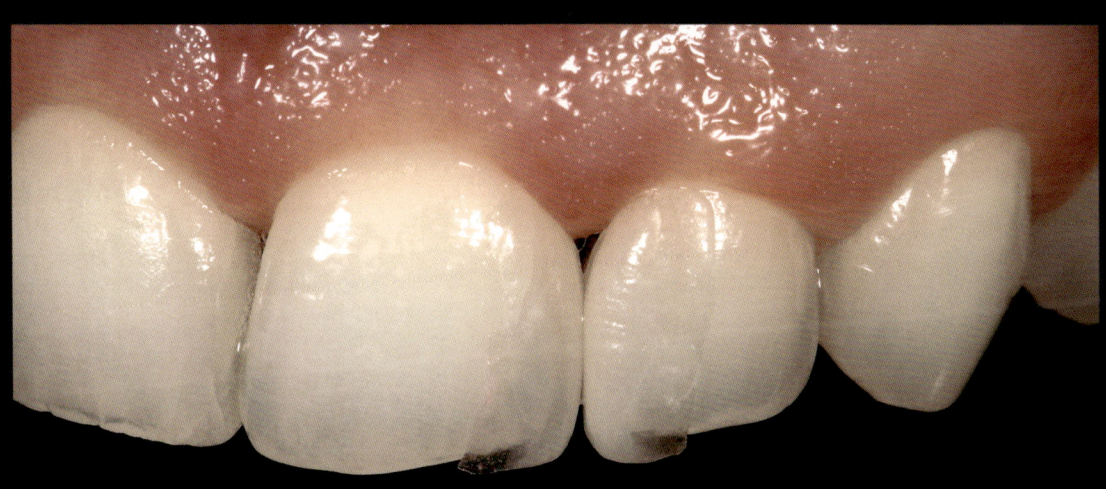

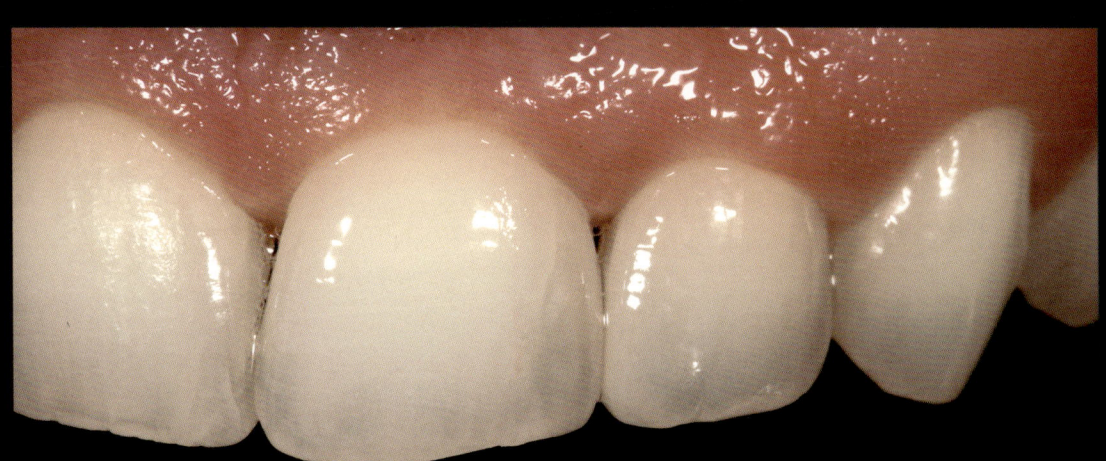

Naoki Aiba, CDT, Oral Design

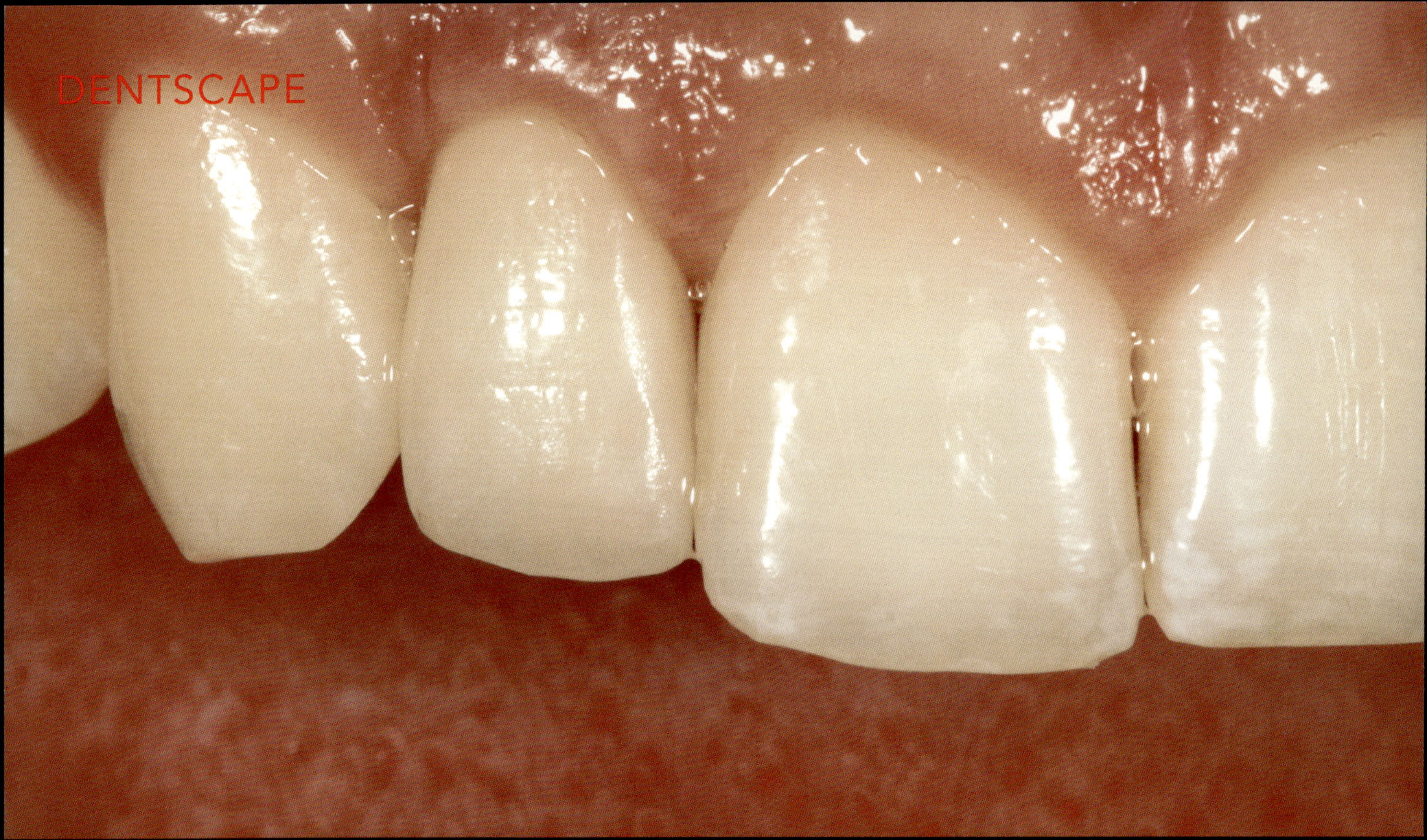

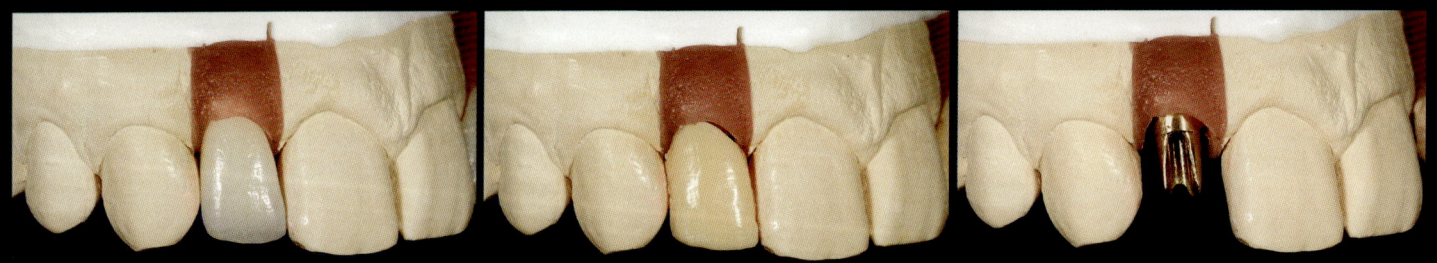

Clinician: Chris E. Lindsey, DDS

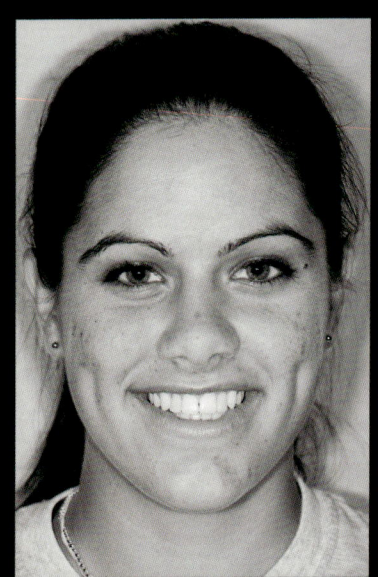

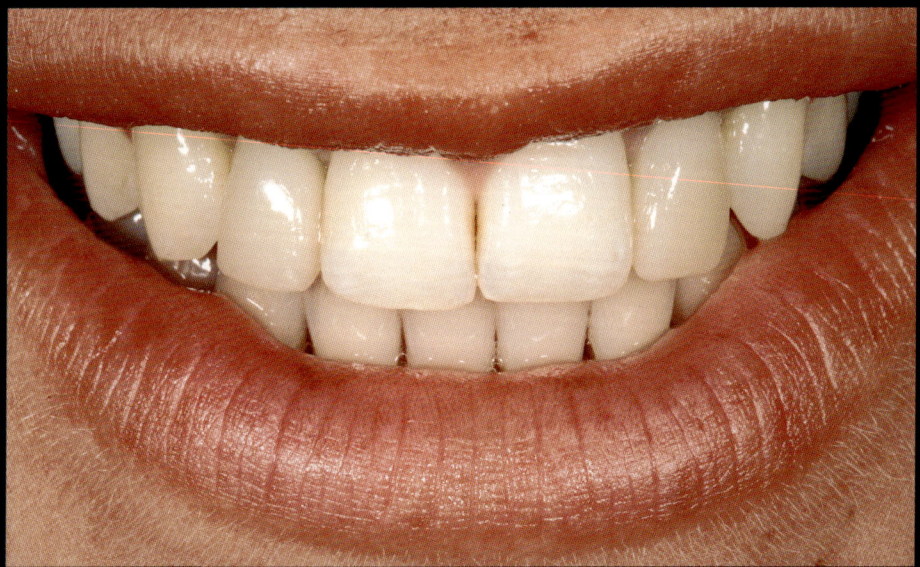

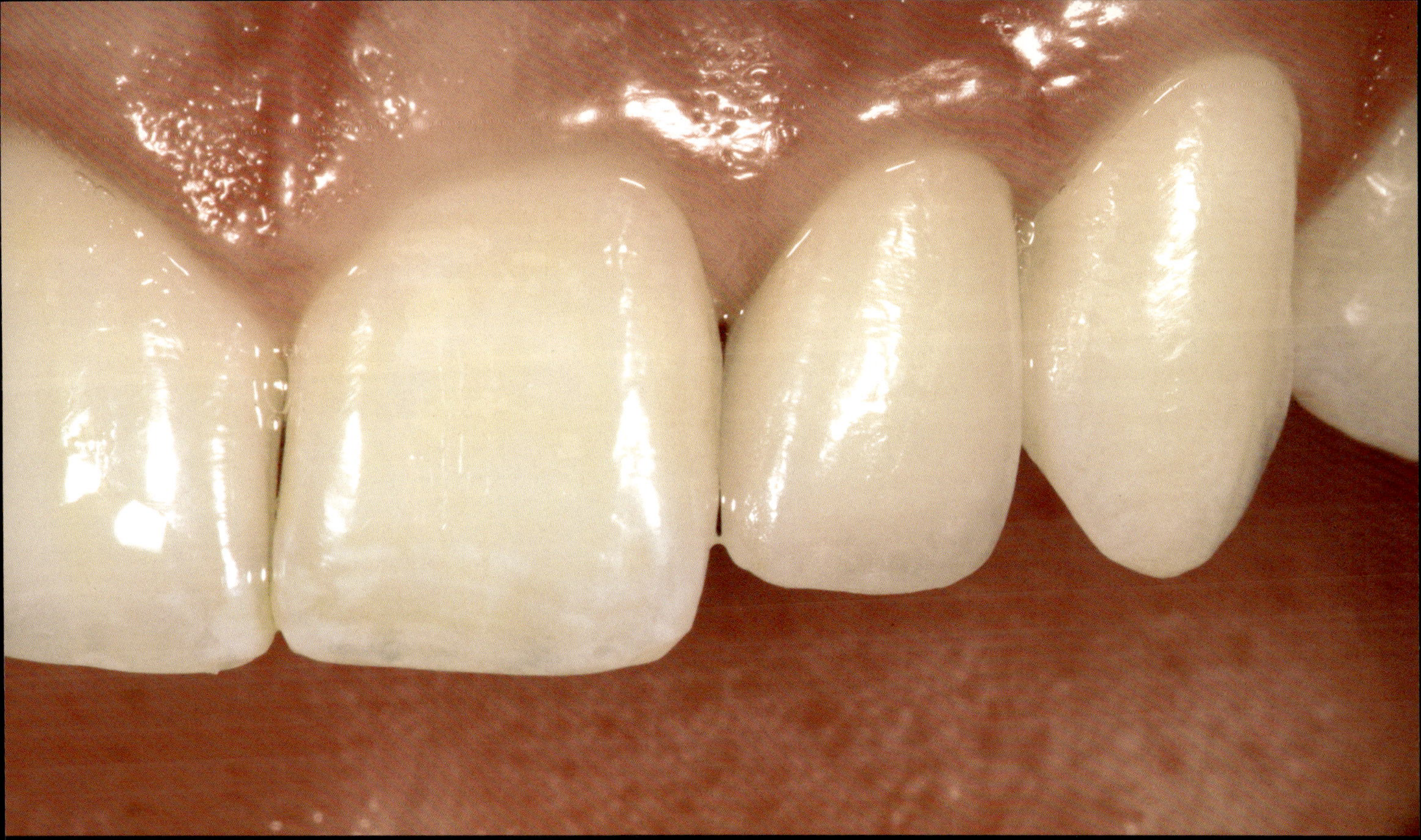

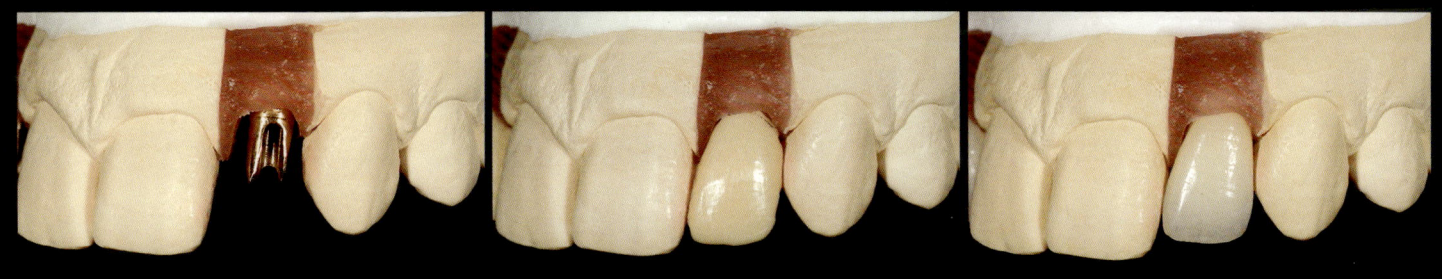

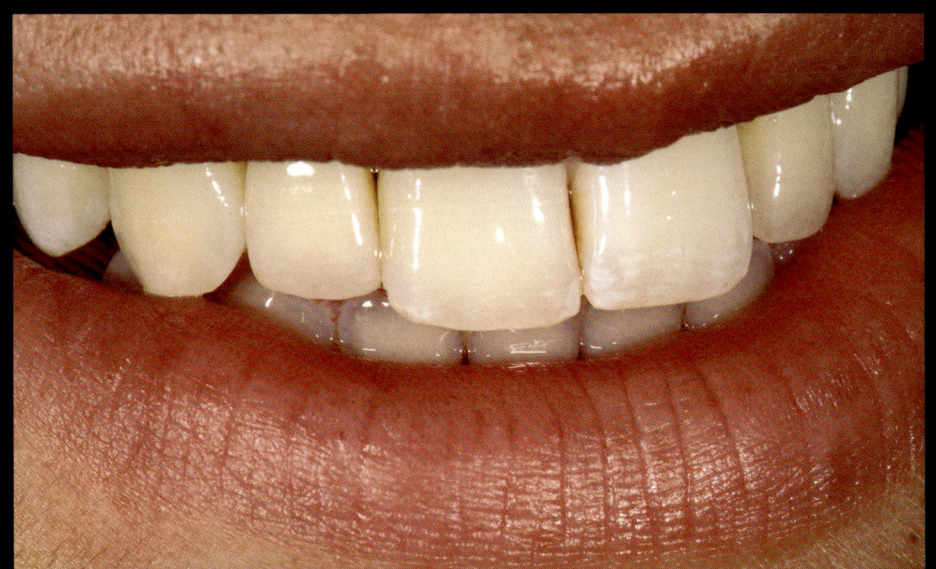

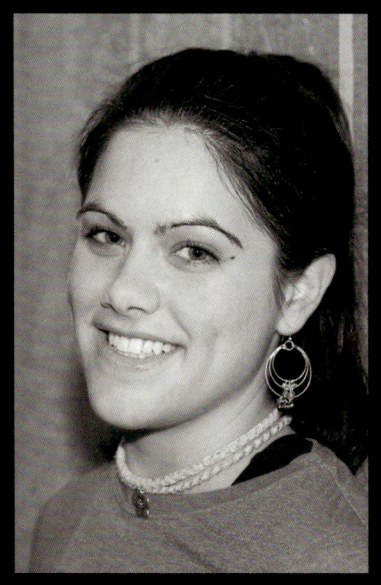

Naoki Aiba, CDT, Oral Design

DENTSCAPE

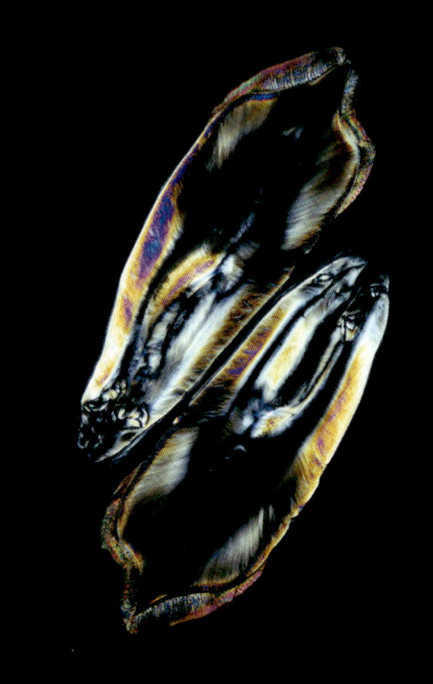

www.naokiaiba.com

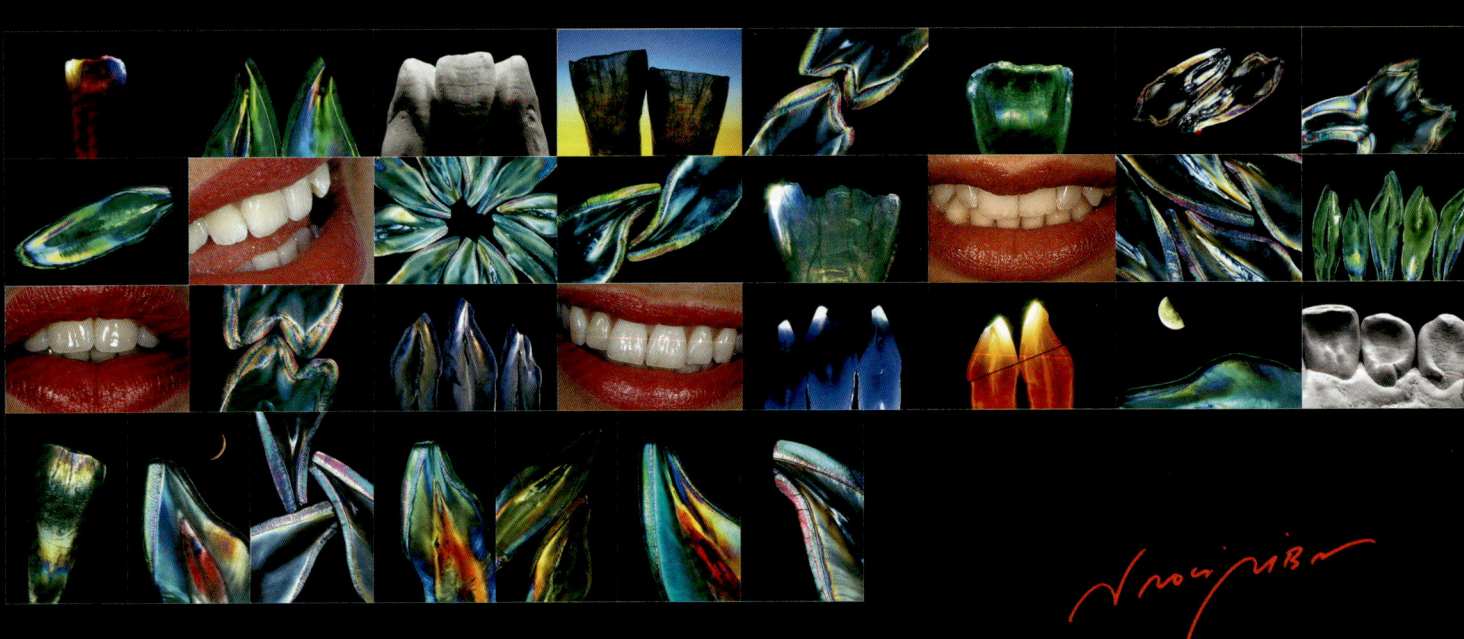

Science Art, Inc./Naoki Aiba Photography   484-B Washington Street, #323, Monterey, California 93940 USA   Phone/Fax: +1 (831) 333-9077

USING ZIRCONIA IN ESTHETIC IMPLANT RESTORATIONS

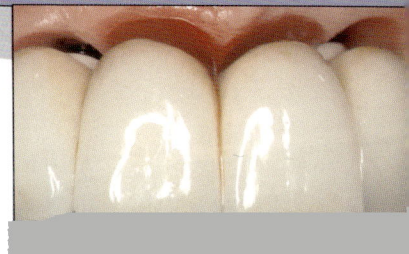

Eric Van Dooren, DDS[1]

During recent years, the treatment options and modalities for achieving optimal functional and esthetic outcomes with implant restorations have clearly changed. There has been a shift toward minimally invasive surgery, with the introduction of concepts such as computer-guided surgery, flapless surgery, and the use of orthodontics (eg, forced eruption) as a tool to guide soft tissue and bone levels.

The introduction of narrow-diameter implants with altered geometry and an improved bone-to-implant contact ratio allows clinicians to manage difficult esthetic cases with unfavorable hard tissue topography without the use of bone grafting, and permits minimally invasive treatments.

Changes in implant design and geometry, as well as in abutment design (eg, concave transmucosal profiles, platform switching), allow for improved soft tissue stability.

As shown by histologic evidence, soft tissue stability and thickness are prerequisites for soft tissue adhesion and improved long-term soft tissue behavior. Clinical observation suggests that improved soft tissue behavior, stability, and adhesion will result in a better seal or barrier.

This seal will protect the bone more efficiently from the external environment (ie, oral cavity) and result in decreased marginal bone resorption. Clinically, this will translate into less soft tissue recession and long-lasting marginal soft tissue levels and esthetics.

However, this soft tissue adhesion is only possible with biocompatible materials. Until now, titanium, aluminum oxide, and zirconium dioxide have proven to be biocompatible materials.

For many years, titanium was the material of choice for abutments; however, with the recent introduction of CAD/CAM-generated technology, new high-strength ceramic materials are becoming the first choice in treating esthetic implant cases. This new technology allows technicians to generate abutments, crowns, and fixed partial prostheses in highly esthetic and biocompatible materials that provide a high strength and excellent fit.

[1]Private practice, Antwerp, Belgium.

Correspondence to: Dr Eric Van Dooren, Tavernierkaai 2, 2000 Antwerp, Belgium. E-mail: vandoorendent@skynet.be

Zirconium dioxide has been shown to be a biocompatible, esthetic, and functional material for long-lasting restorations. This high-strength ceramic material allows for light transmission at the critical interface between marginal gingival tissue and prosthetic components. Clinical observation has shown clearly favorable esthetic outcomes and better translucency compared to ceramometallic restorations.

This article describes the use of zirconia in different clinical situations, from abutments to single crowns to short- and long-span fixed partial dentures, on both implants and natural teeth.

CASE 1

A 40-year-old patient presented with a canine agenesis in the left maxilla. Positive soft tissue architecture and a thick biotype were observed (Figs 1 and 2). The radiographs showed sufficient bone for primary implant stabilization and immediate implant placement and loading (Fig 3). However, a closer radiologic evaluation with tomography revealed minimal thickness of the bone in the critical coronal zone (Fig 4).

In order to be minimally invasive and avoid bone augmentation, a narrow-platform implant was placed (Speedy Groovy, Nobel Biocare, Göteborg, Sweden) (Fig 5). The improved geometry and osteoconductive surface characteristics of the implant, with extra bone-to-implant contact (30%), provided high primary stability (45 Ncm) at placement and consequently allowed for immediate "pseudo-loading."

Because there was no real extraction socket, implant placement was comparable to placing an implant in a healed site, and primary stability was obtained.

In cases using narrow-platform implants at the sites of canines or central incisors, the difficulty is using a concave transmucosal abutment design while achieving a normal canine cross-section diameter at the marginal gingival level.

A Procera Zirconia CAD/CAM-generated abutment (Nobel Biocare) was secured (Fig 6). The abutment had a concave transmucosal profile, which resulted in extra soft tissue thickness in this critical zone (Fig 7). The abutment can be designed on a cast before surgery, or, preferably, the surgeon should have a collection of CAD/CAM-generated abutments with different diameters, collar heights, and angulation at his or her disposal. This way, the proper abutment can be selected for different clinical situations.

Care must be taken to preserve the critical material thickness to avoid fractures of the zirconia abutment after loading. A predictable way to combine material strength and concave design while avoiding fractures is to scan the modified abutment a second time on the Procera three-dimensional scanner (Nobel Biocare), to make sure that the dimensions fall within the safety zone (indicated by a red dot on the computer screen).

The abutment was prepared with a high-speed handpiece with water cooling. Next, a provisional crown was adapted. When using concave transmucosal profiles in extraction sockets, it is important not to press resin into this area.

After initial incisal positioning and adaptation of the provisional crown with resin composite on the abutment intraorally, extraoral adaptation and polishing of the provisional restoration on the abutment is recommended and preferable. It is mandatory, however, that after any extraoral manipulation of the abutment, the zirconia abutment surface is cleaned or sterilized for optimal soft tissue adhesion.

The final form of the abutment must always be duplicated (silicone impression). This allows the technician to make a die and transfer cap (Pattern Resin, GC America, Alsip, IL, USA) (Fig 8) and facilitates final impression taking by avoiding retraction cord placement and allowing for minimally invasive prosthetic handling and treatment.

Before cementation (Temp Bond, Kerr, Orange, CA, USA) of the provisional crown (Fig 9), the abutment was secured at 35 Ncm.

It is advisable, whenever possible, to avoid contact with the antagonist in centric and excur-

CASE 1 (Figs 1 to 18)

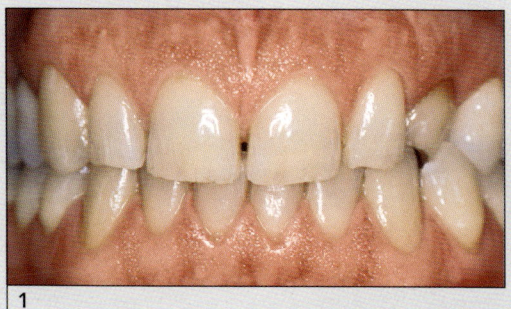

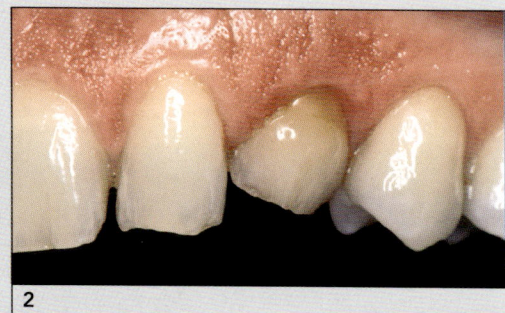

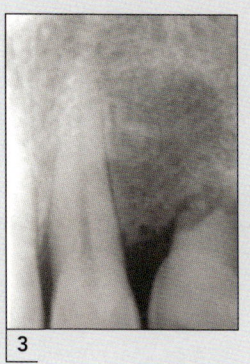

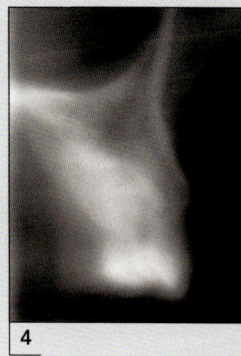

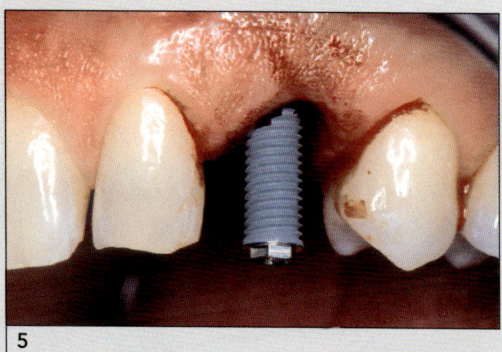

Figs 1 and 2 Preoperative views.

Figs 3 and 4 Initial radiographs *(left)* showed sufficient bone for implant stabilization; however, further radiographs with tomography *(right)* revealed minimal bone thickness in the cortical zone.

Fig 5 A narrow-platform implant was inserted.

Figs 6 and 7 A CAD/CAM-generated abutment was secured to the implant.

Fig 8 Custom abutment coping and die for the taking of final impressions.

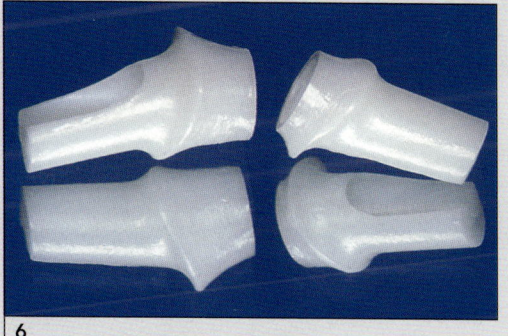

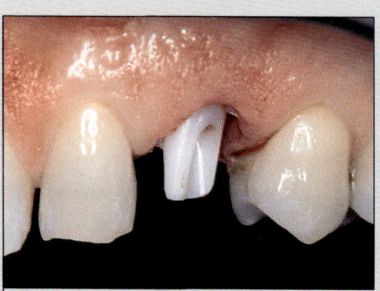

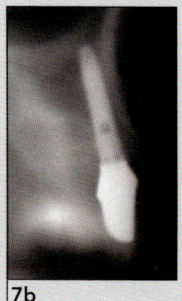

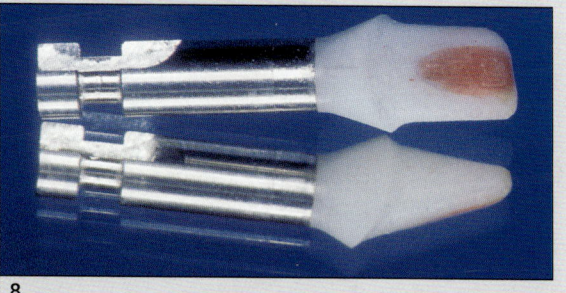

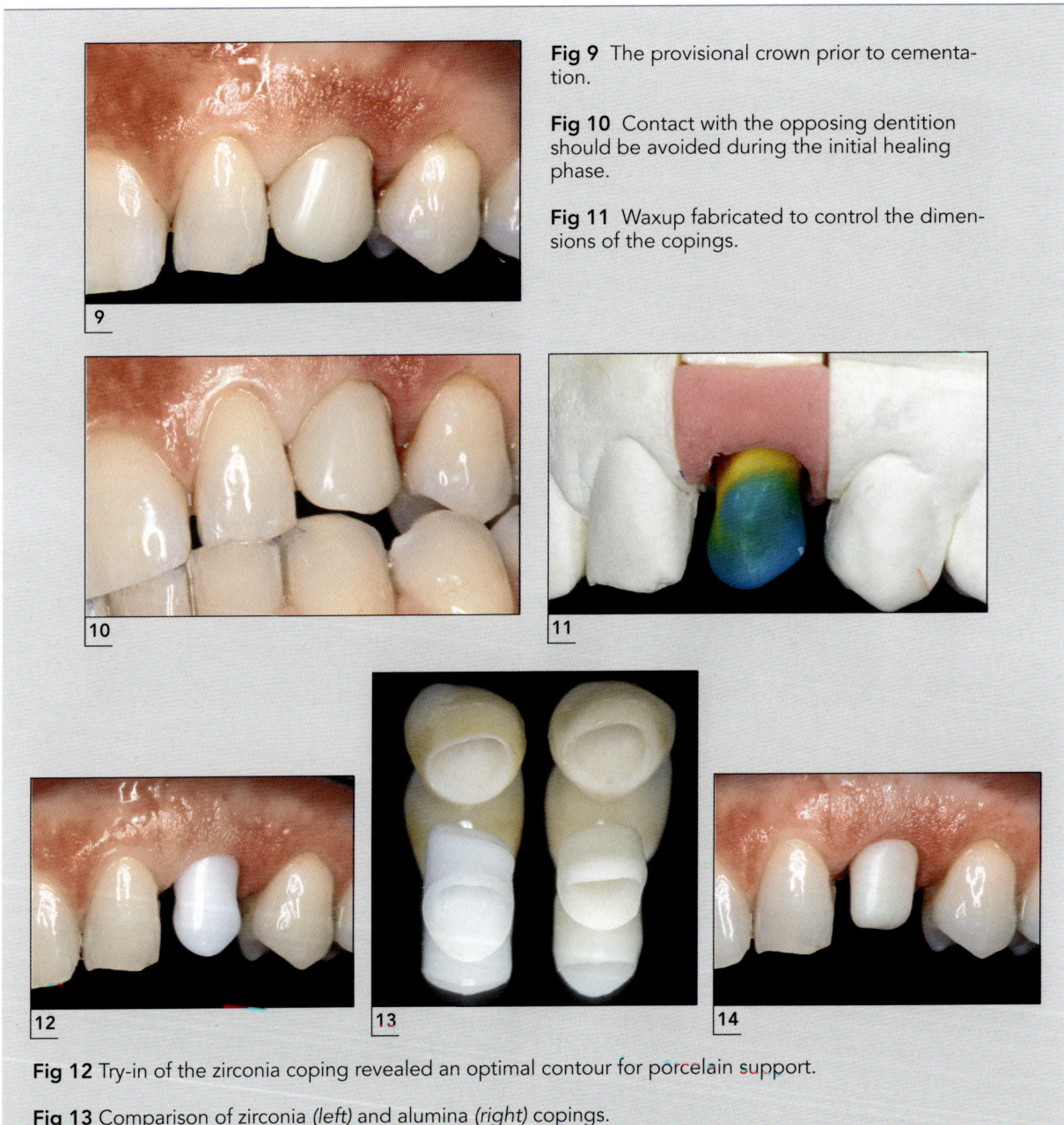

Fig 9 The provisional crown prior to cementation.

Fig 10 Contact with the opposing dentition should be avoided during the initial healing phase.

Fig 11 Waxup fabricated to control the dimensions of the copings.

Fig 12 Try-in of the zirconia coping revealed an optimal contour for porcelain support.

Fig 13 Comparison of zirconia (left) and alumina (right) copings.

Fig 14 Try-in of the alumina coping revealed improper porcelain support.

sive movements during the intitial healing phase (Fig 10).

After 12 weeks, the provisional restoration was removed and the soft tissue contours were evaluated. Soft tissue maturation was evident and final impressions were taken. Casts were fabricated, and

after a full waxup for ideal tooth form and position, a labial silicone index was made.

This allows for visual control of the coping dimensions related to the final tooth form, in order to provide proper porcelain support (Fig 11). The double-scan technique is generally the best solu-

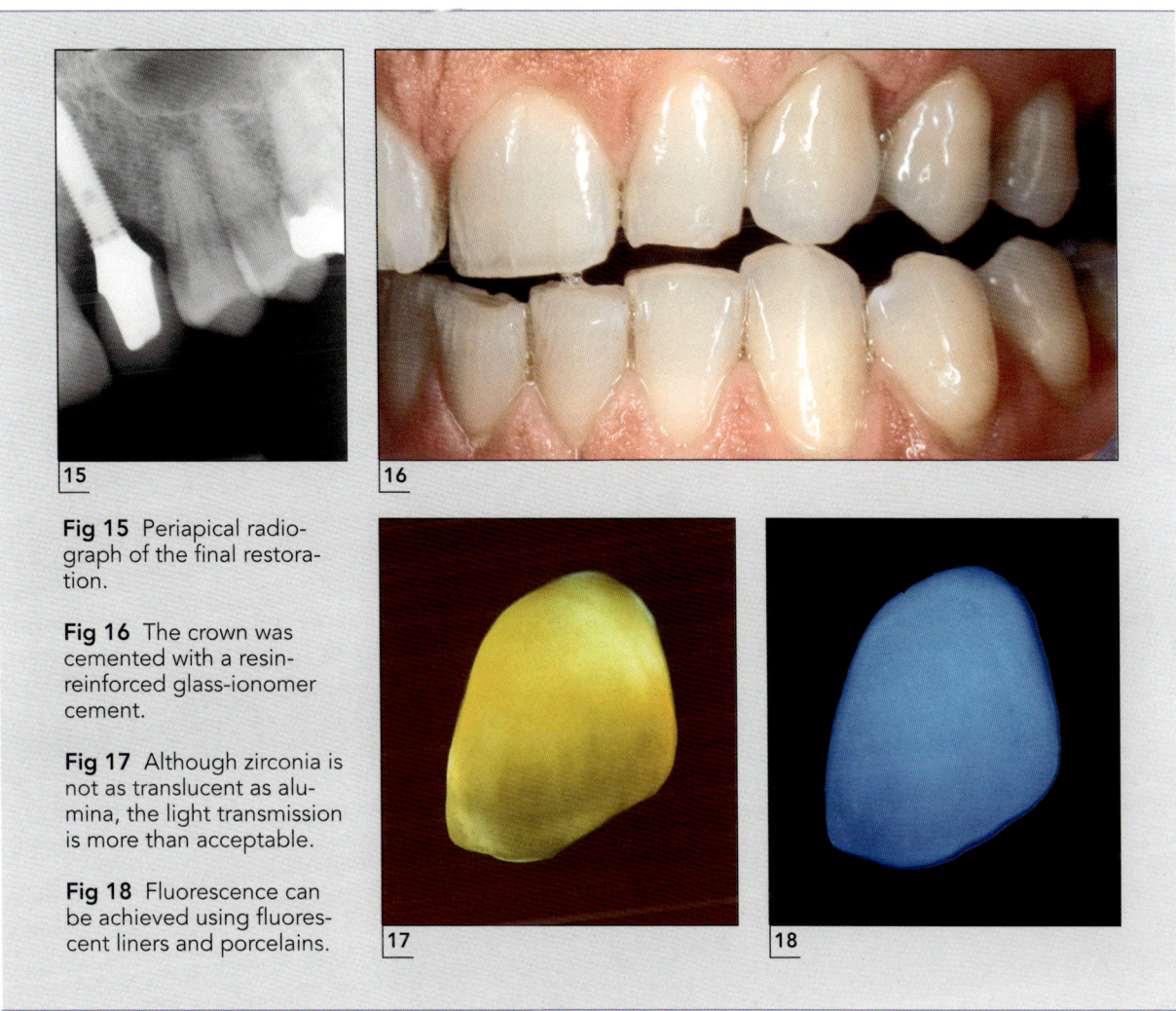

Fig 15 Periapical radiograph of the final restoration.

Fig 16 The crown was cemented with a resin-reinforced glass-ionomer cement.

Fig 17 Although zirconia is not as translucent as alumina, the light transmission is more than acceptable.

Fig 18 Fluorescence can be achieved using fluorescent liners and porcelains.

tion to obtain proper coping dimensions, since a uniform, standard coping thickness will in most cases not provide optimal support. The most common error and reason for failures and porcelain fractures is improper porcelain support. The Procera system allows the clinician to choose between different ceramic materials (aluminum oxide and zirconium dioxide) with different physical and optical properties and thicknesses (Figs 12 to 14). In cases using a zirconia coping with insufficient space for porcelain layering, the coping can eventually be reduced in thickness (from 0.7 mm to 0.4 mm) to allow for proper layering and an optimal esthetic outcome. After reducing or sandblasting the zirconia coping, it is necessary to place the coping for 15 minutes at 1,000°C to restore the

tetragonal structure of the zirconia and avoid porcelain cracks during the porcelain layering.

After final glazing and tightening of the zirconia abutment at 32 Ncm (Fig 15), the crown was cemented with a resin-reinforced glass-ionomer cement (Fuji Plus, GC, Tokyo, Japan) (Fig 16). It is important to decontaminate the inner surface of the crown before cementation (ultrasonic etching in isopropylic alcohol for 5 minutes).

The literature suggests that zirconia is not as translucent as alumina; however, clinical observation shows that that the light transmission is more than acceptable (Fig 17). Although alumina and zirconia copings are not fluorescent, fluorescence is obtained by using fluorescent liners and porcelains (Nobel Rondo, Nobel Biocare) (Fig 18).

CASE 2 (Figs 19 to 32)

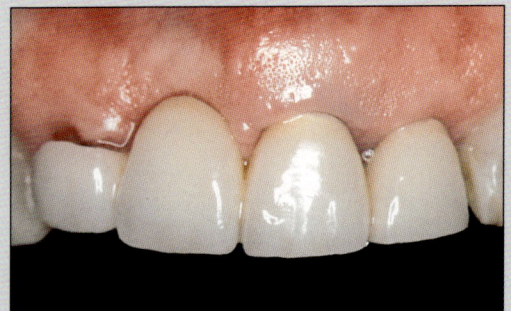
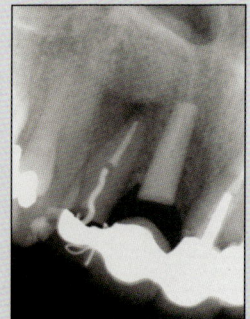

Fig 19 Preoperative view.

Figs 20 and 21 Periapical radiographs of the failing fixed partial denture.

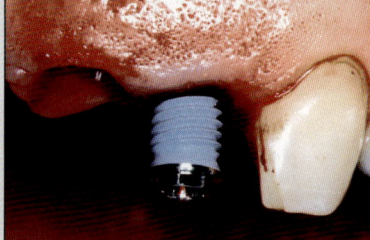
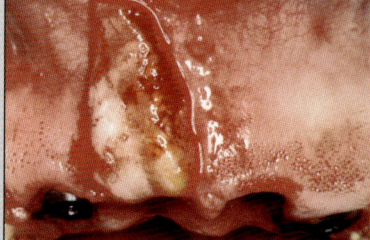
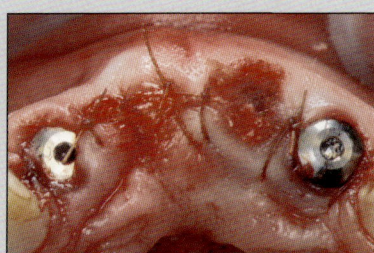

Fig 22 Implants were placed at the right and left lateral incisor sites.

Fig 23 The extraction socket of the left central incisor was filled with Bio-Oss.

Fig 24 Ridge augmentation was performed at the right central incisor.

CASE 2

A 50-year-old female patient presented with a failing four-unit maxillary anterior ceramometallic restoration (Fig 19). Clinical and radiologic evaluations revealed extensive decay, and it was decided to extract the three remaining incisors (Figs 20 and 21). The treatment plan was to place a four-unit fixed partial denture on two implants and to bond feldspathic facings on the right and left canines and right first premolar. Implants (15-mm Brånemark Mark IV, Nobel Biocare) were placed at the time of extraction at the right and left lateral incisor sites (Fig 22). The extraction socket of the left central incisor was filled with Bio-Oss (Geistlich Pharma, Wolhusen, Switzerland) (Fig 23) to prevent excessive tissue collapse, and ridge augmentation was performed at the right central incisor with a subepithelial connective tissue graft (Fig 24).

Clinical observation has shown that with a proper concept for implant placement (eg, flapless surgery, atraumatic extraction, palatal implant placement, use of filler material), immediate implant placement is most likely the treatment of choice for minimizing tissue resorption.

However, it is also the author's opinion and clinical observation that in these immediate implant placement cases, immediate loading of the implants is *not* the best treatment option. Clinical observation has shown decreased osseointegration rates for implant placement in extraction sockets with immediate loading compared to implant placement and loading in healed sites. This is especially true for patients with thin biotypes. In this case, a removable partial prosthesis was the treatment of choice.

After 10 weeks, impressions were made and casts were fabricated. It is important to make two sets of casts. The first cast should be made with

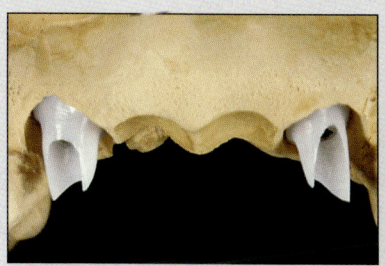

Fig 25 Custom zirconia abutment fabricated on the cast.

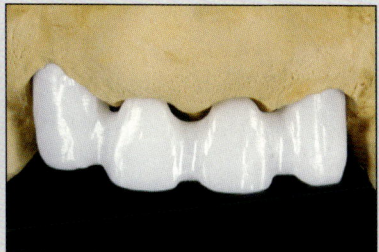

Fig 26 Prosthetic gingival pontic design prepared on the cast with the zirconia framework in place.

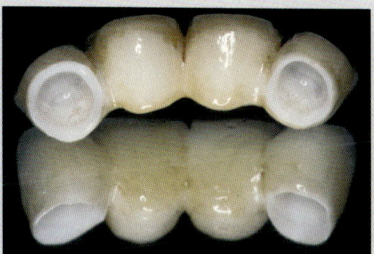

Fig 27 The porcelain was fired on the framework. Note the polished surfaces in the pontic areas.

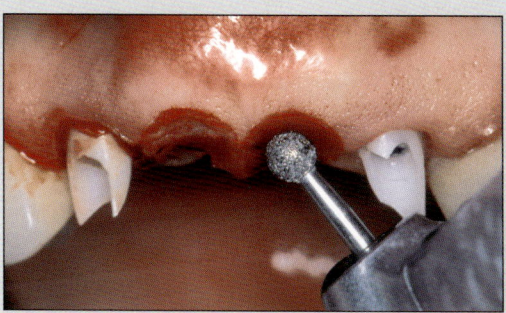

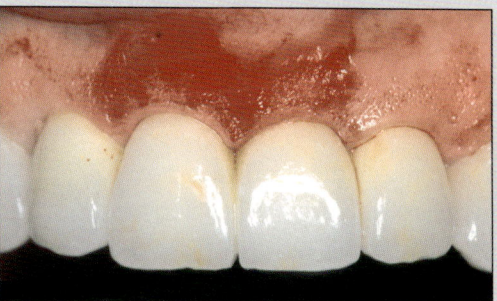

Figs 28 and 29 The tissue was plastied to create a smooth surface and eliminate scar tissue.

silicone soft tissue mask and the second with gypsum. On the first cast, two zirconia abutments were made in relation to the full waxup and silicone index. At this stage, before designing the fixed partial denture framework, it is important to sculpt the soft tissue on the second cast. Ultimately, the final clinical gingival scalloping will be a copy or reflection of the prosthetic gingival pontic design that was prepared on the cast (Fig 25).

A Pattern Resin prototype (GC America) was made and scanned. The fixed partial denture was milled from a zirconia block (Procera Zirconia, Nobel Biocare).

It is very important to observe the minimum dimensions for the connectors (3 × 2 mm) to avoid fractures of the material (Fig 26). It has been established that if minimum connector dimensions are followed, the mean load to fracture is high. This number should be related to the maximum occlusal force for a young dentate patient (maximum around 665 N for molars and 220 N for incisors).

Clinically, the marginal fit of the prosthesis was very good. This clinical observation is confirmed by the literature, which generally shows the marginal fit to be between 30 and 70 µm.

Porcelain was fired on the framework (Nobel Rondo), and care was taken to obtain the proper gingival prosthetic support and highly polished surfaces in the pontic areas (Fig 27).

Intraorally, the abutments were placed and secured at 32 Ncm, and the pontic areas were reduced and sculpted with a coarse diamond bur to create the illusion of a scalloped gingival design. On the labial aspect, the tissue was plastied to create a smooth surface and eliminate scar tissue (Figs 28 and 29).

The prosthesis was cemented with provisional cement (Temp Bond, Kerr) for 8 to 12 weeks for evaluation of the soft tissue design and maturation.

Optimal soft tissue health, color, and texture were obtained, and the prosthesis was cemented with resin-reinforced glass-ionomer cement (Fuji Plus, GC). Excellent light transmission and an optimal

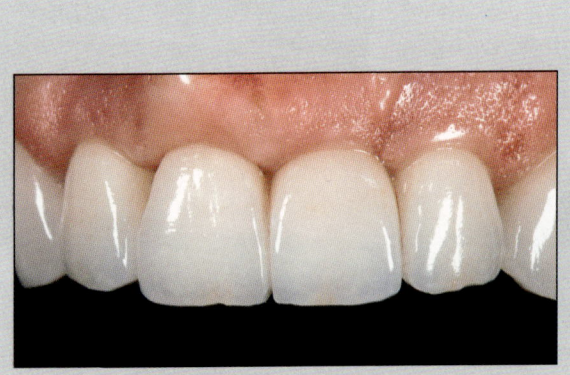

Fig 30 The final result. An excellent esthetic outcome was achieved.

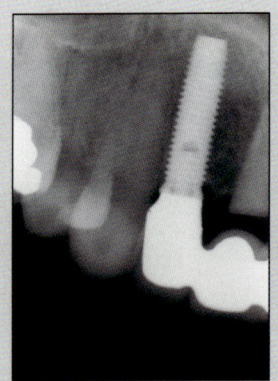
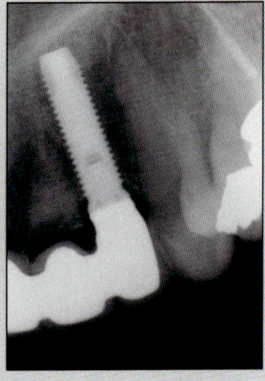

Figs 31 and 32 Radiographs after 18 months revealed minimal bone remodeling.

esthetic outome at the gingiva-prosthesis interface were achieved (Fig 30). Radiologic evaluation at 18 months revealed minimal bone remodeling after loading (Figs 31 and 32).

CASE 3

A 64-year-old female patient presented with an esthetically and functionally failing maxillary and mandibular full-arch ceramometallic restoration (Fig 33 and 34). After periodontal and radiologic evaluations, and after observing multiple teeth with recurrent decay, it was decided to extract all maxillary teeth and make a full-arch implant-supported restoration. In these cases, it is often preferable to keep three or four strategically located abutment teeth for provisionalization with a fixed metal-reinforced construction. This allows for immediate implant placement after extraction of the remaining teeth (not supporting the provisional fixed prosthesis) without immediate loading. After initial healing and osseointegration of these implants, the natural teeth that supported the provisional fixed prosthesis can be extracted. In the lab, the provisional fixed prosthesis can subsequently be turned into an implant-supported fixed prosthesis. This allows for optimal soft tissue healing and high osseointegration success rates.

After final soft tissue contouring and impression making, a full waxup and silicone index were made (Fig 35). For zirconia frameworks, a plaster cast is necessary, since these frameworks cannot be sectioned and soldered.

A Pattern Resin prototype (GC America) was sculpted, observing the ideal form for optimizing strength, esthetics, and porcelain support. Care was taken to maximize the connector height and respecting connector width (Fig 36).

At this point, it was decided to make a screw-retained zirconia fixed prosthesis. The maximum size of these prototype prostheses was limited by the available zirconia block size at that time (30 or 60 mm). This explains why the maxillary restoration was split into a four- and eight-unit zirconia screw-retained fixed prosthesis. The Duralay pattern (Reliance Dental, Worth, IL, USA) was scanned, and a copy in zirconia was milled (Procera Zirconia, Nobel Biocare). Minor adjustments were necessary to obtain ideal forms (Figs 37 and 38).

Porcelain was fused to the framework (VITA VM9, VITA Zahnfabrik, Bad Säckingen, Germany), and optimal function and esthetics were obtained. Care was taken to leave an untreated biocompatible zirconia surface in the transmucosal areas. This allowed for optimal soft tissue integration. Removal of the prosthesis for soft tissue evaluation after 12 weeks clearly showed optimal soft tissue health.

CASE 3 (Figs 33 to 41)

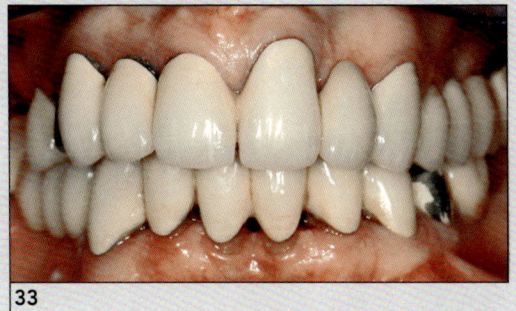

33

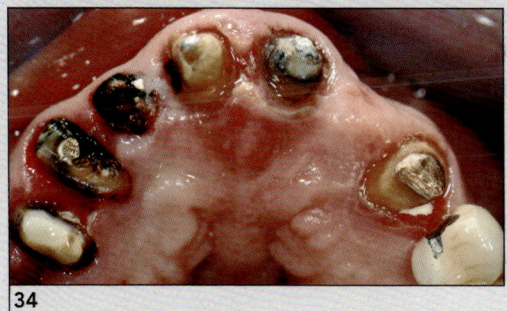

34

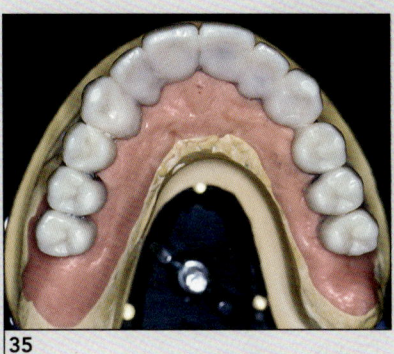

35

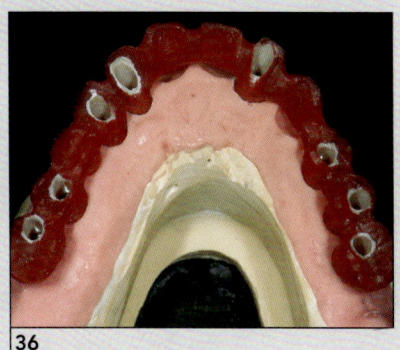

36

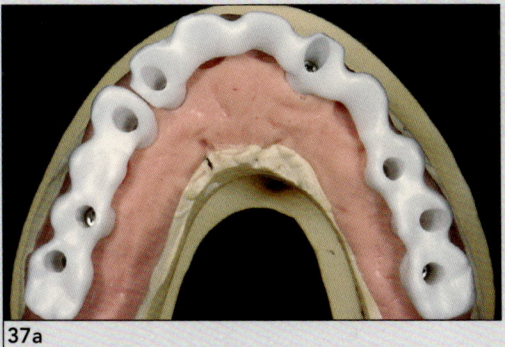

37a

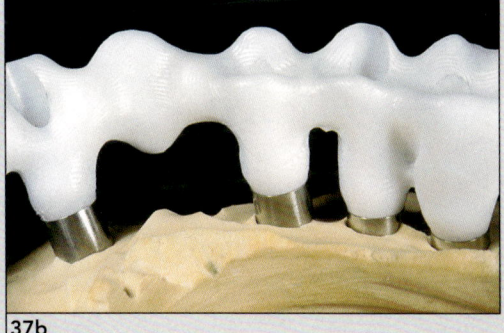

37b

Figs 33 and 34 Preoperative views with the existing restoration in place *(left)* and removed *(right)*.

Fig 35 Soft tissue contouring was performed with the impression coping in place.

Fig 36 Full contoured waxup to create the silicone matrices.

Figs 37a and 37b The milled framework. Note the excellent fit of the zirconia substructure.

Figs 38 Occlusal view after soft tissue conditioning. Note the specific soft tissue arch.

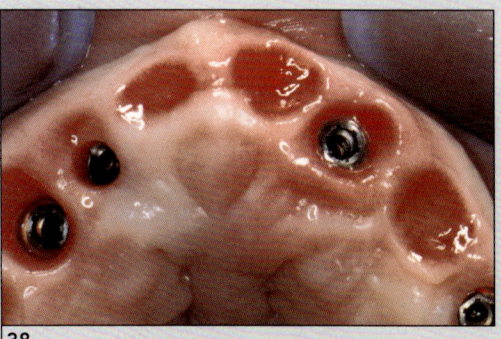

38

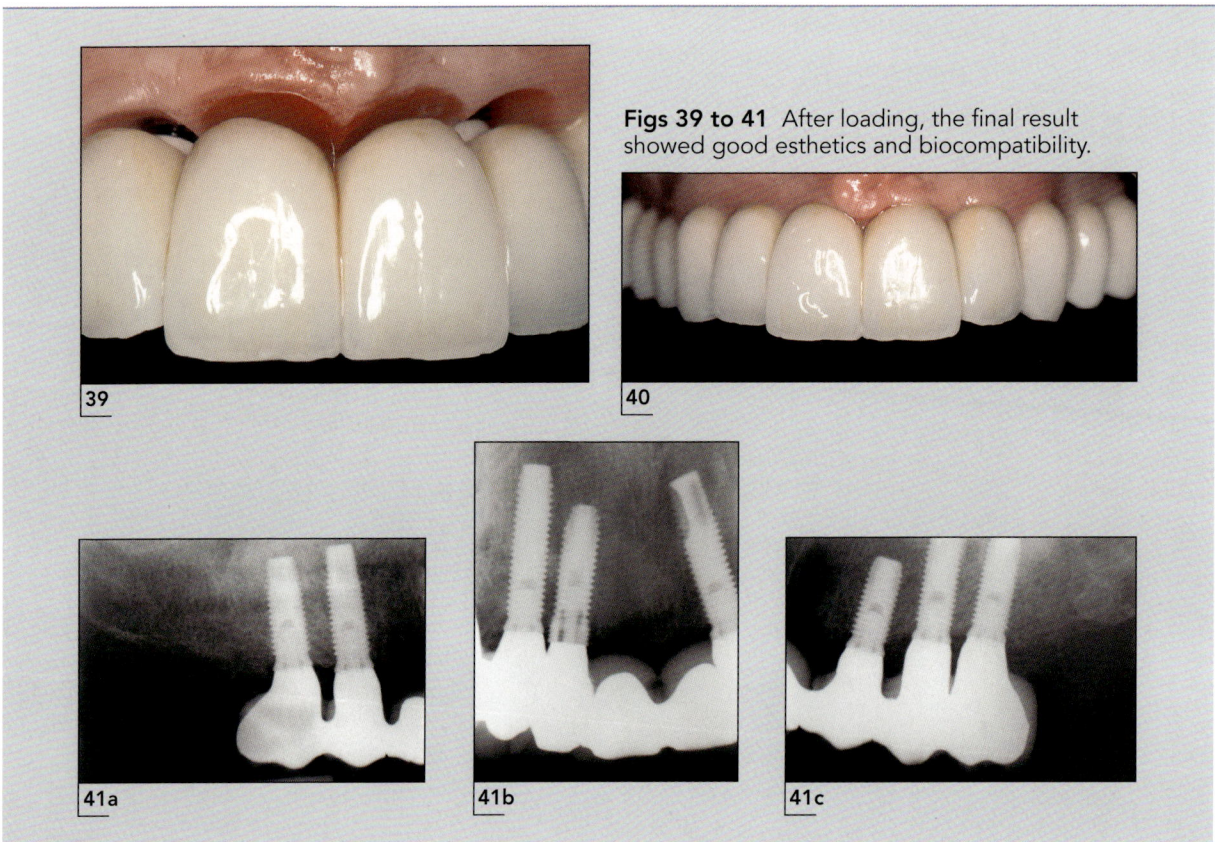

Figs 39 to 41 After loading, the final result showed good esthetics and biocompatibility.

39

40

41a

41b

41c

CONCLUSION

The optical and physical properties, strength, fit, and biocompatibility make CAD/CAM-generated zirconia frameworks a very promising alternative for conventional ceramometallic prosthetic work (Figs 39 to 41).

ACKNOWLEDGMENTS

The author thanks Patrick and Luk Rutten, Dental Team, Tessenderlo, Belgium, and Stefano Inglese, Tandartsenpraktijk Tavernierkaai, Antwerp, Belgium, for the laboratory fabrication of the restorations presented in this article.

BIBLIOGRAPHY

Allen EP. Use of mucogingival procedures to enhance esthetics. Dent Clin North Am 1998;32:307–330.

Chiche G, Pinault A. Esthetics of Anterior Fixed Prosthodontics. Chicago: Quintessence, 1993.

Degidi M, Artese L, Scarano A, Perrotti V, Gehrke P, Piattelli A. Inflammatory infiltrate, microvessel density, nitric oxide synthase expression, vascular endothelial growth factor expression, and proliferative activity in peri-implant soft tissues around titanium and zirconium oxide healing caps. J Periodontol 2006;77:73–80.

Fontijn-Tekamp FA, Slagter AP, Van Der Built A, et al. Biting and chewing in overdentures, full dentures, and natural dentitions. J Dent Res 2000;79:1519–1524.

Kohal RJ, Weng D, Bachle M, Strub JR. Loaded custom-made zirconia and titanium implants show similar osseointegration: An animal experiment. J Periodontol 2004;75:1262–1268.

Lu YC, Tseng H, Shih YH, Lee Sy. Effects of surface treatments on bond strength of glass-infiltrated ceramic, J Oral Rehabil 2001:28:805–813.

Nevins M, Camelo M, De Paoli S. A study of the fate of the buccal wall of extraction sockets of teeth with prominent roots. Int J Periodontics Restorative Dent 2006;26:19–29.

Rimondini L, Cerroni L, Carrassi A, Torricelli P. Bacterial colonization of zirconia ceramic surfaces: An in vitro and in vivo study. Int J Oral Maxillofac Implants 2002;17:793–798.

FULL-MOUTH REHABILITATION OF THE HOPELESS DENTITION: TREATMENT CONSIDERATIONS

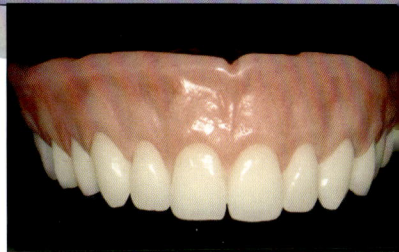

Alexander Shor, DMD, MSD[1]
Yoshihiro Goto, DDS, MSD[2]
Darrin Rapaport, BDS, MSD[3]
Kavita Shor, BDS, MSD[3]

Despite the fact that the rate of edentulism is declining in some industrialized countries, epidemiologic data for the United States indicate that a significant number of the population is edentulous or will become edentulous in the future.[1,2] It is obvious that the dentition of every edentulous patient experienced a terminal state from which it was transitioned into edentulism. Although dental literature does not provide a precise definition for this state, the authors consider the term *hopeless dentition* appropriate.[3]

At the level of the individual tooth, dental caries and periodontal disease have been de-scribed as the leading causes of tooth loss.[4,5] On the other hand, the causative factors for the loss of the whole dentition have not been presented in the dental literature. Nevertheless, it seems probable that plaque-induced diseases are the most common etiology of the hopeless dentition. It is also evident that congenital disorders, various forms of tooth wear, and traumatic injuries can contribute to tooth loss, thus rendering the dentition into a hopeless state.

Management of the hopeless dentition represents a unique and challenging practice in dentistry. In addition to the purely mechanistic aspect of the treatment, which is difficult in its own right, clinicians must attend to the emotional and physical handicaps commonly associated with the hopeless dentition and the edentulous state.

Critical aspects in the management of the hopeless dentition include treatment options and prosthetic design, along with a strategy for the patient's transition into a definitive prosthesis. A brief overview of these aspects follows.

[1]Affiliate Assistant Professor, School of Dentistry, University of Washington; private practice, Seattle, Washington, USA.
[2]Clinical Assistant Professor, University of Southern California; private practice, Los Angeles, California, USA.
[3]Private practice, Seattle, Washington, USA.

Correspondence to: Dr Alexander Shor, 1500 Fairview Avenue East, Suite 300, Seattle, WA 98102, USA. Fax: 206-323-6273. E-mail: alexshor38@hotmail.com

TREATMENT OPTIONS

Since the hopeless dentition represents a transitional state toward edentulism, the available treatment options are analogues to the rehabilitation of an edentulous patient. These options include a tissue-supported removable complete denture and a dental prosthesis retained or supported by implants.[6-8] The success of these options greatly varies in the mandible and maxilla; the available treatment alternatives regarding the individual arch therefore must be considered separately.

Because of their poor retention and stability, conventional mandibular complete dentures are often not well accepted by patients and are considerable physical and mental handicaps.[9-13] Alternatively, the literature is unequivocal regarding the advantages of dental implants in the rehabilitation of the edentulous mandible. Comparative studies of conventional complete dentures and implant-stabilized prostheses consistently show a significant improvement in the quality of life and patient satisfaction for the latter.[14,15] Based on these findings, implant prostheses are recommended as the treatment of choice for the rehabilitation of the mandible.[16]

On the other hand, maxillary complete dentures show good patient acceptance. Studies comparing conventional complete dentures with implant-stabilized prostheses are scarce. The available data, although limited, indicate comparable satisfaction between these treatment alternatives.[17] Based on these findings, and taking into account the complexity and high cost of implant treatment, it can be concluded that conventional maxillary complete dentures remain a viable treatment alternative. However, implant prostheses should be considered as the treatment of choice for maladaptive patients whose clinical presentation includes a hyperactive gag response or an atrophic maxilla, or for patients who are psychologically unwilling to accept a removable complete denture.

PROSTHETIC DESIGN

The complete denture is a well-accepted design, and its fabrication and maintenance are relatively straightforward.[6] On the other hand, the design of an implant prosthesis can be executed in several different ways, and some controversy still exists regarding its design and indications. A brief review of the available options is presented below. For additional information, readers are referred to two articles by Zitzmann and Marinello.[7,8]

In its general form, the design of implant prostheses has evolved as a modification of the conventional removable denture or fixed prosthesis. The available options may be classified as follows: an implant-retained and soft tissue–supported removable overdenture, an implant-supported removable overdenture, or an implant-supported fixed prosthesis.[7,8] The most critical factors that influence the selection of the appropriate design include the patient's expectations, anatomic and morphologic presentation, and treatment cost.[7,8]

All aforementioned designs have been successfully used in the rehabilitation of the edentulous mandible. The limited comparative research indicates that patients usually prefer a more stable design, such as an implant-supported prosthesis.[18] One study that evaluated patients' preferences between the implant-supported fixed or removable prosthesis reported that some patients favored fixed while others favored a removable design.[19]

In terms of the prosthetic design, the situation is somewhat different in the maxilla. Most of the available clinical research has evaluated the performance of the implant-supported fixed or removable designs.[20-24] The available data indicate that these options show an acceptable performance. As in the mandible, there is no distinct superiority of the fixed or removable prosthesis, and patients may favor either design.[25] Information on the clinical performance and patient satisfaction of the implant-retained and tissue-supported removable overdenture is scarce, and its use in clinical practice is still somewhat experimental.[26,27] It is also plausible that in the maxilla, this design may not provide significant advantages over the removable complete denture.

Special consideration should be given to clinical scenarios in which both arches will be restored with an implant-supported prosthesis. Long-term data are mostly available for designs that use prefabricated acrylic resin denture teeth and veneering acrylic resin. A high incidence of restorative material failure in the form of denture tooth wear, denture tooth fracture, and veneering resin fracture have been reported.[20,28,29] Alternatively, veneering dental ceramics have also been used for this type of restoration.[30–32] However, long-term data on the performance of this type of material are not available. It is plausible that dental ceramics may also be susceptible to high fracture rates when used for implant-supported prostheses.[33] Therefore, it appears that implant-supported designs for both arches present a high risk of restorative complications, and these risks should be clearly communicated to the patient. It is also clear that further optimization is required for this type of restoration to be successfully used in clinical practice.

TRANSITION STRATEGY

The transition protocol for the hopeless dentition varies depending on the chosen definitive prosthesis. In situations where the definitive prosthesis includes a complete denture or an implant-retained/implant-supported overdenture, the most common transition protocol involves fabrication of an immediate denture.[34,35]

For the complete denture treatment, the immediate denture can be converted into the definitive prosthesis via a reline procedure. If, however, the immediate denture is deemed inadequate, a new complete denture is fabricated following appropriate soft and hard tissue healing. For the overdenture treatment, a new definitive prosthesis is usually constructed following appropriate healing time.

For the implant-supported fixed prosthesis, transition of the hopeless dentition can be carried out using several different protocols. Similar to the overdenture protocol, immediate denture prostheses can be used. Upon completion of the surgical treatment, the fabrication of a fixed provisional restoration is usually required, followed by the fabrication of the definitive restoration. An alternative protocol involves fabrication of a fixed provisional restoration supported by strategically selected remaining teeth or immediately loaded dental implants.[36,37] In this manner, a transitional removable prosthesis is avoided. The main advantages of this approach include the potential for the preservation of soft tissue architecture and tooth landmarks for the implant placement surgery, as well as superior patient acceptance. However, compared to the immediate denture transition strategy, this approach is more technique sensitive, since it requires careful selection of the abutment teeth and implant sites, and also must include provisions for potential implant failure. In addition, increased structural demands for the fixed provisional restoration should be taken into account with this approach.

The following case presentation illustrates the concepts mentioned above and provides some technical solutions for the treatment of this type of case.

CASE PRESENTATION

A 46-year-old female patient was referred for prosthodontic rehabilitation of her dentition. The patient's recent dental history showed comprehensive restorative treatment of her compromised dentition. This treatment included removal of the hopeless teeth, root canal treatment, foundation restorations, crown-lengthening surgery, and full-mouth provisional restorations. Because of the compromised state of her dentition, definitive restorations were not completed, and the patient still had provisional restorations (Fig 1).

A standard comprehensive examination was performed to evaluate the patient's dental condition and develop a new restorative treatment

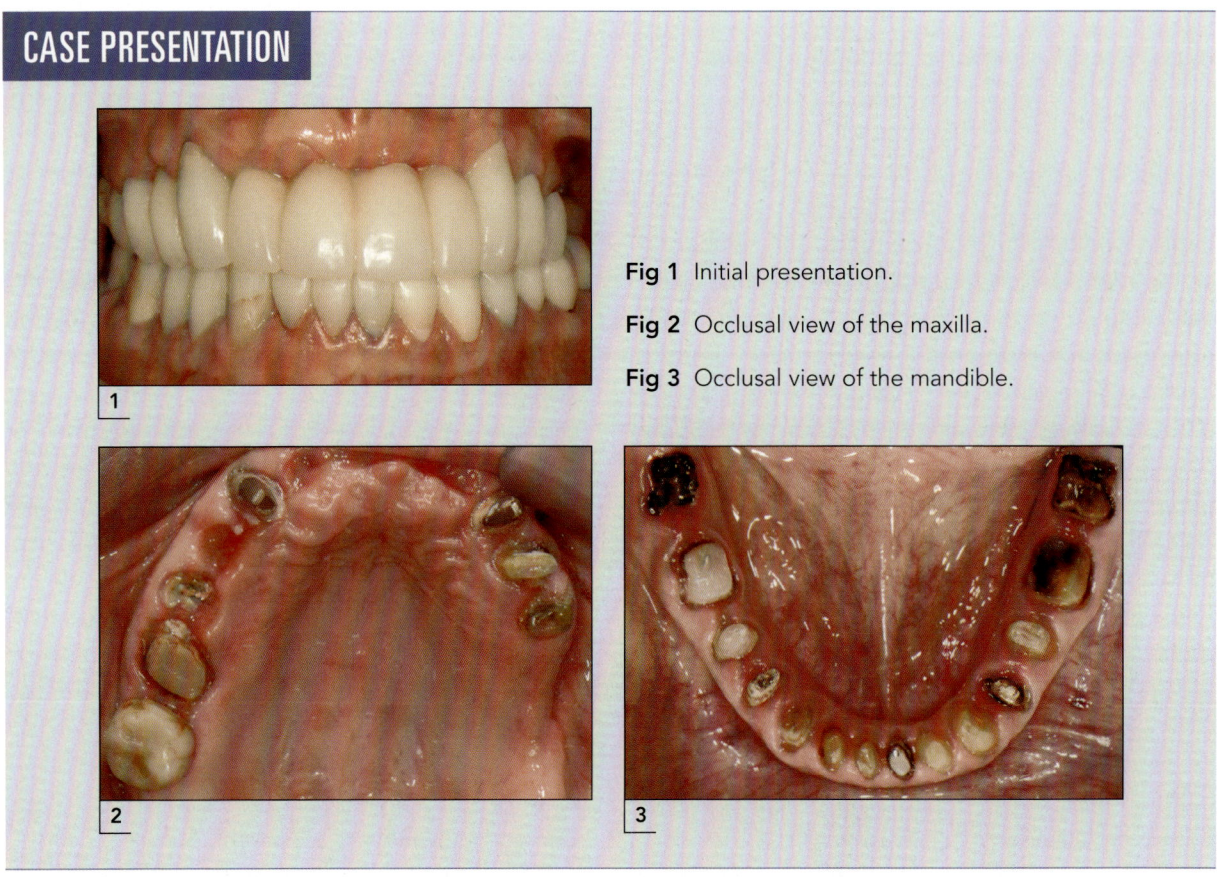

CASE PRESENTATION

Fig 1 Initial presentation.

Fig 2 Occlusal view of the maxilla.

Fig 3 Occlusal view of the mandible.

plan. Clinical and radiographic examinations revealed a failing dentition. The remaining teeth showed extensive caries lesions, numerous root canal fillings, and a mild to moderate degree of attachment loss. Diagnostic removal of the provisional restorations revealed gross caries lesions on all remaining teeth and significant loss of tooth structure on most teeth (Figs 2 and 3). A treatment plan was prepared following the standard protocol, which took into consideration the patient's desires, risk factors, treatment alternatives, and treatment cost. In the maxilla, the treatment plan included removal of all remaining teeth and fabrication of a complete denture. In the mandible, the treatment plan included removal of all remaining teeth and their replacement with an implant-supported fixed prosthesis. The planned prosthetic design included a segmented ceramometal prosthesis. The decision was also made to transition the patient's mandibular dentition into definitive restorations via immediate implant

placement and an immediate loading protocol, thus avoiding immediate denture treatment.

Mandibular Fixed Provisional

The existing mandibular provisional restoration had been fabricated in several segments, and exhibited numerous fractures and marginal discrepancies. It was obvious that a new provisional restoration was required. In the process of dentofacial and occlusal examinations, important diagnostic landmarks such as tooth dimensions and positions, location of the incisal-occlusal plane, and the occlusal relationship of maxillary and mandibular teeth, were evaluated and determined to be within an acceptable range (Fig 4). Therefore, the decision was made not to fabricate a new diagnostic waxup, but rather to duplicate the contour and form of the existing mandibular provisional restorations. A polyvinyl siloxane index was fabricated over the mandibular

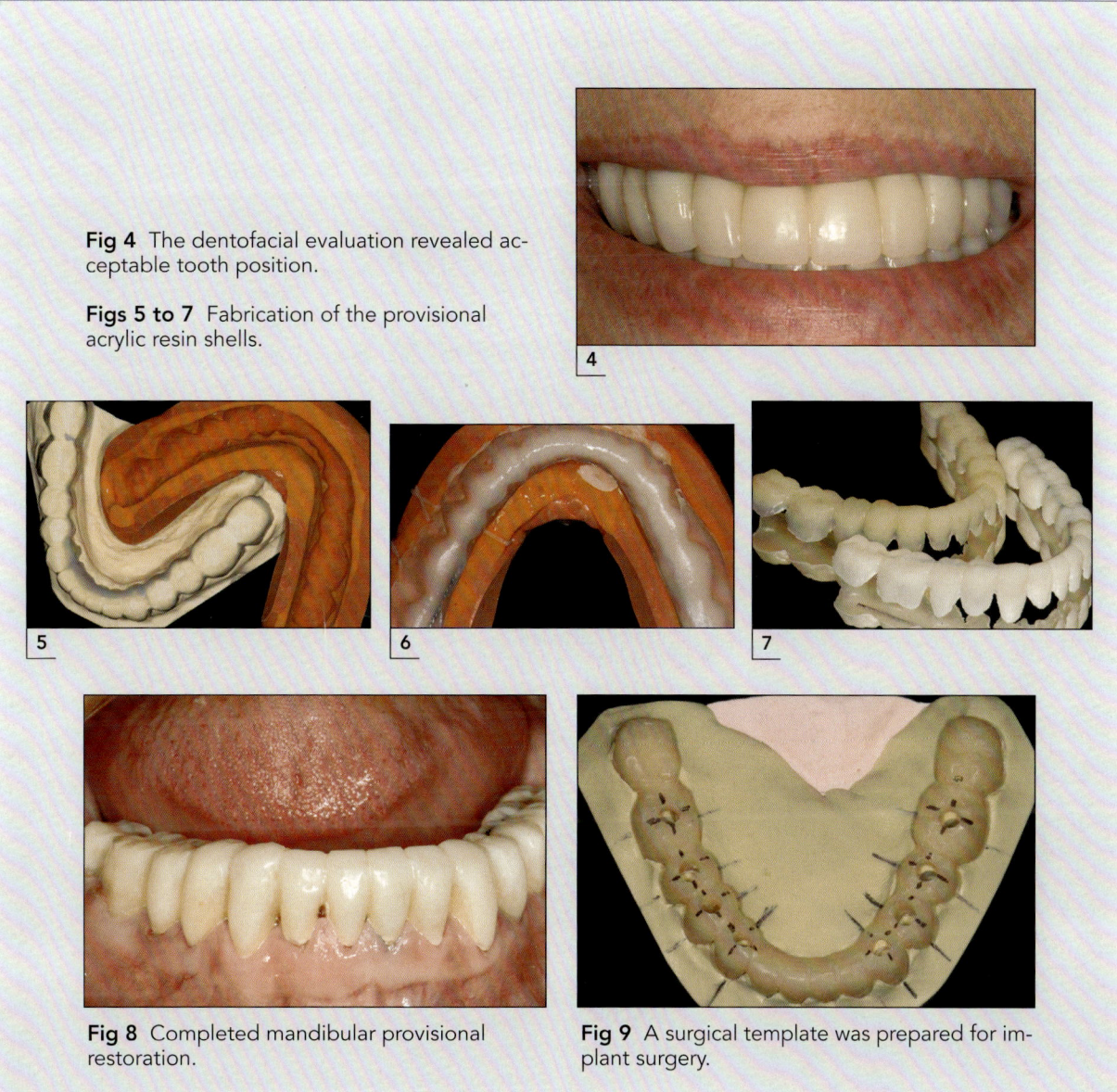

Fig 4 The dentofacial evaluation revealed acceptable tooth position.

Figs 5 to 7 Fabrication of the provisional acrylic resin shells.

Fig 8 Completed mandibular provisional restoration.

Fig 9 A surgical template was prepared for implant surgery.

teeth on the diagnostic cast (Fig 5). A twisted stainless steel wire was secured in the index. Autopolymerized acrylic resin was poured into the index, and complete polymerization was carried out in a pressure pot under controlled vacuum and pressure conditions (Fig 6). The excess material beyond the margins was trimmed away. The intaglio surface of the provisional prosthesis was also trimmed to form a uniform shell-like structure with a thickness of 0.5 to 1.00 mm. For the construction of the surgical template, a second acrylic resin shell was fabricated in a similar fashion (Fig 7). Intraorally, the acrylic resin shell was relined with an autopolymerized acrylic resin. The finished mandibular one-piece provisional prosthesis was cemented with temporary cement (Fig 8). The second acrylic shell was prepared for the implant surgery. Upon intraoral reline and finishing, it was seated into the polyvinyl siloxane putty. Holes measuring 2 mm in diameter were placed to correspond to the center of each proposed implant location (Fig 9).

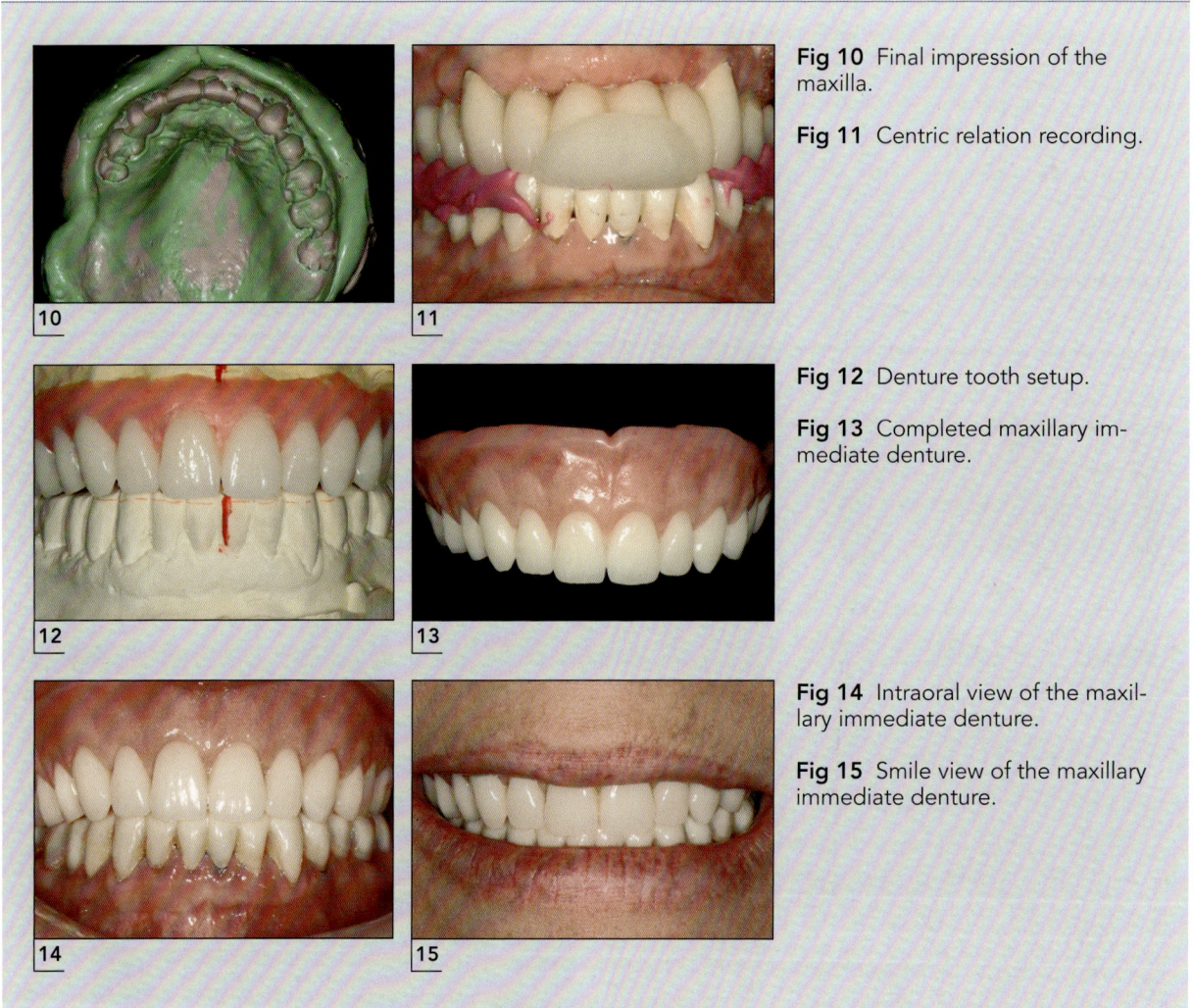

Fig 10 Final impression of the maxilla.

Fig 11 Centric relation recording.

Fig 12 Denture tooth setup.

Fig 13 Completed maxillary immediate denture.

Fig 14 Intraoral view of the maxillary immediate denture.

Fig 15 Smile view of the maxillary immediate denture.

Maxillary Immediate Denture

In preparation for the maxillary final impression, a custom tray was fabricated on the maxillary diagnostic cast. Maxillary final impressions were taken with a low-viscosity polyvinyl siloxane impression material injected over the teeth and a high-viscosity polyvinyl siloxane impression material placed into the custom tray (Fig 10). A maxillary master cast was fabricated using type III dental stone. The centric relation was recorded with the help of an anterior jig (Fig 11). Maxillary and mandibular casts were articulated with the centric relation record and arbitrarily mounted to a semiadjustable articulator. A maxillary denture tooth mold was selected based on the dimensions of the existing teeth, and the maxillary tooth shade was approved by the patient. The setup was completed following removal of the stone teeth on the master cast (Fig 12). The references provided by the original teeth served as a guide in the placement of the denture teeth. It was also noted that an adequate amount of vertical space was present for the tooth length and denture thickness. Thus, alveoloplasty was not required in the maxilla. Maxillary denture waxup, processing, and finishing were completed using standard prosthodontic protocols (Fig 13).

The maxillary denture was delivered immediately following removal of the remaining maxillary teeth. The intaglio surface of the denture was relined with a soft reline material (Lynal, Dentsply,

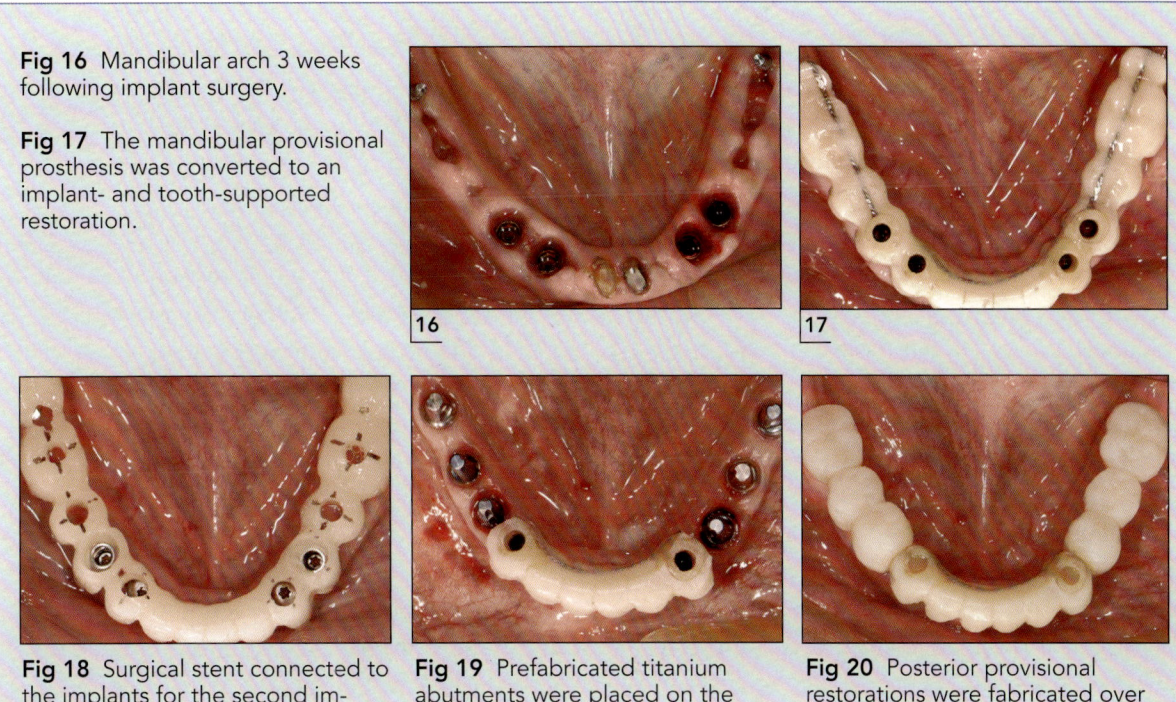

Fig 16 Mandibular arch 3 weeks following implant surgery.

Fig 17 The mandibular provisional prosthesis was converted to an implant- and tooth-supported restoration.

Fig 18 Surgical stent connected to the implants for the second implant surgery.

Fig 19 Prefabricated titanium abutments were placed on the posterior implants.

Fig 20 Posterior provisional restorations were fabricated over the abutments.

York, PA, USA). During the healing phase, the maxillary denture was relined several times to compensate for the soft tissue shrinkage. The patient expressed satisfaction with the denture (Figs 14 and 15). Approximately 3 months following removal of the maxillary teeth, the intaglio surface of the denture was relined chairside with a hard reline material (Astron LC, Astron Dental, Lake Zurich, IL, USA).

Implant Placement Surgery

For the mandibular implant-supported prosthesis, eight implants were used. The chosen implant sites corresponded bilaterally to the first molars, first and second premolars, and canines. Because of the close proximity of the mandibular canal to the roots of the second premolars and first molars, immediate placement of the dental implants was contraindicated for these sites. Therefore, it was decided to proceed with implant surgery in a staged approach.

The first implant surgery included extraction of all mandibular teeth, with the exception of central incisors, and placement of dental implants (Straumann, Basel, Switzerland) at the sites of the first premolars and canines bilaterally. For additional distal support of the provisional restoration, one provisional mini-implant (Nobel Biocare, Göteborg, Sweden) was placed in the interproximal bone area between the maxillary first and second molars bilaterally (Fig 16). Immediately following surgery, the tooth-supported provisional restoration was converted to an implant- and tooth-supported provisional restoration (Fig 17). In preparation for the second implant surgery, the mandibular surgical template was connected to the implants via nonengaging titanium temporary abutments (Fig 18).

Three months later, the patient returned for a second implant surgery. Implants were placed in the sites of second premolars and first molars bilaterally. Implant placement was performed with the help of the surgical template. The remaining teeth and mini-implants were extracted 2 months following the second implant surgery and upon confirmation of successful osseointegration of all dental implants.

No complications were encountered during the surgical stage, and the patient presented for fabrication of the provisional restorations for the remaining dental implants. The final abutments for a definitive cemented prosthesis were selected at this treatment stage, taking into account implant angulation and soft tissue height around the implants. As a result of the minimal soft tissue thickness and good parallelism, prefabricated titanium abutments were used for the first and second premolars and first molars bilaterally. The selected solid abutments were placed on the implants and torqued to the manufacturers' recommended values (Fig 19). Because of the considerable soft tissue height, individual custom abutments were fabricated for implants in the canine sites. The posterior teeth were sectioned from the existing provisional restoration, thus resulting in an individual screw-retained anterior provisional segment. Acrylic shells were fabricated for the posterior provisional restorations in the previously described silicone index. Prefabricated acrylic copings were placed on the abutments, and provisional shells were relined with an autopolymerized acrylic resin. The finished provisional restorations were cemented with temporary cement (Fig 20). Approximately 4 months following delivery of the provisional prosthesis, the patient presented for the fabrication of the definitive restorations.

The Definitive Prosthesis

Reevaluation of the tooth position in the immediate denture and mandibular fixed provisional restorations revealed certain deviations from the desired goals (Fig 21). These deviations probably resulted from the numerous denture and provisional relines. Therefore, a new maxillary denture was fabricated. Rather than proceed with a standard protocol for denture fabrication, a duplicate acrylic resin denture was fabricated for the simultaneous impression and dentofacial evaluation pro-

cedures. A two-part, top and bottom polyvinyl siloxane mold was fabricated for the duplication of the existing denture (Fig 22). Upon completion of the mold, the top and bottom parts were secured to each other with rubber bands. Autopolymerized clear acrylic resin (Orthodontic Resin, Dentsply) was poured into the mold (Fig 23). The complete polymerization of the acrylic resin was carried out in the pressure pot. The intaglio surface of the duplicate denture was relieved by several millimeters, with the exception of the central area of the hard palate, and numerous holes were created for the retention of the impression material (Fig 24).

A combination of low- and high-viscosity polyvinyl siloxane impression materials was placed inside the duplicate denture for the final impression (Fig 25). During the impression procedure, care was taken to center the denture during seating. Following completion of the impression procedure, the duplicate denture was reinserted into the mouth and the tooth position was evaluated (Fig 26). The ideal location of the incisal-occlusal plane and maxillary midline was marked on the duplicate with an indelible ink pen. In addition, a standard series of photographs was taken to facilitate denture tooth setup in the laboratory.

For the mandibular final impression, pickup-type impression copings were used for the posterior implants. For the canine sites, transfer-type impression copings were attached to the implants. These impression copings were connected to each other with a light-polymerized resin composite material (Fig 27). The final impression was taken in a stock plastic tray using a combination of a low-viscosity polyvinyl siloxane injected around the copings and high-viscosity polyvinyl siloxane placed into the impression tray. Implant analogs were attached to the impression copings and the case was returned to the laboratory (Fig 28).

Standard protocols were used for fabrication of the maxillary and mandibular master casts. The maxillary duplicate denture repositioned on the master cast was mounted to the articulator (PCH, Panadent, Grand Terrace, CA, USA) as follows (Fig 29). Smile photographs of the patient with the duplicate denture were used in the evaluation of

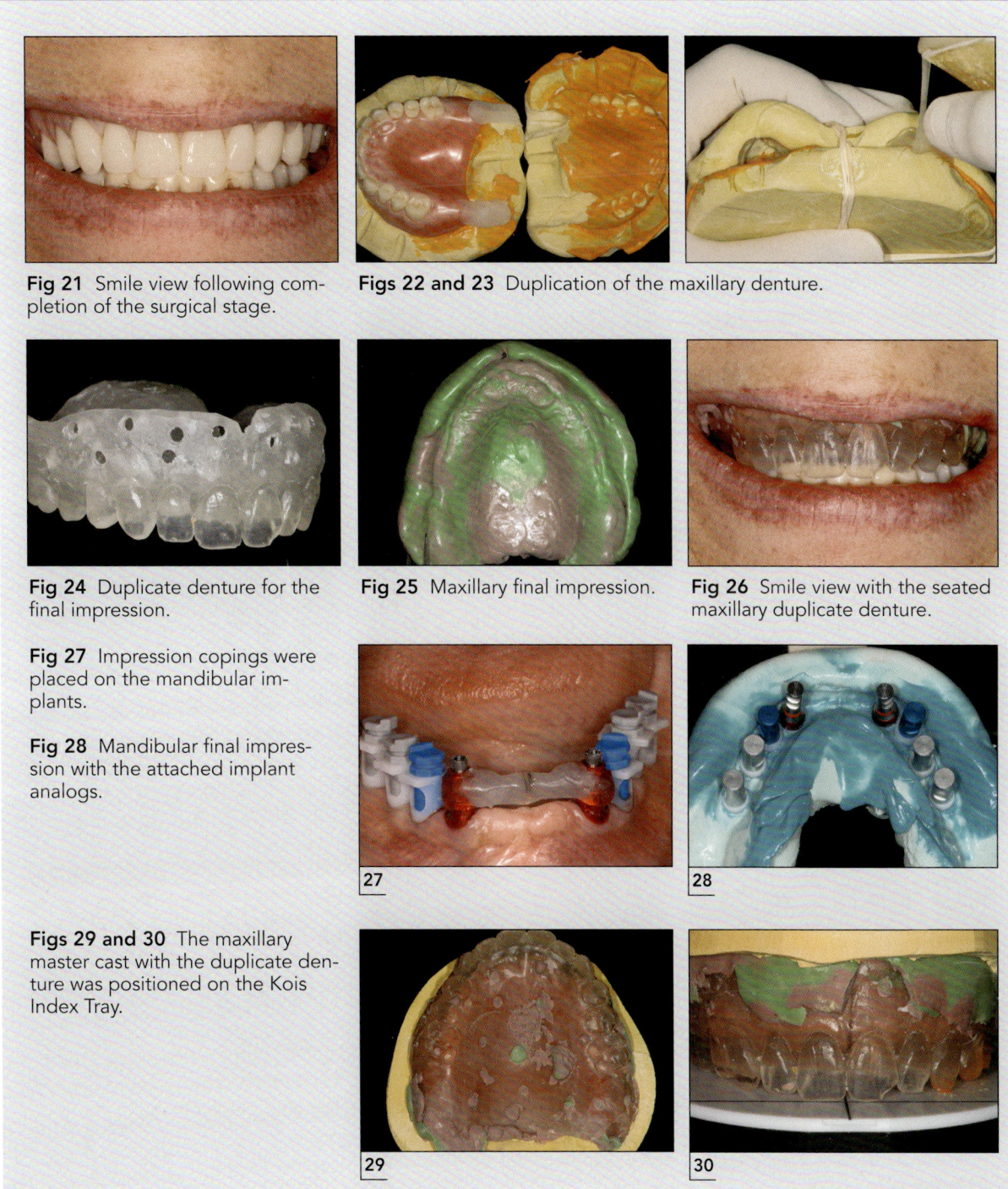

Fig 21 Smile view following completion of the surgical stage.

Figs 22 and 23 Duplication of the maxillary denture.

Fig 24 Duplicate denture for the final impression.

Fig 25 Maxillary final impression.

Fig 26 Smile view with the seated maxillary duplicate denture.

Fig 27 Impression copings were placed on the mandibular implants.

Fig 28 Mandibular final impression with the attached implant analogs.

Figs 29 and 30 The maxillary master cast with the duplicate denture was positioned on the Kois Index Tray.

incisal-occlusal plane. Slight canting of the incisal-occlusal plane in the area of the posterior teeth was corrected via the addition of a sticky wax to the ideal level. The duplicate denture with the master cast was positioned on the flat plane of the Kois Index Tray seated on the Kois Adjustable Platform (Panadent). Care was taken to ensure that the location of the determined midline corresponded to the midline of the index tray (Fig 30). The maxillary cast was then mounted to the upper

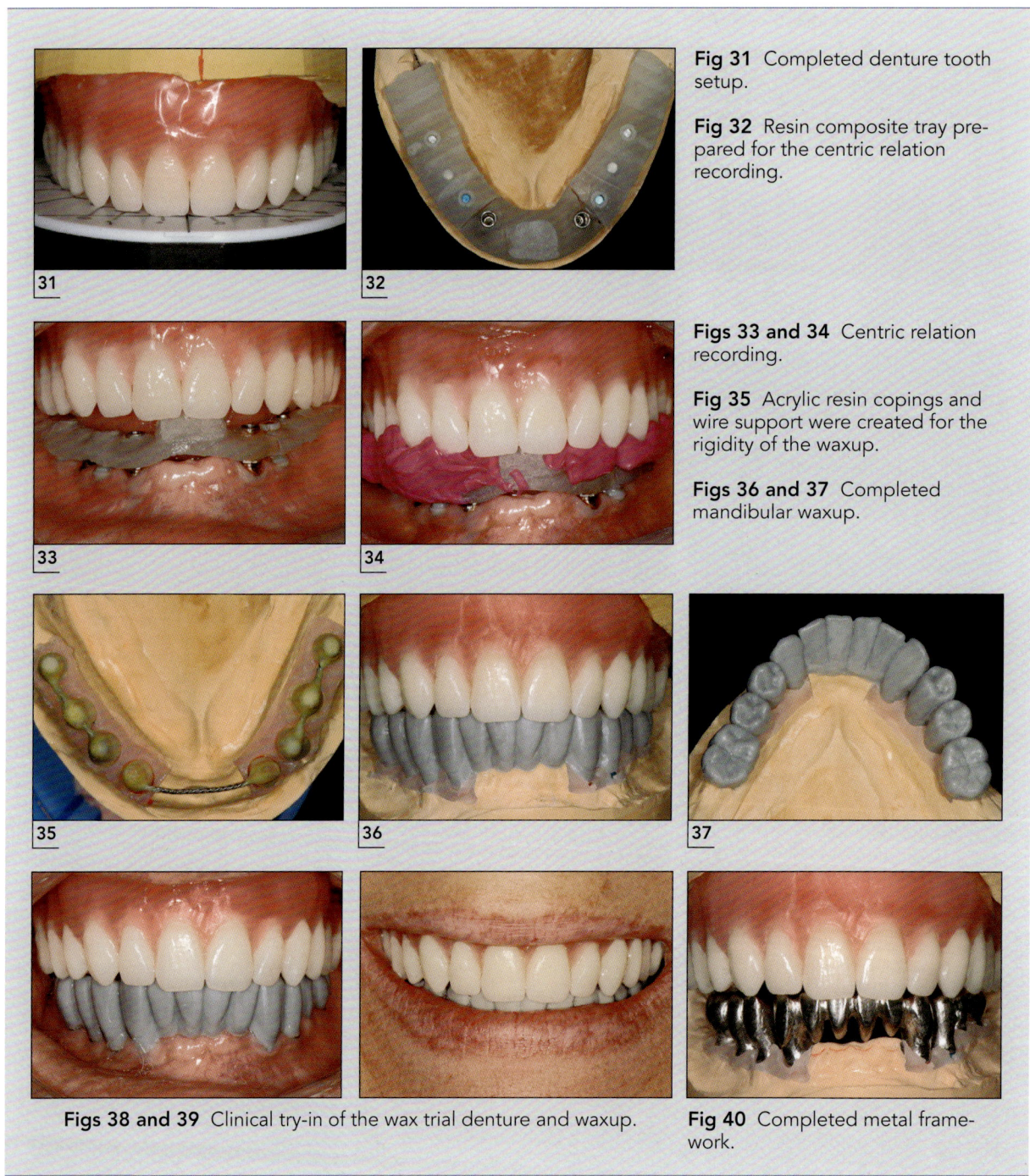

Fig 31 Completed denture tooth setup.

Fig 32 Resin composite tray prepared for the centric relation recording.

Figs 33 and 34 Centric relation recording.

Fig 35 Acrylic resin copings and wire support were created for the rigidity of the waxup.

Figs 36 and 37 Completed mandibular waxup.

Figs 38 and 39 Clinical try-in of the wax trial denture and waxup.

Fig 40 Completed metal framework.

member of the articulator. The corresponding location of each maxillary tooth was marked on the index tray. In preparation for a denture tooth setup, an autopolymerized acrylic resin record base was fabricated on the maxillary master cast. The master cast with record base was reposi-tioned to the upper member of the articulator against the index tray. The maxillary denture tooth setup was completed using the references provided by the index tray (Fig 31). The same denture tooth mold used for the immediate prosthesis was selected for the definitive denture.

For the centric relation recording, a light-polymerized resin composite tray (Triad Trutray, Dentsply) with the attached temporary abutments was fabricated on the mandibular master cast. For ease of seating, the tray was sectioned in the interproximal area between the mandibular canines and first premolars. In addition, a vertical extension of the tray was fabricated in the area of mandibular central incisors in a cone-like shape. This extension of the tray was fabricated in the same light-polymerized resin composite material (Fig 32).

In the clinic, the maxillary wax trial denture was evaluated using traditional prosthodontic protocols. Proposed changes to the position of the denture teeth were recorded, and photographs of the patient's smile were taken with the denture in place. For the centric relation recording, the anterior segment of the resin composite tray was seated over the implants. Baseplate wax was added to the denture, lingual to the maxillary anterior teeth, in the shape of a flat plane, to provide contact with the opposing anterior extension of the tray during closure of the arch (Fig 33). The height of the wax plane was adjusted to the desired level of the vertical dimension of occlusion, which was determined using standard prosthodontic protocols. The posterior segments of the tray were attached to the implants, and care was taken to ensure that no contact occurred between these segments and opposing denture teeth. The centric relation record was obtained by placing the polyvinyl siloxane occlusal registration material onto the posterior areas of the tray and guiding the patient's mandible into closure (Fig 34).

In the laboratory, the maxillary master cast was articulated with the mandibular master cast using the centric relation record, and the mandibular master cast was mounted to the lower member of the articulator. Because of the changes in the tooth position, a decision was made to evaluate the mandibular diagnostic waxup intraorally, simultaneously with the maxillary wax trial denture. To provide rigidity for the mandibular waxup, individual autopolymerized acrylic resin copings were fabricated over the implant/abutment analogs. In addition, copings were connected to each other

with a twisted stainless steel wire, resulting in an armature-like support for the waxup (Fig 35). The desired changes were made to the position of the maxillary denture teeth and the mandibular waxup was completed (Figs 36 and 37).

The wax trial denture and mandibular waxup were returned to the clinic for a try-in (Figs 38 and 39). Tooth position, phonetics, and occlusion were evaluated following standard prosthodontic protocols. The denture tooth position was shown to the patient and approved. The case was returned to the laboratory for the fabrication of the definitive restorations.

The next laboratory step included fabrication of the definitive mandibular restorations. Polyvinyl siloxane putty indices were fabricated around the contours of the mandibular waxup. Custom screw-retained abutments for the canine sites were fabricated in a gold alloy using the standard lost-wax production technique. The finish line of the abutments was placed just below the gingival margin for the ease of cement removal. Following application of a die spacer, the final framework was waxed in three segments. Silicone putty indices were used in the process of the framework waxup. The framework was cast in a ceramometal alloy using the standard lost-wax production technique (Fig 40). Following metal finishing, the framework was returned to the clinic for try-in. The framework fit was determined to be acceptable using standard visual, tactile, and radiographic tests.

The ceramometal restorations were completed using standard laboratory protocols (Figs 41 and 42). Upon completion of the mandibular restorations, waxup of the maxillary denture, processing, and finishing were completed. The definitive restorations are shown in Figs 43 and 44.

At the delivery appointment, custom abutments at the canine sites were attached to the implants and retaining screws were tightened following manufacturer's recommended torque values. Screw access holes were closed with a polyvinyl siloxane impression material, and mandibular restorations were cemented with temporary cement (Temporary Cement, Temrex, Freeport, NY, USA). Standard prosthodontic protocols were used for

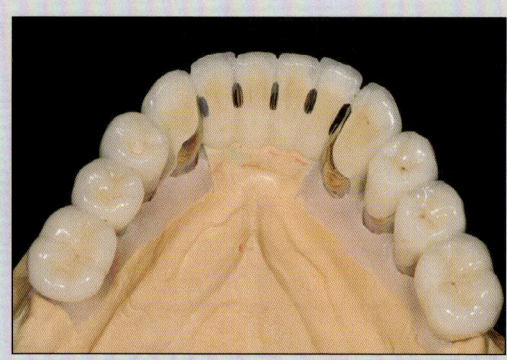
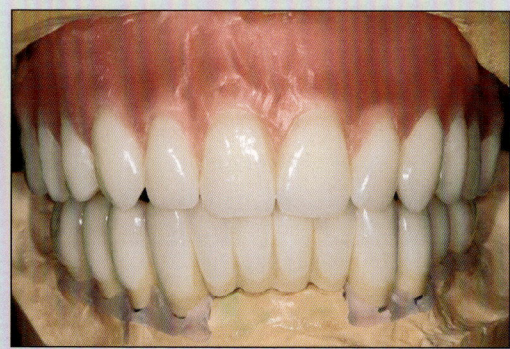

Figs 41 and 42 Completed mandibular ceramometal restorations.

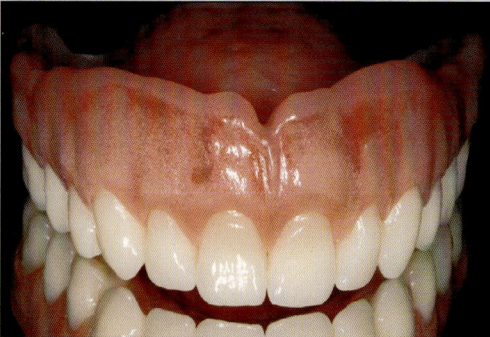

Fig 43 The definitive maxillary restoration.

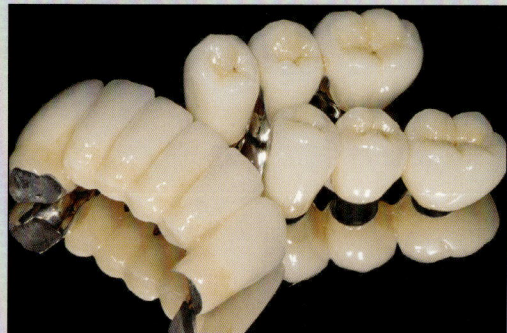

Fig 44 The definitive mandibular restoration.

the denture delivery. The patient received maintenance instructions, and a recall schedule was established. At the subsequent recall appointment, the patient expressed satisfaction with the treatment. Figures 45 to 51 show the final restorative result.

CONCLUSION

This article discussed some of the critical aspects in the management of the hopeless dentition, such as treatment options, prosthetic designs, and transition strategies. The presented case highlights these considerations and provides an example of how to manage these types of cases.

ACKNOWLEDGMENTS

The authors would like to thank Steve McGowan, CDT, for the fabrication of the ceramic restorations and Ruth E. Bourke, LBIST, for the processing of the dentures.

REFERENCES

1. Osterberg T, Carlsson GE, Sundh W, Fyhrlund A. Prognosis of and factors associated with the dental status in the adult Swedish population, 1975–1989. Community Dent Oral Epidemiol 1995;23:232–236.

2. Douglass CW, Shih A, Ostry L. Will there be a need for complete dentures in the United States in 2020? J Prosthet Dent 2002;87:5–8.

3. The glossary of prosthodontic terms. J Prosthet Dent 2005;94:10–92.

4. Richards W, Ameen J, Coll AM, Higgs G. Reasons for tooth extraction in four general dental practices in South Wales. Br Dent J 2005;198:275–278.

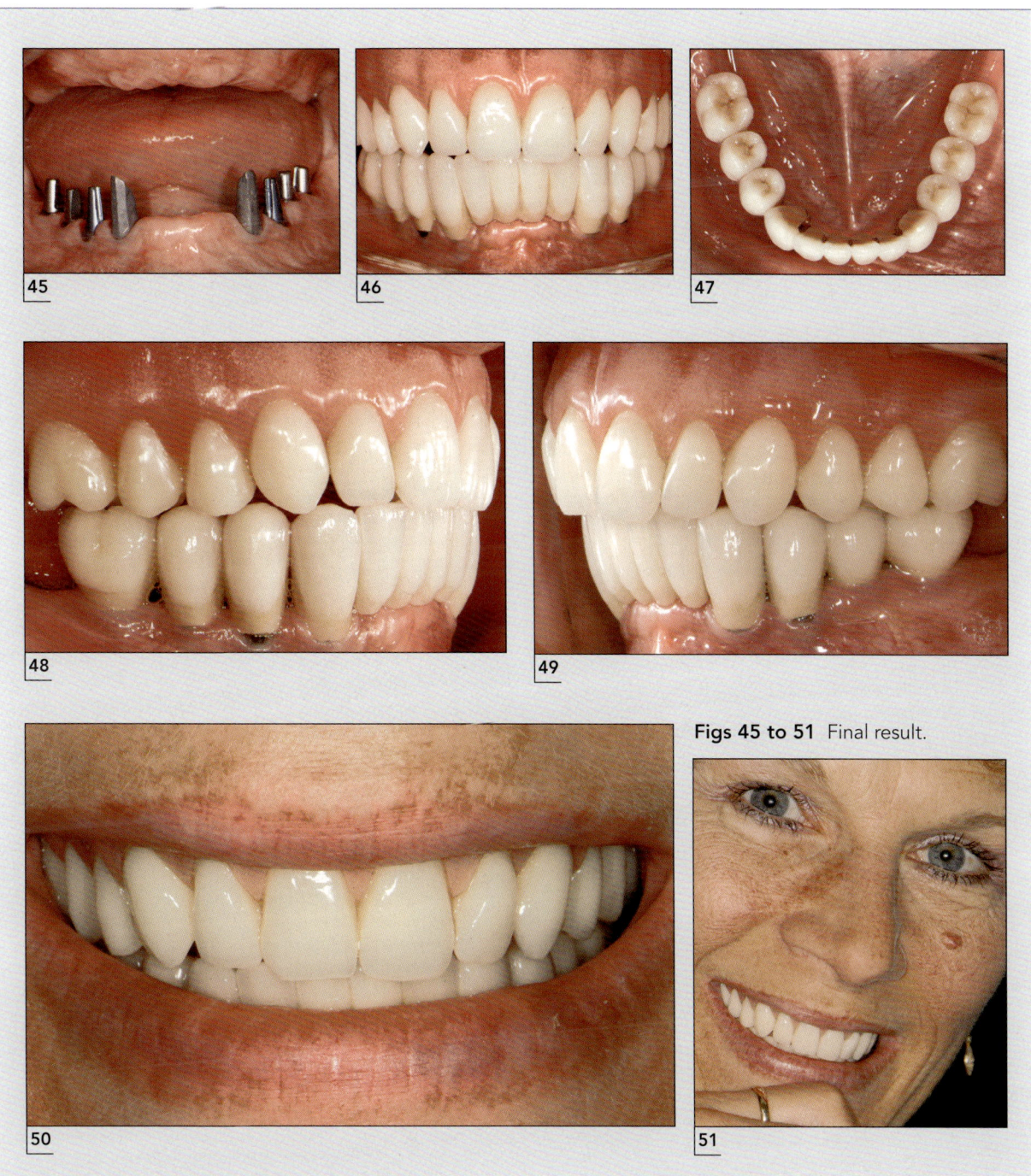

Figs 45 to 51 Final result.

5. Murray H, Locker D, Kay EJ. Patterns of and reasons for tooth extractions in general dental practice in Ontario, Canada. Community Dent Oral Epidemiol 1996;24:196–200.

6. Carlsson GE. Facts and fallacies: An evidence based for complete dentures. Dent Update 2006;33:134–136, 138–140, 142.

7. Zitzmann NU, Marinello CP. A review of clinical and technical considerations for fixed and removable implant prostheses in the edentulous mandible. Int J Prosthodont 2002;15:65–72.

8. Zitzmann NU, Marinello CP. Fixed or removable imlant-supported restorations in the edentulous maxilla: Literature review. Pract Periodontics Aesthet Dent 2000;12:599–608.

9. Awad MA, Feine JS. Measuring patient satisfaction with mandibular prostheses. Community Dent Oral Epidemiol 1998;26:400–405.

10. Morin C, Lund JP, Sioufi C, Feine JS. Patient satisfaction with dentures made by dentists and denturologists. J Can Dent Assoc 1998;64:205–208, 210–212.

11. Allen PF, McMillan AS, Walshaw D. Patient expectations of oral implant-retained prostheses in a UK dental hospital. Br Dent J 1999;186:80–84.

12. Berg E. The influence of some anamnestic, demographic, and clinical variables on patient acceptance of new complete dentures. Acta Odontol Scand 1984;42:119–127.

13. Berg E. A 2-year follow-up study of patient satisfaction with new complete dentures. J Dent 1988;16:160–165.

14. Melas F, Marcenes W, Wright PS. Oral health impact on daily performance in patients with implant-stabilized overdentures and patients with conventional complete dentures. Int J Oral Maxillofac Implants 2001;16:700–712.

15. Awad MA, Lund JP, Dufresne E, Feine JS. Comparing the efficacy of mandibular implant-retained overdentures and conventional dentures among middle-aged edentulous patients: satisfaction and functional assessment. Int J Prosthodont 2003;16:117–122.

16. Feine JS, Carlsson GE, Awad MA, et al. The McGill consensus statement on overdentures. Mandibular two-implant overdentures as first choice standard of care for edentulous patients. Montreal, Quebec, May 24–25, 2002. Int J Oral Maxillofac Implants 2002;17:601–602.

17. de Albuquerdue Jr RF, Lund JP, Tang L, et al. Within-subject comparison of the maxillary long-bar implant-retained prostheses with and without palatal coverage: Patient-based outcomes. Clin Oral Implats Res 2000;11:555–565.

18. Tang l, Lund JP, Tache R, Clokie CM, Feine JS. A within-subject comparison of mandibular long-bar and hybrid implant-supported prosthesis: Psychometric evaluation and patient preference. J Dent Res 1997;76:1675–1683.

19. Feine JS, de Grandmont P, Boudrias P, et al. Within-subject comparison of implant-supported mandibular prostheses: Choice of prosthesis.

20. Jemt T, Johansson J. Implant treatment in the edentulous maxilla: A 15 year follow-up study on the 76 consecutive patients provided with fixed prosthesis. Clin Implant Dent Relat Res 2006;8:61–69.

21. Fortin Y, Sullivan RM, Rangert BR. The Marius implant bridge: Surgical and prosthetic rehabilitation for the completely edentulous jaw with moderate to severe resorption: A 5-year retrospective clinical study. Clin Implant Dent Relat Res 2002;4:69–77.

22. Bergkvist G, Sahlholm S, Nilner K, Lindh C. Implant-supported fixed prostheses in the edentulous maxilla. A 2-year clinical and radiological follow-up of treatment with non-submerged ITI implants. Clin Oral Implants Res 2004;15:351–359.

23. Zitzmann NU, Marinello CP. Treatment outcomes of fixed or removable implant-supported prostheses in the edentulous maxilla. Part I: Patients' assessments. J Prosthet Dent 2000;83:424–433.

24. Zitzmann NU, Marinello CP. Treatment outcomes of fixed or removable implant-supported prostheses in the edentulous maxilla. Part II: Clinical findings. J Prosthet Dent 2000;83:434–442.

25. Heydecke G, Boudrias P, Awad MA, De Albuquerque RF, Lund JP, Feine JS. Within-subject comparisons of maxillary fixed and removable implant prostheses: Patient satisfaction and choice of prosthesis. Clin Oral Implants Res 2003;14:125–130.

26. Narhi TO, Hevinga M, Voorsmit RA, Kalk W. Maxillary overdentures retained by splinted and unsplinted implants: A retrospective study. Int J Oral Maxillofac Implants 2001;16:259–266.

27. Watson CJ, Tinsley D, Sharma S. Implant complications and failures: The complete overdenture. Dent Update 2001;28:234–238, 240.

28. Davis DM, Packer ME, Watson RM. Maintenance requirements of implant-supported fixed prostheses opposed by implant-supported fixed prostheses, natural teeth, or complete dentures: A 5-year retrospective study. Int J Prosthodont 2003;16:521–523.

29. Eliasson A, Palmqvist S, Svenson B, Sondell K. Five-year results with fixed complete-arch mandibular prostheses supported by 4 implants. Int J Oral Maxillofac Implants 2000;15:505–510.

30. Zitzmann NU, Marinello CP. Clinical and technical aspects of implant-supported restorations in the edentulous maxilla: The fixed partial denture design. Int J Prosthodont 1999;12:307–312.

31. Gallucci GO, Bernard JP, Belser UC. Treatment of completely edentulous patients with fixed implant-supported restorations: Three consecutive cases of simultaneous immediate loading in both maxilla and mandible. Int J Periodontics Restorative Dent 2005;25:27–37.

32. Mitrani R, Vasilic M, Bruguera A. Fabrication of an implant-supported reconstruction utilizing CAD/CAM technology. Pract Proced Aesthet Dent 2005;17:71–78.

33. Bragger U, Aeschlimann S, Burgin W, Hammerle CH, Lang NP. Biological and technical complications and failures with fixed partial dentures (FPD) on implants and teeth after four to five years of function. Clin Oral Implants Res 2001;12:26–34.

34. Arbree NS. Immediate dentures. In: Zarb GA, Bolender CL, Eckert S, Jacob R, Fenton A, Mericske-Stern R (eds). Prosthodontic Treatment for Edentulous Patients: Complete Dentures and Implant-Supported Prostheses. St Louis: Mosby, 2003:123–159.

35. Shor A, Goto Y, Shor K. Immediate denture prosthesis for the rehabilitation of hopeless dentition: clinical and laboratory considerations. Quintessence Dent Technol 2006;29:157–170.

36. Waliszewski M, Janakievski J. Sequencing patients to implant-supported, full mouth reconstructions: A case report. Pract Proced Aesthet Dent 2005;17:267–272.

37. Mitrani R, Beerli M. Full-mouth rehabilitation of teeth and osseointegrated implants Quintessence Dent Technol 2006;29:113–126.

DEVELOPING IDEAL IMPLANT TISSUE ARCHITECTURE AND PONTIC SITE FORM

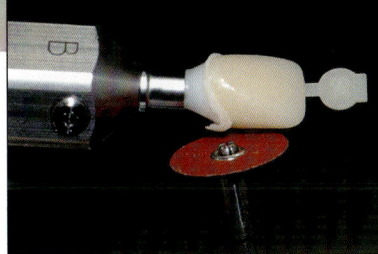

Sonia S. Leziy, DDS, Dipl Perio[1]
Brahm A. Miller, DDS, Dipl Pros[1]

With the development of implant therapy, there are now highly successful treatment options to replace missing teeth or teeth planned for extraction. When tooth extraction is planned, clinicians must decide when to extract, how to manage the extraction sockets to minimize ridge remodeling, and what method of tooth replacement will be used. This treatment planning is necessary to minimize the need for extensive hard and soft tissue reconstructive efforts, which rarely result in an ideal balance between tooth form and the surrounding hard and soft tissue ridge architecture. The residual or reconstructed ridge is generally the weak link in an esthetic oral rehabilitation.

The appropriate timing of tooth extraction is important. It should be noted that many traditional resective periodontal and endodontic surgical procedures have a potentially negative impact on the hard and soft tissue volume. Figures 1a to 1c show the negative impact of prior surgical and orthodontic treatment on the ridge anatomy in the maxillary anterior dentition. The right central incisor is at high risk for coronal or root fracture because of the minimal remaining coronal tooth structure and the wide, short post. The radiograph (Fig 1a) shows several potential problems for future implant placement at the right central incisor, including malpositioned teeth as a result of postorthodontic treatment relapse, a root proximity problem between the right lateral and central incisors, and previous apical surgery on the right central incisor. These kinds of therapies only complicate future tooth replacement, particularly with implant therapy, where starting an ideal ridge anatomy is essential for a highly esthetic outcome.

Further, it is crucial to recognize when a tooth has a poor long-term prognosis and when it should be extracted. Pleasing the patient by restoring a tooth with a significant amount of loss of radicular dentin, a large post, and an inadequate ferrule to direct forces along the long axis of the tooth, can result in vertical root fracture and subsequent bone loss. Again, the negative effect on hard tissue

---
[1]Associate Clinical Professor, University of British Columbia, British Columbia, Canada; private practice, North Vancouver, British Columbia, Canada.

Correspondence to: Dr Sonia Leziy, 401-221 West Esplanade, North Vancouver, British Columbia, Canada V7M 3J3. E-mail: sonia@imperio.ca

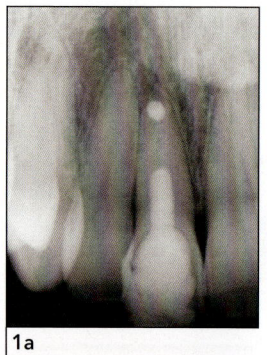

1a

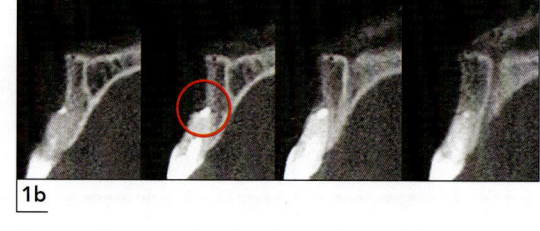

1b

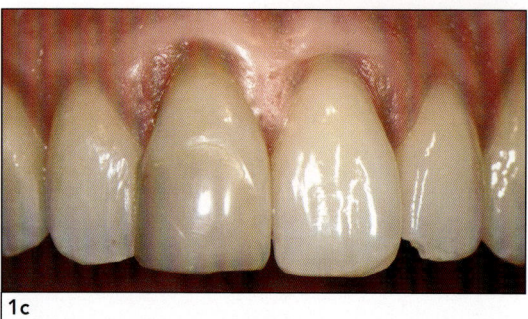

1c

Fig 1a Periapical radiograph of the right central incisor.

Fig 1b Cross-sectional tomographic images showing the areas of concern. Note the thin or absent buccal bone over the incisor and significant facial bone loss at the apex of the right central incisor caused by the previous apical surgery.

Fig 1c The extensively restored right central incisor and buccal recession developing over the unfavorably positioned roots.

would necessitate procedures that would not have been required with earlier proactive extraction.[1] Unfortunately, this kind of mistake occurs far too often. Figures 2a to 2f show a case originally referred for crown lengthening and restoration of the left central incisor. Extraction of this tooth was the only reasonable plan because of the lack of tooth structure necessary for predictable crown retention and the high risk for root fracture because of the overprepared post space. Immediate implant placement and loading was the optimal method for preservation of the ridge anatomy and soft tissue form.

It is the clinician's responsibility to guide patients in the decision-making process by informing them about the pros and cons of various treatment options based on data regarding success rates, a critical appraisal of the dental literature, and personal clinical experiences. It seems reasonable to advise patients to choose extraction and implant therapy, because this treatment modality shows very high success rates.[2,3] Indeed, comparing the success rates of implant therapy versus extensively restored teeth (eg, endodontic treatment, posts and cores, apical surgery, crown lengthening) is necessary in the informed-consent process.[4] From a financial perspective, it is often more reasonable to consider ex-

traction and implant therapy compared to an interdisciplinary treatment approach to save a tooth.

Although the high success rate of implant integration is well documented, the esthetic result also plays a crucial role in a successful outcome.[5] Along with a pleasing and esthetic appearance, it is equally important to create harmony between the restoration and the remaining dentition and soft tissue framework. Therefore, a considerable amount of the authors' treatment efforts focus on enhancing the balance of pink and white esthetics using a combination of surgical and restorative treatments. Creating such a balance is usually easy, as long as the various stages of treatment are appropriately timed. It must be considered that when something is lost or removed, there is always a biologic consequence. This often means that a soft and hard tissue deficiency will develop following the loss of a tooth. Ideally, the goal should be to never let this occur; however, in reality, this remains a significant challenge. Clinicians must condition themselves to think comprehensively and with a broad perspective. Figures 3a to 3e illustrate the characteristic remodeling that develops following extraction and the typical efforts necessary to enhance the hard and soft tissue framework.

Fig 2a Preoperative view of an esthetically compromised anterior dentition, with metal margin display on the right lateral incisor, discolored restorations, and worn and displeasing incisal edge positions. Note the ideal soft tissue architecture and tissue quality.

Fig 2b Radiograph showing the compromised state of the left central incisor. Note that the root form is tapering with an excessively prepared post space, resulting in extensive loss of radicular dentin. This increases the chance of future root fracture.

Fig 2c After removing the existing restoration, a minimal amount of residual coronal tooth structure remains, thus rendering it nonrestorable, even with procedures such as crown lengthening or extrusion. Extraction is the only reasonable alternative.

Figs 2d and 2e Preservation of ridge anatomy and soft tissue form is best accomplished with extraction and immediate implant placement. Following a 3-month integration period, a custom zirconia abutment was fabricated for the Replace Select 5.0-mm implant at the left central incisor and Procera Alumina crowns on all 4 incisors.

Fig 2f Three-year posttreatment radiograph shows ideal bone levels around the implant.

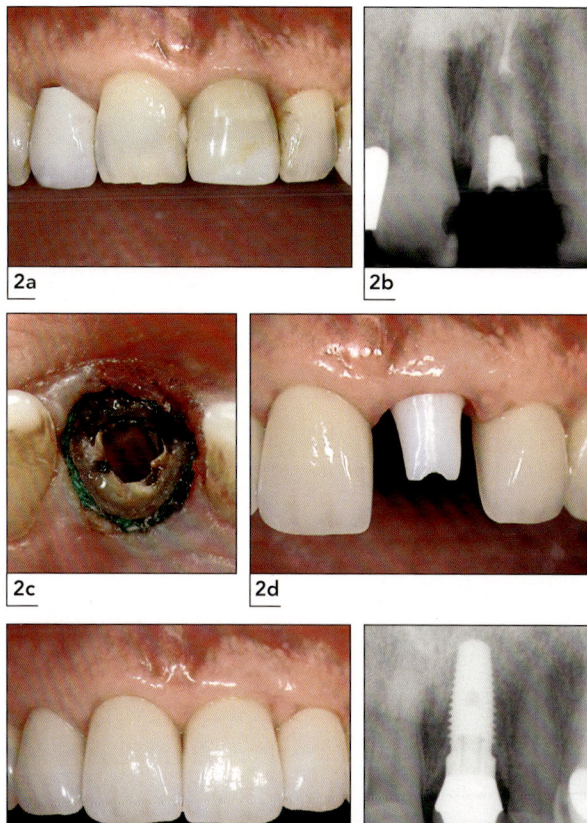

Fig 3a Typical postextraction ridge resorption. Despite attempts to guide the soft tissue form with a removable partial denture, hard tissue preservation was not considered when the left central incisor was extracted.

Figs 3b to 3d Following placement of a scalloped implant, the site is augmented with the bone substitute Bio-Oss (Osteohealth, Shirley, NY, USA) and the bone graft is confined with a Bio-Gide membrane (Osteohealth).

Fig 3e Ideal tissue form around the abutment/implant 6 months postsurgery highlights the important role of correct three-dimensional implant positioning, bone grafting, and provisionalization to guide the soft tissue architecture.

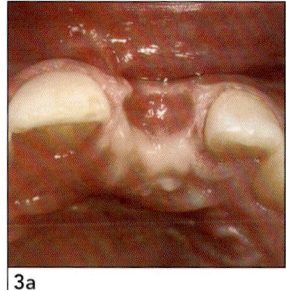
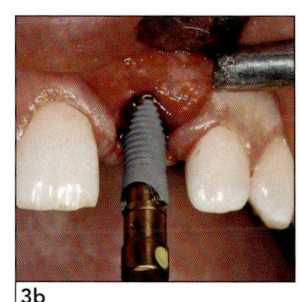
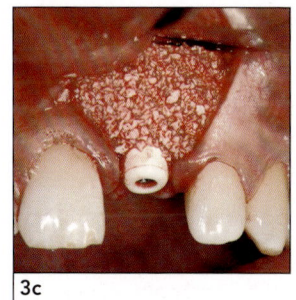
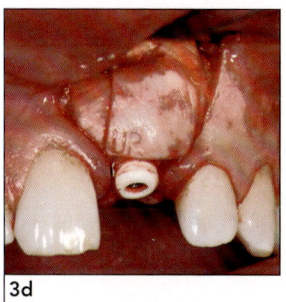

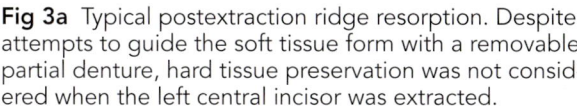

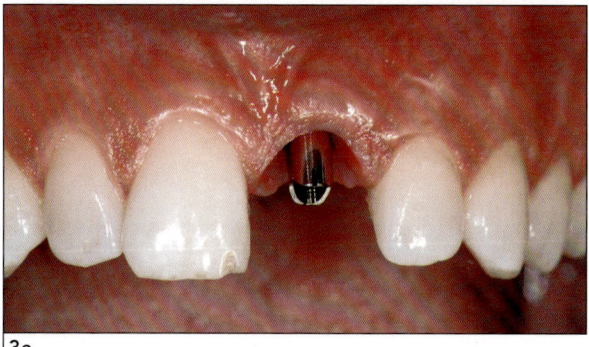

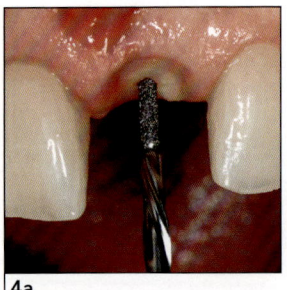
4a

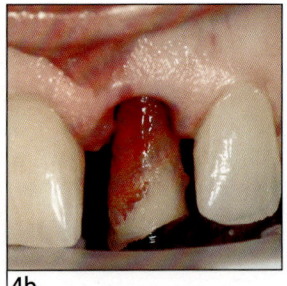
4b

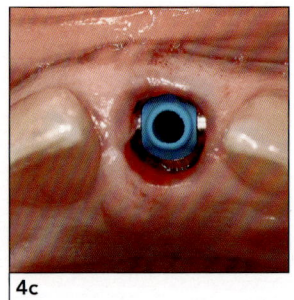
4c

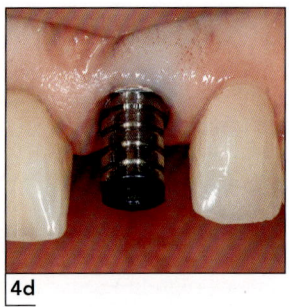
4d

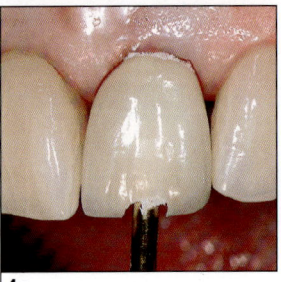
4e

Fig 4a The left central incisor is fractured to the free gingival margin and an extraction post is inserted into the root canal. Based on the clinical and radiographic appearance, this is an optimal site for immediate implant placement and restoration using a flapless or minimally invasive surgical approach.

Fig 4b The left central incisor is extracted using a vertical root extraction system to eliminate the risk of damage to the typically thin facial cortical bone in this area.

Fig 4c Wide-diameter scalloped implant placed with a standard preparation protocol using an incisionless approach. Not shown is the application of a bone-grafting product into the residual buccal horizontal defect and a buccal connective tissue graft to enhance the gingival biotype.

Fig 4d Provisional titanium abutment prior to modification.

Fig 4e Screw-retained provisional restoration fabricated by fusing a polycarbonate crown shell to the modified provisional abutment using acrylic resin.

It is essential to consider treatment strategies and sequencing to prevent or minimize the unfavorable ridge remodeling that generally occurs after extraction.[6] With this in mind, there are several hard tissue preservation and regeneration procedures and implant placement strategies that have been developed to enhance esthetic treatment outcomes:

1. *Immediate implant placement:* Extraction and immediate implant placement is viewed by many clinicians as an ideal treatment strategy for conservation of hard and soft tissue ridge anatomy when the clinical situation presents a favorable pretreatment framework.[7]

2. *Flapless surgery:* There is also increasing interest in surgical procedures that are minimally invasive, such as flapless surgery, because they can minimize the unfavorable soft tissue changes often induced by surgical procedures using a flap approach.[8,9]

3. *Immediate implant placement and loading:* The concept of immediate implant placement and restoration/loading is gaining acceptance

because many studies have reported high success rates. Bearing in mind that appropriate case selection is essential, this strategy allows the clinician to engineer both bone and soft tissue simultaneously (see Figs 2a to 2f).[10,11] Figures 4a to 4e illustrate the concept of immediate placement and loading. This treatment strategy is effective if the initial hard and soft tissue framework is ideal or close to ideal and when conservative surgical procedures like flapless implant placement are meticulously executed. The clear benefit of this approach is evident in the clinical appearance of the gingival tissues throughout treatment.

4. *Delayed implant placement:* At times, immediate implant placement is not possible because of the extent of existing bone loss and/or the severity of an active infection, and ridge preservation or regeneration are necessary to allow future implant placement.

5. *Orthodontic treatment:* In some cases, orthodontic site development prior to tooth extraction is indicated to nonsurgically improve the hard and soft tissue ridge topography (Figs 5a to 5e).[12] Al-

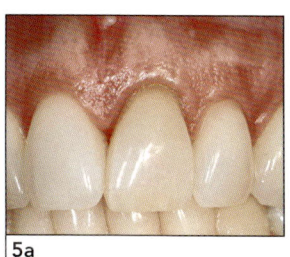

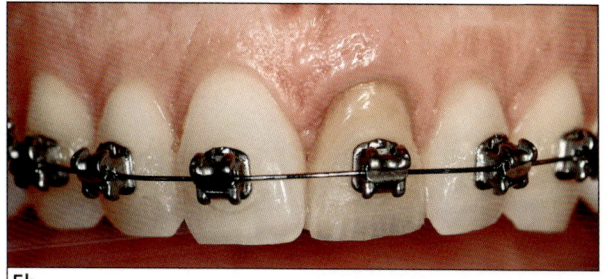

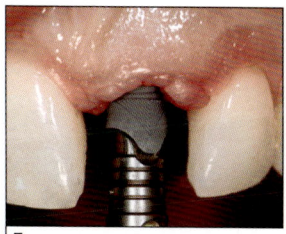

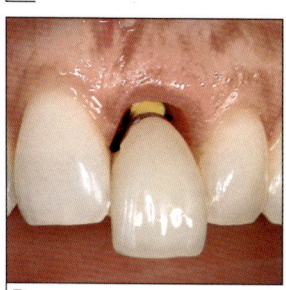

5a

5b

5c

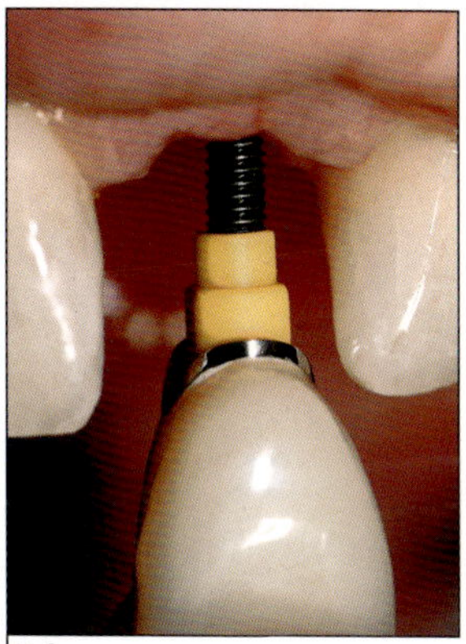

5d

5e

Fig 5a Preoperative photograph. Note the unfavorable buccal gingival tissue margin position on the left central incisor and, more importantly, the blunted papilla between the central incisors.

Fig 5b The extrusive procedure optimally developed the previously deficient papilla and resulted in a slight excess of buccal tissue. This sets the framework for predictable esthetic implant placement and restoration.

Fig 5c Immediate implant placement.

Fig 5d Immediate implant restoration/loading.

Fig 5e Four-month postsurgical view of the developed gingival architecture clearly shows the important role of hard and soft tissue integration.

though implant placement and correction of the buccal marginal recession with a connective tissue graft is often possible, correction of vertical hard and soft tissue deficiencies is unpredictable using conventional surgical techniques.

Regardless of the implant approach, several issues are of paramount importance to an ideal treatment outcome: *(1)* atraumatic extraction techniques, *(2)* ideal three-dimensional implant placement, *(3)* supplemental ridge augmentation when necessary, and *(4)* adjunctive soft tissue regenerative augmentation to enhance the soft tissue biotype and tissue volume.

In the authors' opinion, provisionalization is arguably the most important step in developing optimal tissue form around implants. However, many clinicians fail to recognize or trivialize the role that provisionalization plays in maintaining or enhancing soft tissue architecture. Although several studies suggest that ideal tissue architecture will ultimately form around implant restorations without provisionalization, this form will not be complete until many months, sometimes years, following

delivery of the definitive restoration.[13] This potentially results in several problems:

1. Difficulty communicating to the technician the optimal form to develop the subgingival prosthetic envelope or emergence profile of the restoration.
2. Increased likelihood of multiple try-ins and modification of the final prosthesis. This in turn increases the probability of porcelain revision and the possible loss of vitality of the ceramic restoration.
3. Possibility that the soft tissue may never form optimally around the finalized restoration.
4. Repeated placement and removal of transmucosal components can potentially contribute to increased crestal ridge remodeling and an apical movement of the connective tissue/epithelial complex.[14]

Developing tissue form using provisional restorations provides distinct advantages for the restoring dentist, technician, and patient. The primary benefit for all involved parties is fewer try-in/

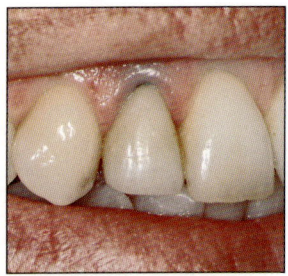

Fig 6a Preoperative view of the right lateral incisor, which is fractured and nonrestorable.

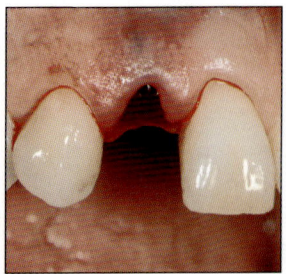

Fig 6b Atraumatic extraction conserving soft and hard tissue anatomy.

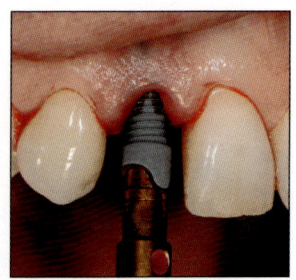

Fig 6c Narrow-diameter scalloped implant insertion.

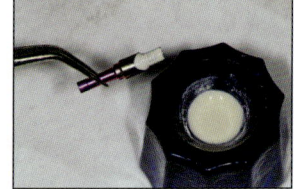

Fig 6d Opaquing the provisional titanium abutment (previously modified extraorally on an implant replica and refined intraorally using profuse irrigation and a titanium bur).

modification appointments with the final prosthesis and preapproval of the tooth form and color as developed in the provisional restoration. From the technician's perspective, provisionalization enhances communication with the dental team regarding optimal tooth contours and decreases the cost and risk of complications associated with guesswork.

PROVISIONALIZATION STRATEGIES

The following provisionalization strategies illustrate typical techniques designed to optimize soft tissue contours:

- Screw-retained implant-level provisional restorations
- Chairside provisionalization of one-piece implants
- Final abutments placed at surgery supporting provisional restorations
- Ovate pontic sites in fixed partial dentures

Screw-Retained Implant-Level Provisional Restorations

To successfully use provisional restorations to define tissue form, materials that are both durable and esthetic should be used. Use of lab-processed restorations reduces chair time and simplifies the transition to the final restoration. Materials such as Cristobal (Dentsply Ceramco, Burlington, NJ, USA), a heat- and light-cured material, can easily withstand many months of use without degradation. Restorations fabricated with material such as this are easily modified chairside, either by adding resin composite or reducing the material bulk/form with abrasive disks or wheels. Fusing resin composite material to a provisional abutment allows the clinician to develop a screw-retained provisional crown or fixed partial denture. The benefits of creating screw-retained provisional restorations include easy removal/replacement, easy retrieval for repairs or alterations to the emergence profile, elimination of subgingival cement entrapment, and avoidance of loss or dislodgement of the restoration between appointments.[15,16]

Chairside provisionalization is a routine treatment method for restoring dentists and is increasingly recognized as an important step by surgeons.[17] A provisional crown can easily be fabricated using a crown shell, relined with acrylic resin, and adapted to a provisional abutment. Provisional crowns can either be cemented to a provisional abutment or, ideally, fused to an abutment while maintaining a screw access. The provisional restoration is torqued to 35 Ncm and the screw access hole is sealed with cotton and Fermit (Ivoclar Vivadent, Amherst, NY, USA) if the access is on the palatal aspect, or with resin composite if the ac-

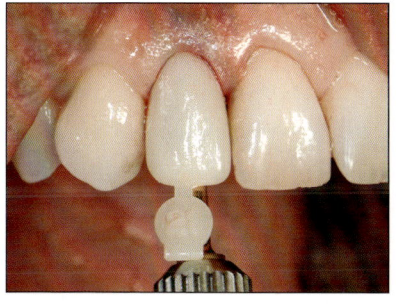
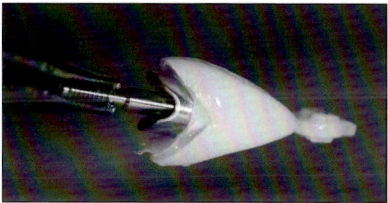
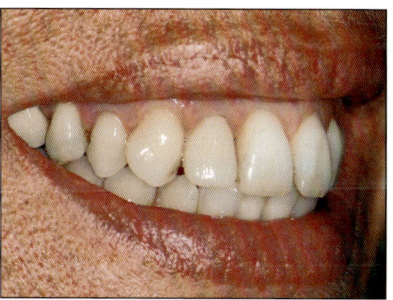

Figs 6e and 6f Crown shell with a screw-access hole is fused intraorally with acrylic resin to the opaqued abutment and then finished extraorally on an implant replica.

Fig 6g The provisional restoration 1 week postsurgery showing favorable early tissue architecture and color.

Fig 7a Preoperative view. A wide-diameter implant was previously placed at the right central incisor. The left central incisor is failing because of external root resorption.

Fig 7b Radiograph confirming the external root resorption at the left central incisor.

Fig 7c Provisionalization with a CAD/CAM-designed restoration (CEREC, Sirona, Charlotte, NC, USA) based on a pre-extraction image of the restoration on the left central incisor and an image of a cast with the implant and prepared abutment. Correlation of the two images allows the design and milling of the provisional restoration.

Fig 7d A provisional crown is milled from a resin composite block.

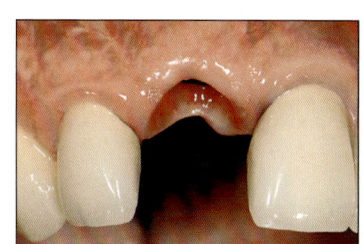
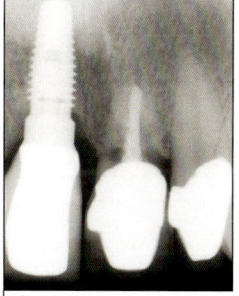

7a   7b

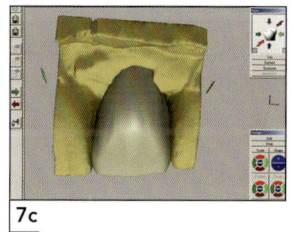
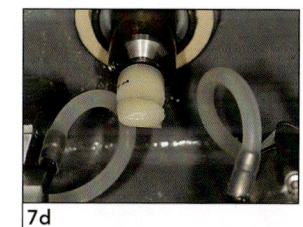

7c   7d

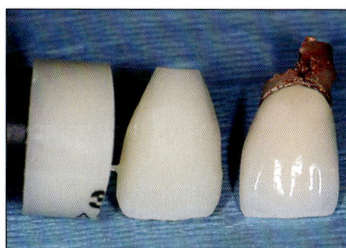
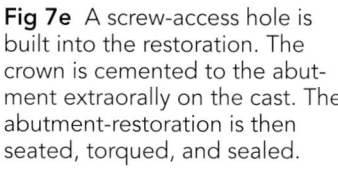
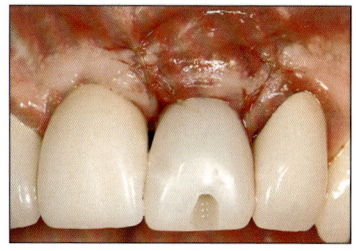
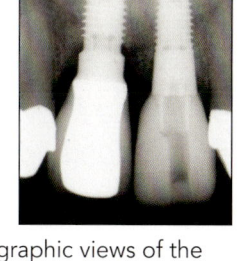

Fig 7e A screw-access hole is built into the restoration. The crown is cemented to the abutment extraorally on the cast. The abutment-restoration is then seated, torqued, and sealed.

Figs 7f and 7g Clinical and radiographic views of the provisional restoration torqued in place at the time of surgery. The facial screw-access hole will be sealed with resin composite.

cess is at the incisal edge or facial aspect. Figures 6a to 6g illustrate a typical chairside technique for fabricating provisional restorations. The drawback of chairside fabrication of provisional crowns is the limitation in shade options. The shade can be improved to some degree by using surface staining systems. An interesting treatment alternative is the use of CAD/CAM provisional crowns fabricated from resin composite blocks, such as Paradigm MZ100 blocks (shade A3.5, 3M ESPE, St Paul, MN, USA) (Figs 7a to 7g).

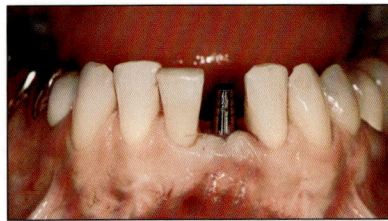

Fig 8a One-piece narrow-diameter implant placed with minimal flap reflection.

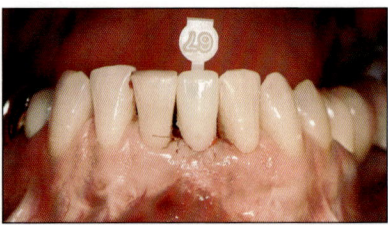

Fig 8b The selected polycarbonate crown form (3M ESPE).

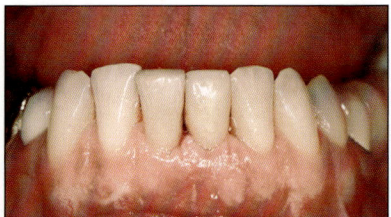

Fig 8c Flap adaptation and cemented provisional crown on the implant at the mandibular left central incisor position 10 days postoperatively. Note the rapid tissue healing and formation of the papilla, guided by the provisional restoration.

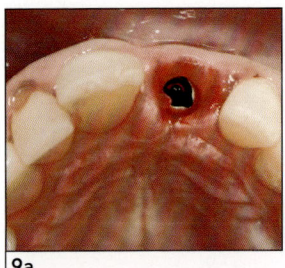

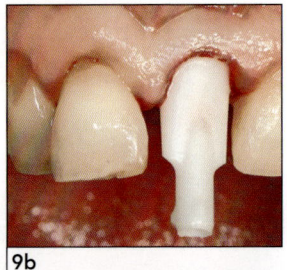

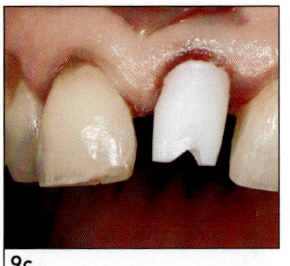

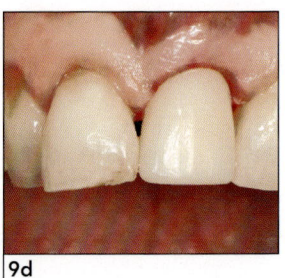

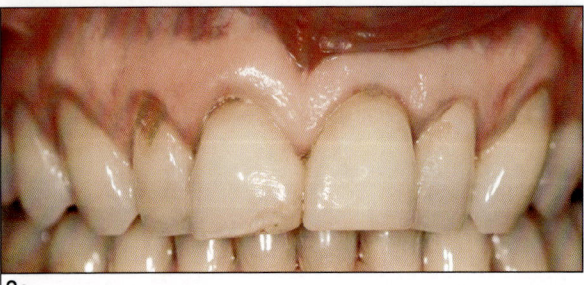

Fig 9a Regular-diameter implant placed at the left central incisor site using a flapless approach.

Fig 9b The prefabricated densely sintered zirconia CAD/CAM abutment.

Figs 9c and 9d Modified abutment is seated and torqued at 35 Ncm, and the provisional restoration is cemented on the abutment.

Fig 9e Final result.

Chairside Provisionalization of One-Piece Implants

When restoring one-piece implants, chairside provisionalization at the time of implant surgery if the primary implant stability is adequate, or following integration, is easily accomplished using either an acrylic resin relined crown shell or a CAD/CAM milled provisional restoration. The developed provisional restoration is cemented to the abutment portion of the implant. Generally, in the early postsurgical period, the restoration margin is kept in a supragingival position, with subsequent apical positioning following integration (Figs 8a to 8c).

Final Abutments Placed at Surgery

A more recent provisionalization strategy in the esthetic zone is to place a final abutment at the time of surgery. Newly available, prefabricated zirconia abutments allow the surgeon or restoring dentist to complete any modifications chairside and deliver the abutment at surgery or following a period of integration. Gross modifications are completed extraorally on an abutment mount. Minor changes can then be finalized intraorally. Reshaping in both instances is accomplished with diamond drills and profuse irrigation (Figs 9a to 9e). Figures 10a to 10c illustrate the process of adapting a crown form to the modified abutment.

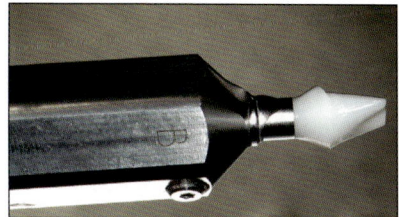

Fig 10a Modified zirconia abutment on the abutment holder.

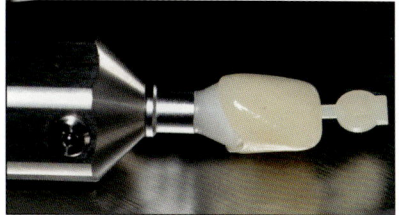

Fig 10b Selected crown form on the abutment.

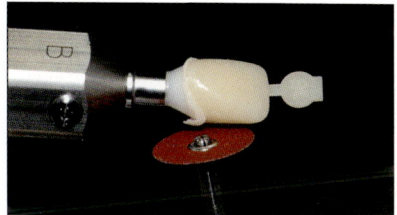

Fig 10c Relining of the provisional crown and adaptation to the abutment is performed intraorally for correct orientation, but finishing is completed extraorally on the abutment mount.

Fig 11a To avoid a graying effect with titanium abutments, the margin must be placed more apically, which increases the risk of cement entrapment.

Fig 11b Modified zirconia abutment. The obvious benefits are control over color and a minimally submerged margin to avoid the risk of cement entrapment.

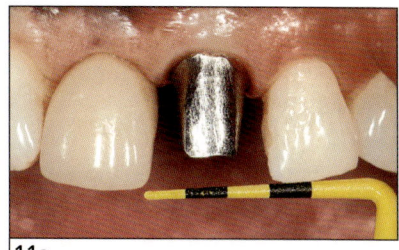

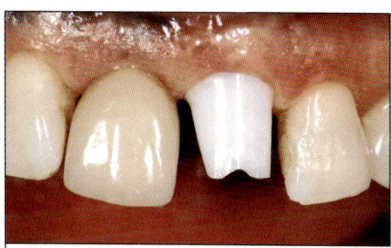

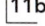

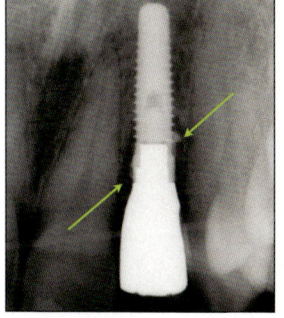

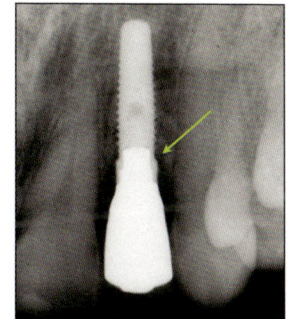

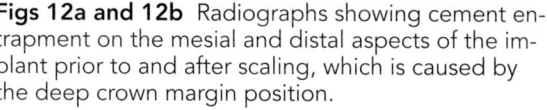

Figs 12a and 12b Radiographs showing cement entrapment on the mesial and distal aspects of the implant prior to and after scaling, which is caused by the deep crown margin position.

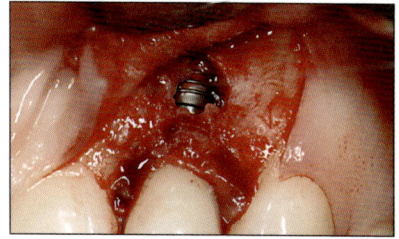

Fig 12c Flap access to remove the residual cement. Significant crestal bone loss has occurred and extensive granulation tissue is evident.

Stock titanium abutments could be used, but the metallic color may be visible at the gingival margin (Figs 11a and 11b). To avoid this, the abutment margin can be placed deeper subgingivally; however, this will increase the likelihood of cement entrapment. This is a potential complication in the esthetic zone, where implants are typically placed 2 to 3 mm apical to the ideal buccal free gingival margin. As a result, the cement line tends to be quite deep in the interproximal areas, making cement removal a challenge. Retained residual cement can have a dramatically destructive effect on the crestal bone and soft tissues (Figs 12a to 12c).

The distinct advantages of using modifiable prefabricated zirconia abutments include more favorable color at the gingival margin, control of the cement line, and enhanced biocompatibility as shown by Rimondini et al (Figs 13a to 13e).[18] The immediate advantage of placing a final abutment at the time of surgery is early engineering of the soft tissue framework. The potential long-term benefit is enhanced crestal ridge stability by avoiding prosthetic reconnection procedures. An animal model study by Abrahamsson et al[14] found that repeated removal and placement of prosthetic components (healing abutments in their

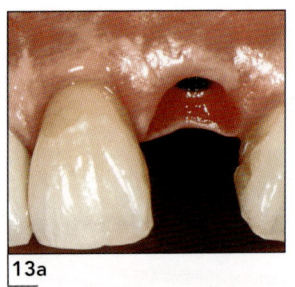
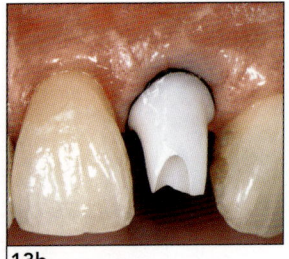
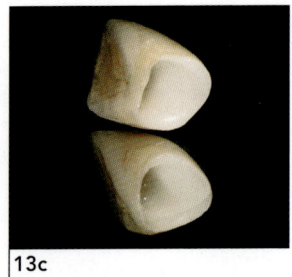
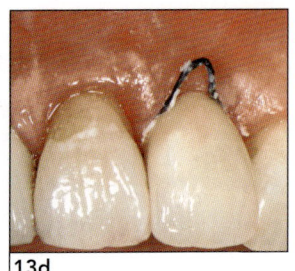

13a 13b 13c 13d

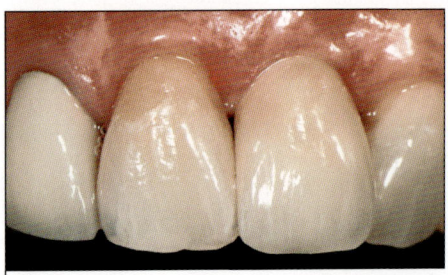

13e

Fig 13a Implant site developed and ready to receive a customized abutment.

Fig 13b Impression cord (No. 000 Ultrapak cord, Ultradent, South Jordan, Utah, USA) gently packed apical to the abutment margin.

Fig 13c Densely sintered alumina CAD/CAM crown.

Fig 13d Easy removal of the cord and excess cement.

Fig 13e Final crown in place with healthy tissue.

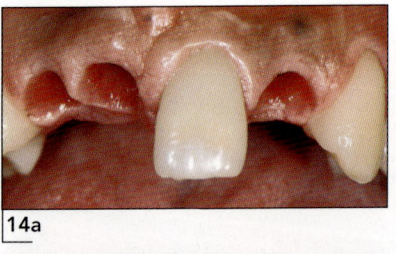
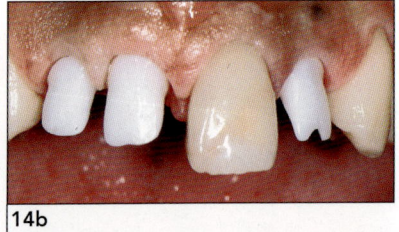
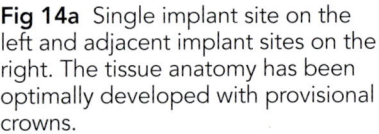

14a 14b

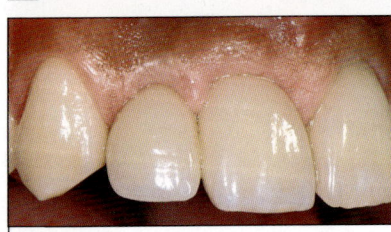
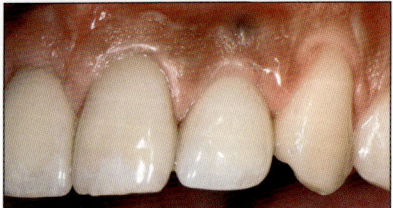

14c 14d

Fig 14a Single implant site on the left and adjacent implant sites on the right. The tissue anatomy has been optimally developed with provisional crowns.

Fig 14b Zirconia abutments are used to control the position of the cement lines and to enhance soft tissue color in the implant-crown transition zone.

Fig 14c Note the characteristic blunted papilla between the implants at the right lateral and central incisor sites, thus requiring a long contact area to mask the tissue deficiency.

Fig 14d Note the ideal papilla architecture around the single implant at the left lateral incisor site.

study) resulted in disruption of the epithelial attachment/connective tissue band. As a result, they noted increased crestal ridge remodeling with the successive interventions in the experimental group compared to the control group, in which healing abutments were not removed throughout the trial. If this holds true in clinical practice, avoiding the removal and replacement of prosthetic components would offer significant advantages by enhancing soft tissue stability through diminished crestal ridge remodeling. This would be particularly important in the restoration of adjacent implants, where clinicians are challenged to conserve optimal papilla anatomy in the interimplant re-

gion. Figures 14a to 14d illustrate the typical inadequate papilla architecture that develops between adjacent implants.

Ovate Pontic Sites in Fixed Partial Dentures

Provisionalization is even more critical when the implant-supported restoration involves a pontic site. Edentulous ridge sites can be modified to architecturally enhance the ridge form, allowing the clinician to convert a flat ridge to a sculpted or anatomic form (Figs 15a to 15d). Ridge-lap pon-

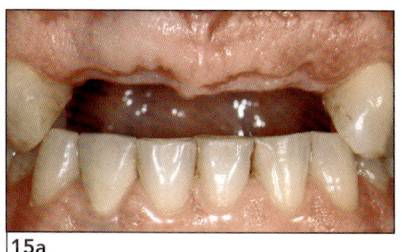
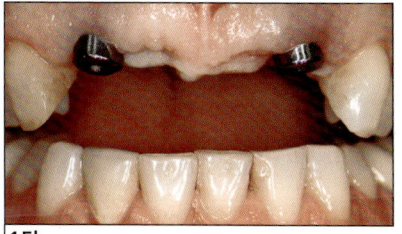
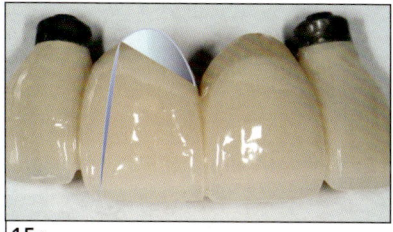

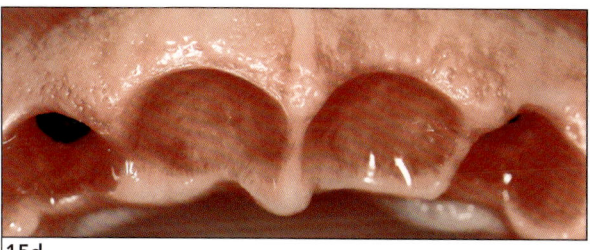

Fig 15a Preoperative view of a long-standing edentulous site spanning the maxillary anterior region.

Fig 15b Narrow-diameter implants placed in the lateral incisor sites.

Fig 15c A lab-processed screw-retained provisional restoration was fabricated and modified chairside through selective recontouring or addition of resin composite to selectively displace the soft tissues.

Fig 15d The flat gingival architecture is converted to a scalloped gingival architecture around the implants and at the pontic sites.

tics lack harmony with the gingival framework and do not effectively stabilize the edentulous ridge site, whereas ovate pontics scaffold and essentially support the gingival framework for long-term esthetic success.

When dealing with pontics supported by teeth or implants, changing a flat ridge form to a scalloped architecture enhances the esthetic outcome by creating the appearance of an intimate relationship between the ridge and the overlying pontic.[19] The goal is to create the illusion that the pontic emerges from the tissue as would a natural tooth.

It is the opinion of the authors that resective shaping in the pontic sites coupled with selective tissue displacement is essential to optimally develop the tissue form. With this in mind, the following should be considered in the development of the pontic site:

1. Soft tissue removal, and if necessary, bone removal, can be accomplished with burs or other resective tools. If tissue recontouring is limited to soft tissue removal only, which is common in the case of a thick gingival biotype, resection can be achieved with burs, lasers, electrosurgery, biopsy punches, or blades.

2. Tissue removal or reshaping should be avoided on the facial aspect of the pontic site. Removing tissue in this region will compromise the esthetic result and is difficult to repair.
3. Tissue removal should be limited to the depth and palatal aspect of the pontic site.

Next, properly designed provisional restorations allow the clinician to move or push tissue into the desired position. That is to say, tissues do not grow; they are relocated (Fig 15c).[20] The following guidelines should be considered:

1. The pontic should enter the tissue a minimum of 2 to 3 mm to properly support the facial and interproximal tissues before transitioning into a rounded form. The pontic form should be elliptical and egg shaped. Polishing and achieving a smooth finish is necessary for development of a healthy subjacent gingiva.[21]
2. The provisional restoration should be left in place for a minimum of 3 months to define the tissue architecture. The pontic area should not be flossed for the first 3 to 4 weeks, until initial epithelization of the peripontic tissue is complete. At that time, flossing under the pontics

can be initiated.[22] Figure 15d illustrates the tissue architecture developed around the implants and at the pontic sites.

Finally, the definitive restoration is typically delivered following a 4- to 6-month provisionalization phase.

CONCLUSIONS

As clinicians are driven and inspired to produce esthetically pleasing implant restorations, adjunctive surgical and restorative procedures become integral components in the planning and treatment process. Subtle but often clinically relevant improvements in soft tissue architecture are more likely to be achieved using refining procedures such as provisionalization. When the goal is to optimize the esthetic outcome, provisionalization is a logical step in this pursuit. The refinement of the soft tissue architecture is a crucial step that simplifies the restoration phase of treatment and enhances communication between the restoring dentist, technician, and patient.

ACKNOWLEDGMENTS

The authors would like to thank Hans Forssander, RDT, and David Choo, RDT, for their exceptional work and dedication in enhancing the esthetic and functional results of our treatment with their progressive and knowledgeable contributions. Their work and their opinions inspire us to always strive for our personal best.

REFERENCES

1. Lewis S. Treatment planning: Teeth versus implants. Int J Periodontics Restorative Dent 1996;16:367–377.
2. Belser UC, Schmid B, Higginbottom F, Buser D. Outcome analysis of implant restorations located in the anterior maxilla: A review of the recent literature. Int J Oral Maxillofac Implants 2004;19(suppl):30–42.
3. Simon JF. Retain or extract: The decision process. Quintessence Int 1999;30:851–854.
4. Mordohai N, Reshad M, Jivraj SA. To extract or not to extract? Factors that affect individual tooth prognosis. J Calif Dent Assoc 2005;33:319–328.
5. Buser D, Martin W, Belser UC. Optimizing esthetics for implant restorations in the anterior maxilla: Anatomic and surgical considerations. Int J Oral Maxillofac Implants 2004;19(suppl):43–61.
6. Schropp L, Wenzel A, Kostopoulos L, Karring T. Bone healing and soft tissue contour changes following single-tooth extraction: A clinical and radiographic 12-month prospective study. Int J Periodontics Restorative Dent 2003;23:313–323.
7. Werbitt MJ, Goldberg PV. The immediate implant: Bone preservation and bone regeneration. Int J Periodontics Restorative Dent 1992;12:207–217.
8. Becker W, Goldstein M, Becker BE, Sennerby L. Minimally invasive flapless implant surgery: A prospective multicenter study. Clin Implant Dent Relat Res 2005;7(suppl):S21–S27.
9. Petrungaro PS. Immediate restoration of implants utilizing a flapless approach to preserve interdental tissue contours. Pract Proced Aesthet Dent 2005;17:151–158.
10. Kan F, Rungcharassaeng K. Immediate placement and provisionalization of maxillary anterior single implants: A surgical and prosthetic rationale. Pract Periodont Aesthet Dent 2000;12:817–824.
11. Saadoun AP. Immediate implant placement and temporization in extraction and healing sites. Compend Contin Educ Dent 2002;23:309–316.
12. Salama H, Salama M. The role of orthodontic extrusive remodeling in the enhancement of soft and hard tissue profiles prior to implant placement: A systematic approach to the management of extraction site defects. Int J Periodontics Restorative Dent 1993;13:312–333.
13. Jemt T. Restoring the gingival contour by means of provisional resin crowns after single-implant treatment. Int J Periodontics Restorative Dent 1999;19:20–29.
14. Abrahamsson I, Berglundh T, Lindhe J. The mucosal barrier following abutment dis/reconnection. An experimental study in dogs. J Clin Periodontol 1997;24:568–572.
15. Cornelini, R, Cangini F, Covani U, Wilson TG Jr. Immediate restoration of implants placed into fresh extraction sockets for single-tooth replacement: A prospective clinical study. Int J Periodontics Restorative Dent 2005;25:439–447.
16. Leziy S, Miller B. Replacement of adjacent missing anterior teeth with scalloped implants: A case report. Pract Proced Aesthet Dent 2005;17:331–338.
17. Moy PD, Parminter PE. Chairside preparation of provisional restorations. J Oral Maxillofac Surg 2005;63(9 suppl 2):80–88.
18. Rimondini L, Cerroni L, Carrassi A, Toricelli P. Bacterial colonization of zirconia ceramic surfaces: An in vitro and in vivo study. Int J Oral Maxillofac Implants 2002;17:793–798.
19. Mitrani R, Phillips K, Kois JC. An implant-supported, screw-retained, provisional fixed partial denture for pontic site enhancement. Pract Proced Aesthet Dent 2005;17:673–678.
20. Jacques LB, Coelho AB, Hollweg H, Conti PC. Tissue sculpturing: An alternative method for improving esthetics of anterior fixed prosthodontics. J Prosthet Dent 1999;81:630–633.
21. Dylina TJ. Contour determination for ovate pontics. J Prosthet Dent 1999;82:136–142.
22. Zitzmann NU, Marinello CP, Berglundh T. The ovate pontic design: A histologic observation in humans. J Prosthet Dent 2002;88:375–380.

INDIVIDUALIZING ESTHETIC TREATMENT OUTCOMES: PLANNING AND FABRICATION

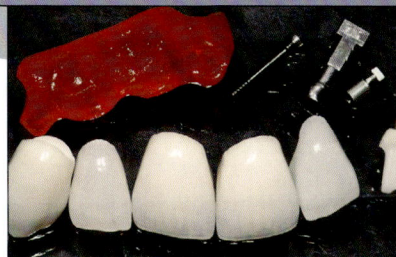

Salvatore Sgrò, CDT[1]
Basil Mizrahi, BDS, MSc, MEd[2]

[1]Dental Technician, Rome, Italy.

[2]Private practice, London, United Kingdom; Clinical Lecturer, UCL Eastman Dental Institute, London, United Kingdom.

Correspondence to: Mr Salvatore Sgrò, 43 Via Baldo degli Ubaldi, Rome 00167, Italy.
E-mail: info@eccellenzaodontotecnica.it

Patients with failing or defective anterior restorations may lose the positional and anatomic features of the teeth and surrounding gingiva. When restoring the natural esthetics of a smile, the specific facial features and characteristics of each patient need to be taken into account. Generic smile design recipes[1-3] serve only as basic guidelines; they do not consider the individual and intrinsic tooth morphology and how it relates to the facial features and characteristics of each patient.

Simply following a generic smile design recipe may lead to restorations that appear artificial and lack individuality. Optimal esthetic and functional results can be achieved only through a good knowledge of the natural anterior tooth morphology and by observing, analyzing, and modifying the provisional restorations over a period of time.

Recreating an esthetic smile in a patient with previous restorations will usually require two sets of provisional restorations. The primary provisional restorations are based on the existing restorations or a simple waxup, and are fitted on the day the teeth are prepared. The aim of this appointment is simply to remove the existing restorations and allow the patient to leave the office and continue his or her life as normal. Once the primary provisional restorations have been fitted, any adjunctive treatment, such as endodontic, periodontal, and/or implant treatment, can be carried out.

After the teeth are definitively prepared and the soft tissues are stable and disease free, an impression is taken of the prepared teeth to allow the definitive provisional restorations to be made in the laboratory. These definitive provisional restorations should be an esthetic and functional blueprint of the final restoration, and are based on information gathered from the primary provisional restorations as well as the definitive waxup. Fabricating the definitive provisional restorations on a cast of the actual tooth preparations has the following advantages:

- Additional space for acrylic resin allows for creation of ideal esthetic and functional form
- Additional bulk of material provides increased durability and strength
- Marginal accuracy of fit allows for good soft tissue response and biologic seal

The functional and esthetic characteristics of the definitive provisional restorations are then observed in the mouth, and if necessary, minor modifications can be made before proceeding with the final restorations.

The following case report illustrates the use of definitive provisional restorations and individualized tooth morphology to recreate a natural and esthetic smile.

CASE REPORT

The patient was a healthy, 38-year-old female (Fig 1) with two existing ceramic-fused-to-metal crowns on the maxillary central incisors. She had a cantilever resin-bonded prosthesis replacing the missing left canine and bonded to the first premolar (Figs 2 to 4). Her primary complaints were the unsightly appearance of the crowns, color mismatch of the pontic at the left canine site, and periodic debonding of the resin-bonded prosthesis.

An esthetic analysis of her smile revealed the following:

- Incorrect intradental proportion of the two anterior crowns
- Incorrect interdental proportion of the six anterior teeth
- Gingival margin disparity caused by recession above the left lateral incisor
- Flat smile line that did not follow the curvature of the lower lip
- Large interlabial space with a large lower lip and thin upper lip (Fig 5)

The treatment plan was as follows:

- Replacement of the existing crowns with all-ceramic crowns
- Placement of ceramic veneers on the lateral incisors
- Replacement of the resin-bonded prosthesis with a dental implant at the left canine site
- Connective tissue graft to improve the recession over the left lateral incisor

Placing the Initial Chairside Provisional Restorations

At the initial appointment, the primary provisional restorations were placed (Fig 6). Soon after, a dental implant was placed at the left canine site and a connective tissue graft was placed over the left laterial incisor and canine regions. The resin-bonded prosthesis was modified by drilling holes through the metal to create macromechanical retention, and then was used as the provisional restoration while the implant integrated.

The implant was exposed 4 months after placement and a healing cap was placed. By this time, the teeth were ready to receive the definitive provisional restorations. A shade was taken and a vinyl polysiloxane impression was made. At this stage, the lateral incisors were not yet prepared for ceramic veneers.

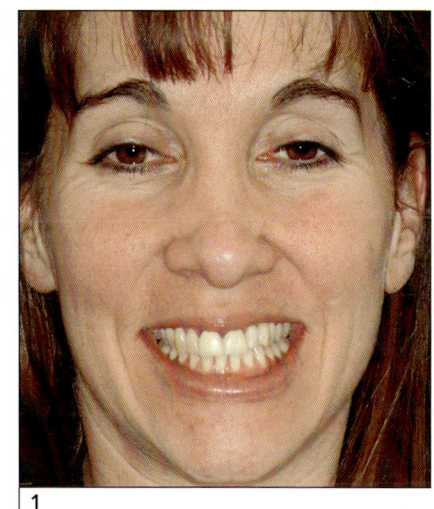

Fig 1 Preoperative facial view.

Fig 2 Preoperative right lateral view.

Fig 3 Preoperative anterior view.

Fig 4 Preoperative left lateral view.

Fig 5 Preoperative smile view.

Fig 6 Initial primary provisionals.

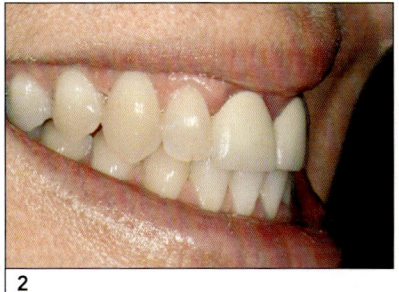

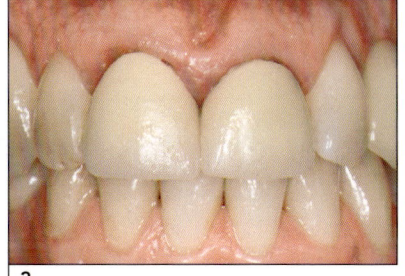

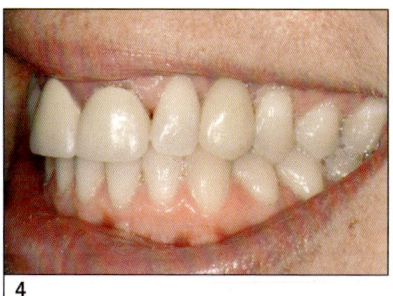

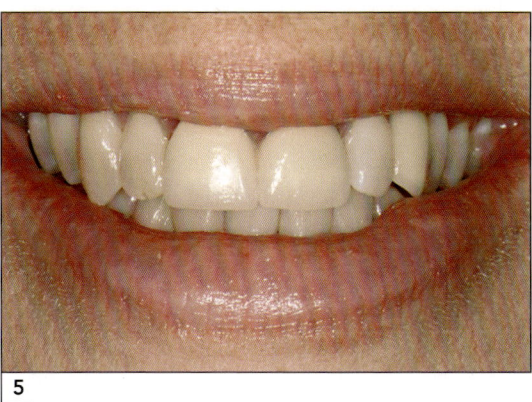

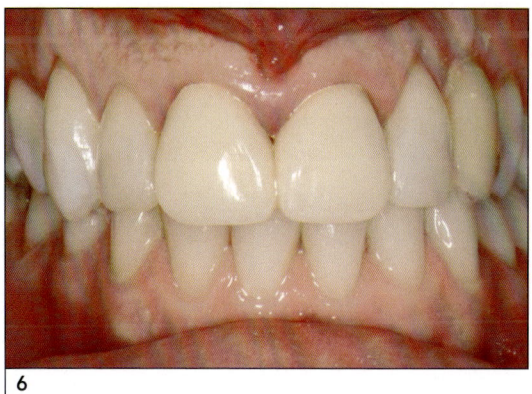

Planning and Fabricating the Definitive Provisional Restorations: Laboratory Procedures

In the laboratory, the dental technician should receive the following from the clinician:

- Three casts showing the following information: *(1)* the original maxillary restorations, *(2)* the mandibular arch, and *(3)* the initial treatment carried out by the clinician (ie, the gingival graft on the left lateral incisor, implant treatment at the left canine site, and the primary provisional restorations on the central incisors and left canine)

- Vinyl polysiloxane impression of the preparations of the central incisors and the implant at the left canine site (Fig 7)

- Facebow record

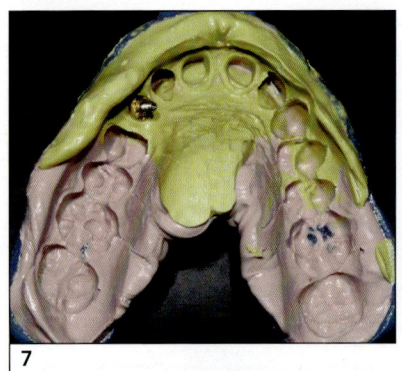

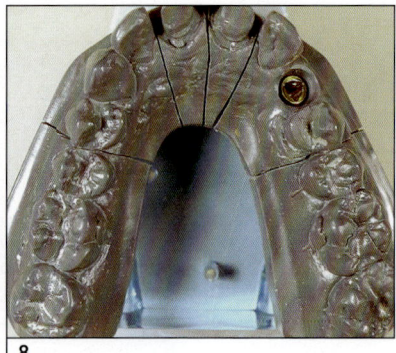

Fig 7 Vinyl polysiloxane impression.

Fig 8 Implant cast fabricated in Metallepox epoxy resin. Note that in this stage, the transmucosal zone is dictated by the shape of a stock implant impression post for a Replace Select regular platform 4.3-mm implant (Nobel Biocare).

- Implant impression post to be modified in the laboratory and given back to the clinician, who will use it to make the final impression
- Disk containing photographs of the patient's face and the initial treatment

An examination of the photographs of the patient's face revealed the following characteristics:

- The face had a rectangular/oval shape[4]
- The upper lip was thinner, indicating less support than the lower lip
- The smile was asymmetrical, because through habit, the patient opened the left side of the mouth to a greater extent, completely exposing the mandibular posterior teeth and gingiva
- The maxillary posterior teeth were below the plane of occlusion

The prescription from the clinician called for the fabrication of a diagnostic waxup, three provisional crowns on the central incisors and left canine, a gold interim implant abutment on the left canine, and two provisional veneers (before tooth preparation) on the lateral incisors.

The philosophy of excellence that underlies every laboratory stage performed by the author is naturally applied to the provisional restorations as well. The need for precision and accuracy is in no way different from that of the definitive restorations. The only difference between the two is the type of materials used.

The impression was disinfected[5] and conditioned[6] so that the impression material did not in-

teract negatively, from a chemical or physical standpoint, with the material used to make the implant cast (Fig 8).[7] The removable dies on this cast were used to contour and fabricate the cervical third of the provisional crowns and to ensure a precise marginal fit with the aid of a microscope. After the implant cast was made, a solid cast was made from the same impression.

Both casts were fabricated using a special epoxy resin, *Metallepox* (product information available from author),[7] which is more stable and durable than gypsum during all stages of the laboratory work.

The mandibular cast, which was made by the clinician, was finished to eliminate the bubbles and creases, and then retrimmed and squared to improve the orientation and make it more visually harmonious.[8-10]

Before mounting in the articulator, a manual control was performed using articulation film (Hanel, Langenau, Germany) to assess the maximum intercuspation between the maxillary and mandibular casts (Fig 9). Selective grinding was performed[11-19] to eliminate errors caused by the impression materials and stomatognathic system (dental intrusion, bone elasticity, meniscus compressibility, etc) (Fig 10).

With the help of a microscope, the exact position of each bite registration record made by the clinician was checked on the casts. The various casts were then cross-mounted on the articulator in all possible combinations that preserved the esthetic and functional information provided by the clinician.

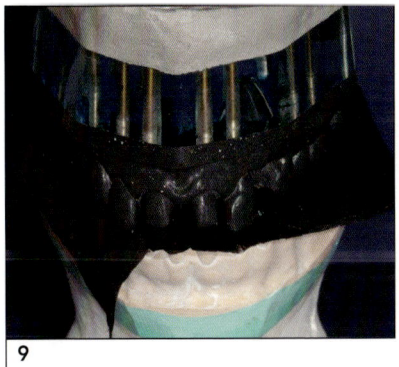 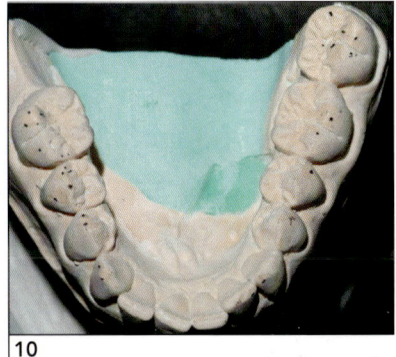

Fig 9 Manual check of the maximum intercuspation using 12-µm double-sided articulation film before mounting in the articulator.

Fig 10 Distribution of occlusal contacts after the selective grinding was performed on the cast.

Fig 11 Waxup of the left canine. Note the difference in shape between the form of the cervical third of the crown and the circumference of the transmucosal zone as created by the stock impression post. (Photographed with a Zeiss OPMI 19-FC stereomicroscope [Zeiss, Thornwood, New York, USA]; magnification ×9.)

Fig 12 Transmucosal zone on the cast, shaped to develop the correct anatomy of the restoration.

Fig 13 Waxup of the left canine perfectly contained within the transmucosal zone of the properly shaped cast.

Fig 14 Reestablishment of correct proportion between the left lateral incisor and canine.

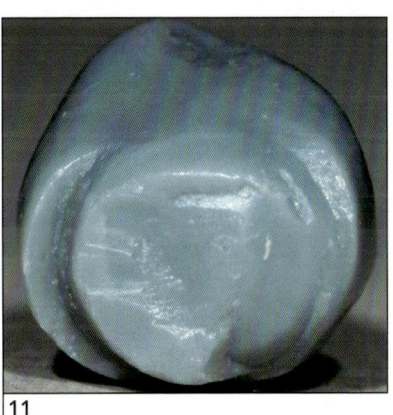

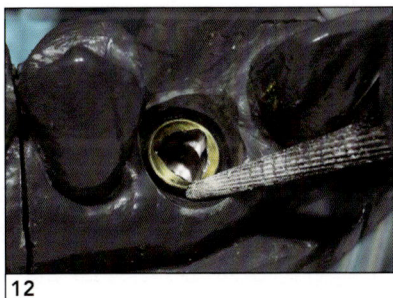 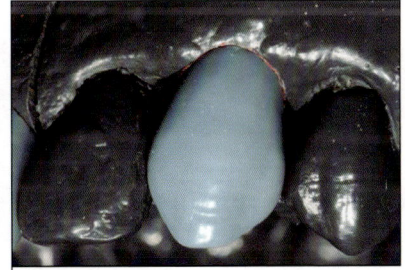 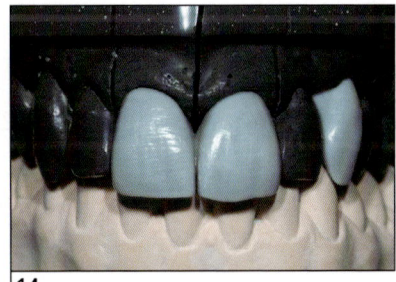

After mounting the casts, a removable waxup of the two central incisors and canine was fabricated. Two anomalies were evident:

1. An anatomic difference between the transmucosal zone and the cervical circumference of the left canine (Fig 11). To correct this, the form of the waxup of this tooth dictated the way in which the transmucosal zone of the cast must be modified for it to fit properly around the perimeter of the crown. This allowed for support of the gingival tissue and conditioned it to take on the correct anatomy by shifting the free gingival tissue in the apical and buccal directions (Figs 12 and 13).

2. A lack of proportion between the anterior teeth. To reestablish a proper proportion, the distal side of the left lateral incisor required slight modification (Fig 14).

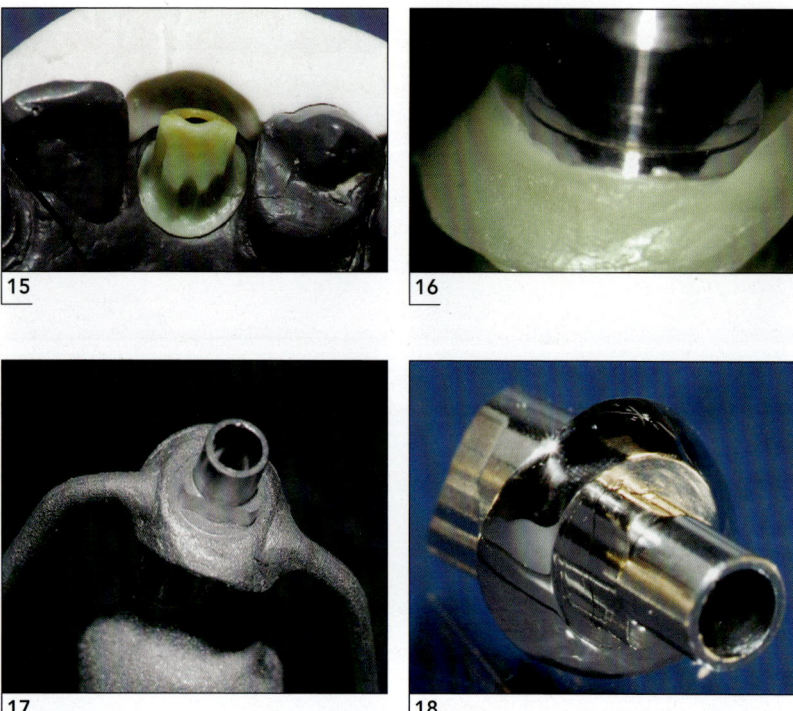

Fig 15 Silicone mask used to evaluate the space needed for the fabrication of the telescopic abutment and the provisional for the left canine.

Fig 16 Separate implant analog with the "cast-to" abutment. The transmucosal zone was molded in wax and then relined in wax for additional precision. (Photographed with a Zeiss OPMI 19-FC stereomicroscope; magnification ×9.)

Fig 17 Casting in gold alloy. Note the cooling channels and the perfect bond between the alloy and the abutment. The melted alloy should not overflow onto the fitting surface of the abutment.

Fig 18 Refinishing, correction, and polishing of the transmucosal zone and fitting surface. (Photographed with a Zeiss OPMI 19-FC stereomicroscope; magnification ×9.)

To allow for the proper geometric design of the implant telescopic abutment,[7] a silicone mask was made on the waxup to evaluate the space taken up by the canine (Fig 15). The transmucosal area was then waxed on a "cast-to" abutment, which was finished later on a separate individual implant analog (Fig 16).

After casting the abutment with gold alloy (Silhouette 65 SF, Leach & Dillon, Cranston, RI, USA) (Fig 17), the telescopic abutment was fitted on a separate implant analog, off the cast. It was then refinished and polished in the transmucosal area (Fig 18) and fitted back on the cast. Next, the geometric design of the telescopic abutment was finalized via milling.

The implant antirotational and positional key[7] was fabricated in heat-polymerizing acrylic resin. Its composition and the heating process were modified to produce more stability and rigidity.

The soft tissues around the end of preparation margins of the central incisors on the cast were removed with a bur, and white wax was used to eliminate all undercuts. The waxup was repositioned on the dies and a silicone impression was made to aid the fabrication of the provisionals.[20–26]

A thin spacer of wax was applied to the axial surfaces of the teeth and implant abutment to eliminate undercuts, provide space for the adhesive cement, and accommodate the polymerization shrinkage of the acrylic resin, which would impede the exact seating of the restorations. The acrylic resin for the provisionals was stratified and processed. The provisionals were then finished, perfecting their anatomy and refining the maximum intercuspal position and all possible protrusive and lateral excursions, until there was a smooth, harmonious movement, free of interference, on the articulator (Figs 19 to 21).[27–29] Additional acrylic resin was added to the margin of the crowns to compensate for the contraction of the polymerized acrylic resin and to achieve perfect marginal closure.

On the cast, the two maxillary lateral incisors were slightly reduced, eliminating the resin composite placed in the mesial area by the clinician when the primary set of provisionals was made. This should be done only after completing the two central incisors and canine with the telescoping abutment, in order to preserve the spatial relationship between the teeth. Very little material was removed from the cast, because the lateral incisors

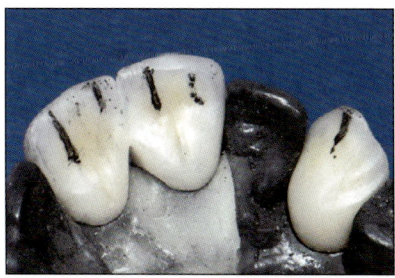

Fig 19 Refinement and careful evaluation of the functional aspects of the provisionals.

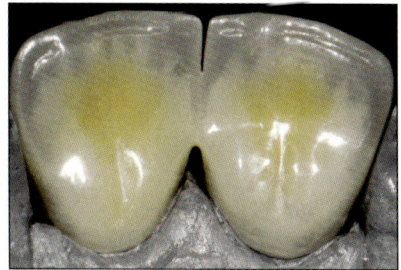

Fig 20 Refinished and polished palatal side of the provisionals on the gypsum cast with the gingival portion intact.

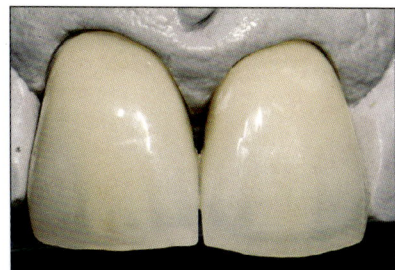

Fig 21 Refinished and polished labial side of the provisionals. Note the translucent acrylic resins, from pure to colored, at the middle third and interproximal areas, and the whitish enamel at the middle of the cervical third.

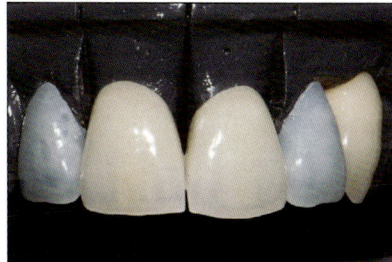

Fig 22 The definitive provisionals.

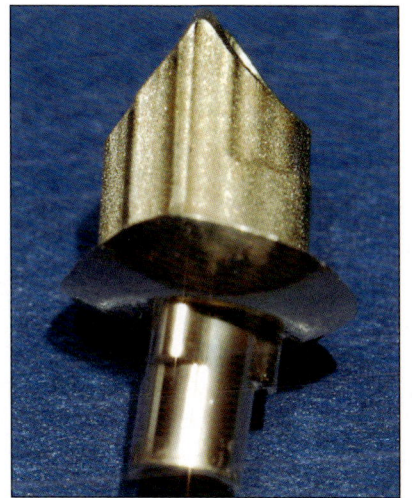

Fig 23 Interim telescopic abutment, electroplated in 99% gold. Note the highly polished transmucosal portion and the emergence profile relative to the fitting surface. The unusual, milled geometry and surface sanding improve adherence with the cement. (Photographed with a Zeiss OPMI 19-FC stereomicroscope; magnification ×6.)

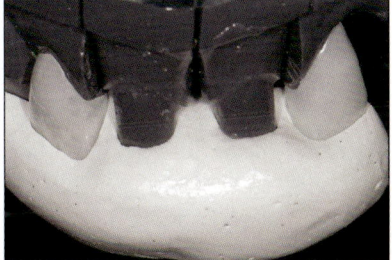

Fig 24 Gypsum key used to transfer the exact spatial position of the veneers to the oral cavity.

were built out labially in relation to the position of the central incisors and canine, so as to provide support for the upper lip and reduce the problem with the lower lip. The veneer facings were modeled in wax and then made entirely of enamel resin (Fig 22). The clinician then adapted them to the patient's teeth and relined them with a dentin resin of the same color used to make the provisionals for the central incisors and canine.

The axial part of the abutment and the interior portion of the provisionals were sandblasted to improve their retention with the provisional adhesive cement. Gold plating of the telescopic abutment was carried out with 99% gold (Fig 23).

A special gypsum transfer and positioning key was made on the cast to allow the exact transfer of the position of the veneers to the oral cavity (Fig 24).

At this point, the transmucosal zone of the implant abutment was copied in acrylic resin on the implant impression post. This way, it could be used by the clinician to make the final impression

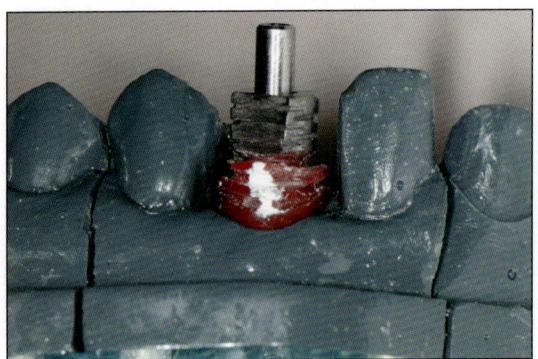

Fig 25 Impression post for the pickup technique with the transmucosal contour copied from the provisional abutment and crown worn by the patient for about 7 months. Note the design, which permits greater retention of the impression material. The buccal position, corresponding to the zenith of the gingival margin, is marked.

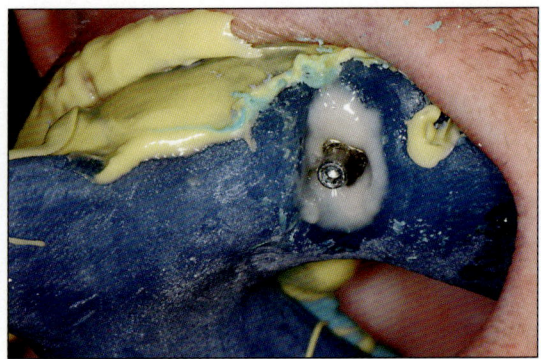

Fig 26 Implant tray. Note the portion of the impression post that protrudes through the tray and is connected by resin composite.

(Fig 25).[30–33] The gingival architecture determined by the cervical-transmucosal margin of the provisional crown and the canine abutment can be transferred onto the definitive cast when the final impression is made. The provisional abutment and crown should be worn by the patient for about 7 months before the clinician makes the final impression.[34,35]

The implant impression tray was made of photopolymerizing resin composite.[24,36–40] A hole was made for the pickup technique, along with occlusal stops and a midline marking for correct positioning inside the mouth. A honeycomb pattern of undercuts was placed on the internal surface to augment the adherence of the impression material.[41,42] Before taking the impression, the clinician painted the impression post and tray with monomer and a bonding agent. When taking the impression, the clinician should unite the impression post and tray with a small amount of resin composite and then perform the photopolymerization (Fig 26). This procedure permits the preservation of the exact spatial positioning of the implant impression post with respect to the teeth, implant, and custom tray. In this way, when the laboratory analog is screwed on, there will be no movement of the impression post, and thus the laboratory analog will accurately transfer the exact position of the implant from the patient's mouth to the final cast.[7]

The acrylic resin provisionals should be made anatomically correct, with a precise marginal fit and a perfect polish, performed with a microscope, to prevent the accumulation of bacterial plaque. In addition, before being sent to the clinician, the provisionals were exposed to a special conditioning treatment, called an *extreme purifying treatment*, which can be applied to all acrylic resins that will be inserted in the oral cavity. The stages of this treatment are as follows:

1. The acrylic resin is placed in a vacuum container for 30 minutes, with the vacuum pump working continuously and immersed in an ultrasonic bath at 132 kHz, at a temperature of 70°C.
2. Hydrogen peroxide (10.8%) is added, and the acrylic resin is left in the same container for another 60 minutes, with the vacuum pump still on and immersed in an ultrasonic bath at 132 kHz, at a temperature of 65°C.
3. The acrylic resin is left to rest in the same container, containing hydrogen peroxide (10.8%), for an additional 2 days.
4. The acrylic resin is placed in a glass container filled with purified, sterile water for 30 minutes, immersed in an ultrasonic bath at 132 kHz at room temperature.
5. The glass container with the acrylic resin and water is placed in a microwave oven at 650

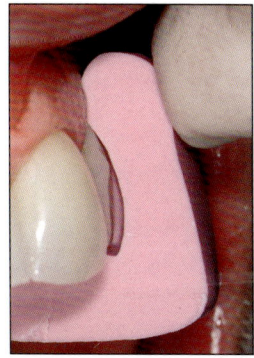

Fig 27 Silicone matrix used as a preparation guide on the left lateral incisor.

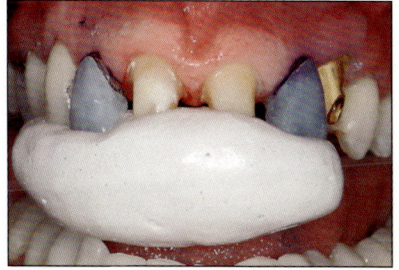

Fig 28 Gypsum key for positioning the provisional veneer shells. Note the interim telescopic abutment in position.

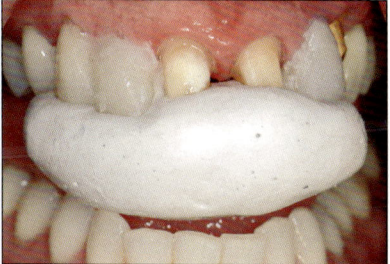

Fig 29 Relining of the provisional veneer shells.

watts for 6 minutes. In case there are any residual metallic components, the prosthesis must first be dried and sealed in a paper/plastic sterilization pouch used for autoclaving instruments. This will prevent any metallic components from sparking and burning the acrylic resin.

6. The acrylic resin is allowed to rest for 2 days in purified, sterile water in the same container.

This treatment significantly reduces the cytotoxicity of the acrylic resins toward the soft and hard tissues[43,44] due to the residual methylmethacrylate monomer and other filterable compounds eluted by the polymerization of the acrylic resin. It also results in an extremely efficient cleaning and disinfection of the acrylic resins,[45] improved mechanical properties,[46] and total saturation, meaning they will not absorb saliva or any other substance in the oral cavity.

After the extreme purification treatment, the acrylic resin prostheses were closed, without drying, in heat-sealed plastic bags to ensure their constant humidity and hygiene before being delivered to the clinician.

The clinician should receive the following from the dental technician:

• Gypsum key for the perfect alignment of the provisional veneers during relining
• Implant key for the exact placement of the telescopic abutment

• Modified impression post for the transfer of the exact morphology of the peri-implant tissues in the final impression to be used for the construction of the definitive restorations
• Provisional restorations for the assessment of osseointegration, function, and esthetics, and to shape the anatomy of the gingival tissues and permit the complete maturation of the peri-implant tissues

Placing the Definitive Provisional Restorations

The lateral incisors were prepared for ceramic veneers using silicone preparation guides based on the definitive provisional restorations (Fig 27).

The telescopic abutment was screwed into place using the implant jig,[7] and the provisional veneer shells were relined with acrylic resin using the gypsum key (Figs 28 and 29). These were relined in the mouth only after verifying that the gypsum key fit perfectly on the patient's teeth and that the veneers did not interfere with the preparations.

The provisional restorations were cemented with non-eugenol–containing cements (Temp-Bond NE and Tempbond Clear, Kerr, Orange, CA, USA) (Fig 30). Once cemented in place, a small amount of acrylic resin was used to lute the provisional veneers to the adjacent provisional

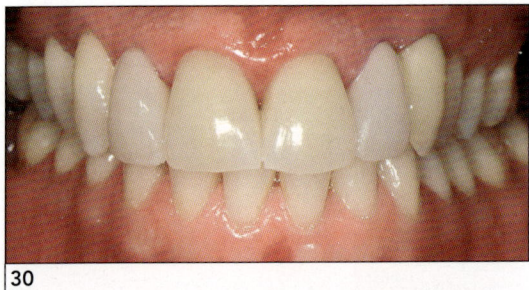

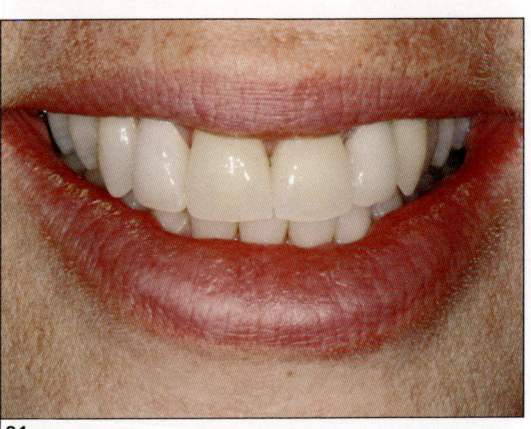

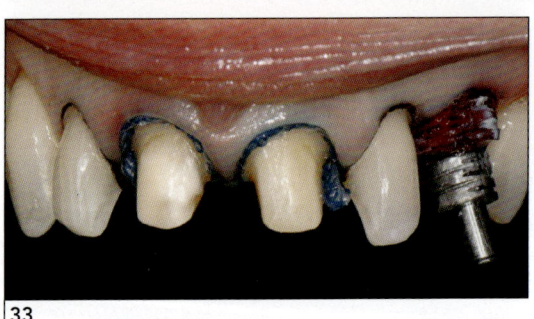

Fig 30 Completed provisional restorations.

Fig 31 Smile view with provisional restorations in place.

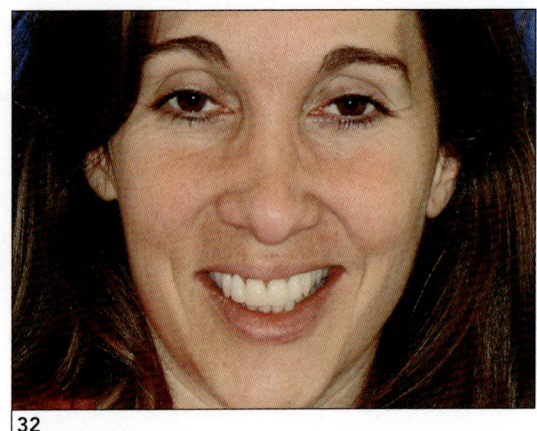

Fig 32 Facial view with provisional restorations in place.

Fig 33 Preparations ready for the definitive impression.

crowns on the palatal aspect. This mechanically locked the provisional veneers in place to increase their retention.

Minor modifications were made to the provisional restorations, and once the esthetic and functional aspects were approved by the patient, clinician, and dental technician (Figs 31 and 32), the final impression was made. The impression was made using a double retraction cord around the crowns and implant and single retraction cord around the veneer preparations (Fig 33). An implant impression tray was used for the implant impression.[7] An impression was made of the provisional restorations, and a maxillomandibular relationship record was made to allow cross-mounting of the cast of the provisional restorations with the cast of the preparations.

Planning and Fabricating the Definitive Restorations: Laboratory Procedures

At this stage, the clinician sent the following to the laboratory:

- Two casts: one of the definitive provisional restorations and one of the mandibular arch (the same used to build the definitive provisionals)

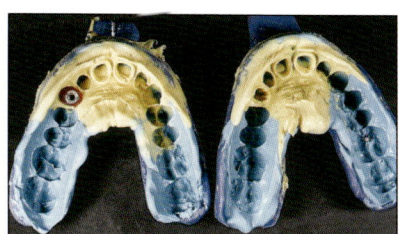

Fig 34 The two impressions received in the laboratory for construction of the definitive restorations.

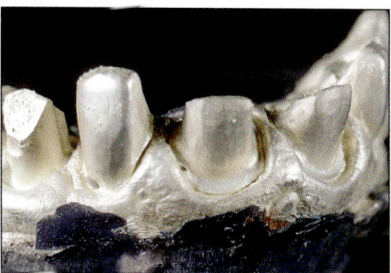

Fig 35 Electroplated cast with Metallepox in the canine-to-canine region. After sectioning, only the two dies of the central incisors were used.

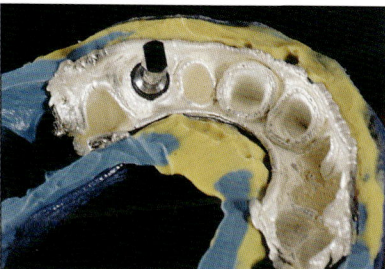

Fig 36 Electroplating of the impression from which the implant cast was developed. Note the electrodeposition around the implant analog, which exactly reproduces the transmucosal contour.

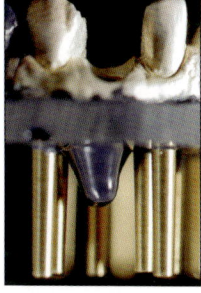

Fig 37 Implant analog embedded in epoxy resin contained in a festooned, truncated, conical excavation in a Plexiglas base (Degussa, Munich, Germany). In addition, this implant analog is held by pins for increased stability.

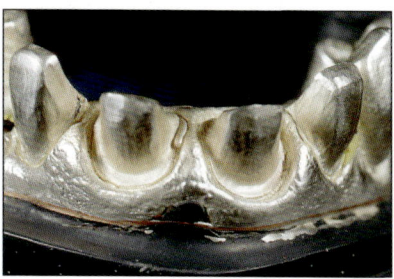

Fig 38 Labial side of the preparations on the implant cast.

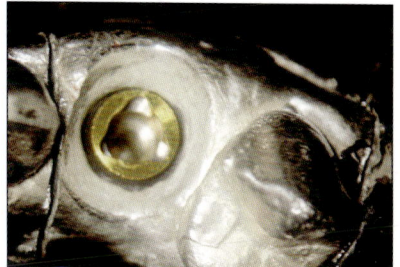

Fig 39 Implant analog in the working cast exactly reproduces the spatial position and geometric design of the implant head. The transmucosal area is created by the interim abutment and provisional crown.

- Two impressions (one had a marginal defect) in vinyl polysiloxane of the preparations of the incisors and the customized impression post on the left canine (Fig 34)

The prescription from the clinician requested the fabrication of the following:

- Three all-ceramic aluminum oxide crowns for the central incisors and left canine
- Two veneers in feldspathic ceramic for the lateral incisors
- An implant abutment in zirconium dioxide at the left canine

The impressions were disinfected,[5] conditioned,[6] and analyzed. Because of a marginal defect in the impression of the palatal aspect of the left central incisor, it was necessary to use both impressions to make the definitive restorations. The accurate impression of the two central incisors was electroplated from canine to canine. Metallepox resin was then placed in the electroplated impression (Fig 35). The accurate impression of the lateral incisors and the implant was electroplated in the region between the first premolars. Metallepox resin was then placed in the electroplated and nonelectroplated parts of the impression, and an implant cast was fabricated (Fig 36).[7] After polymerization was complete—which takes 48 hours for any epoxy resin, not 6 to 8 hours as claimed by various manufacturers—the implant cast was refinished only by eliminating the bubbles and the creases from the entire arch, without trimming the gingival tissue portion (Figs 37 to 39).

Before mounting the cast in the articulator, the maximum intercuspation between the maxillary and mandibular casts was checked manually using

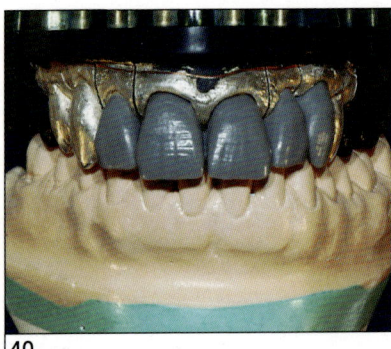

Fig 40 Detailed anatomic waxup of the definitive provisional is transferred onto the implant cast through cross mounting.

Fig 41 Waxup of the antirotational "cast-to" abutment for the definition of the geometric design of the telescopic abutment.

Fig 42 Silicone mask made from the waxup showing the space available around the zirconium abutment for the definitive alumina crown. Note the geometric design of the milling.

Fig 43 Densely sintered zirconia telescopic abutment.

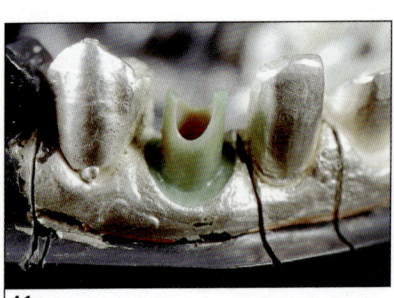

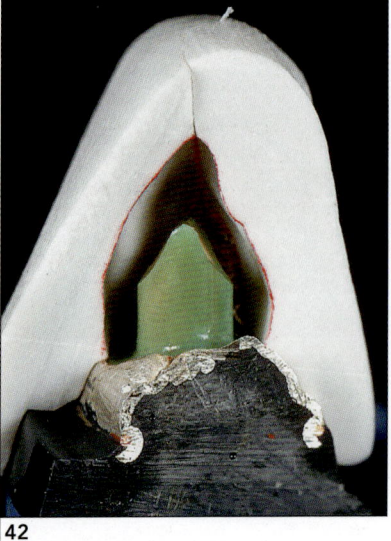

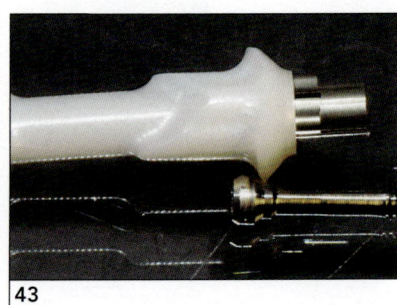

articulation film. With the use of a microscope, selective grinding was performed on the maxillary cast only, since the mandibular cast was the same one used for the fabrication of the definitive provisional restorations. The inclination of the condylar guidance of the articulator (Denar Mark II, Waterpik, Newport Beach, CA, USA) was set at 50 degrees. The various casts were cross-mounted, maintaining the esthetic-functional relationships established by the clinician. Next, the condylar guidance was then changed to 25 degrees for fabrication of the restorations.

The electroplated dies were developed from the accurate impression of the two central incisors and then sectioned and finished. These dies were used to make the alumina copings and perfect the marginal closure. Later, the alumina copings were transferred and fitted on the dies of the implant cast, using a microscope, to build up the ceramic crowns.

The entire gingival portion of the implant cast was left intact. On this cast, the teeth were waxed up (Fig 40), the crowns were built up with ceramic, and the final static and dynamic functioning check was performed using a microscope.

A silicone mask of the waxup was made to evaluate the space occupied by the canine and to allow the execution of the correct geometric design of the telescopic abutment (Figs 41 and 42).[7] After scanning the implant abutment, the data were sent via modem to the Nobel Biocare production facility in Sweden, where the abutment was reproduced in zirconium dioxide modified with yttrium (Fig 43).[47–50] The adaptation of the telescopic abutment was verified on a separate implant laboratory analog. It was then transferred to

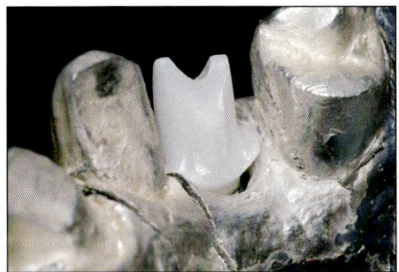

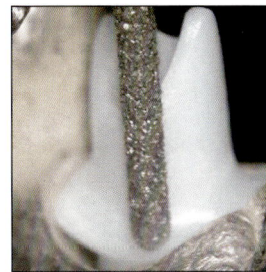

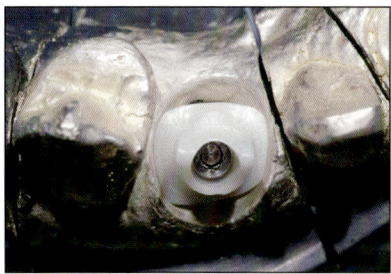

Fig 44 Telescopic abutment perfectly positioned on the implant analog in the cast, without interferences along the transmucosal contour.

Fig 45 Refining the milled geometric design using diamond-tipped burs and jets of water and air to prevent overheating, which could damage the abutment's structural integrity. (Photographed with a Zeiss OPMI 19-FC stereomicroscope; magnification ×6.)

Fig 46 Portions of the abutment shoulder in the transmucosal zone not manufactured by the CAD/CAM system because the angle of emergence of the transmucosal portion of the abutment is greater than 30 degrees.

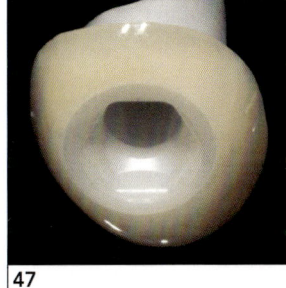

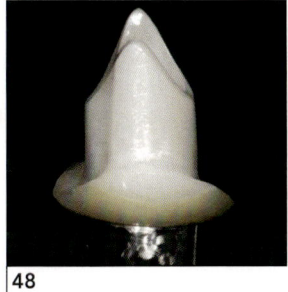

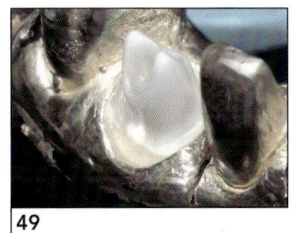

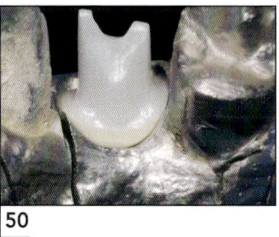

Fig 47 Portions of the shoulder in the transmucosal zone rebuilt using the compatible laminating zirconia shoulder ceramic. Note the finish and polish of the ceramic, which promotes integration with the surrounding tissues. The abutment is manufactured to fit on an externally hexed implant. A titanium antirotational element is then attached to the abutment and converts the external connection into an internal connection. (Photographed with a Zeiss OPMI 19-FC stereomicroscope; magnification ×9.)

Fig 48 Geometric design of the axial portion and the emergence profile of the transmucosal portion of the telescopic abutment. (Photographed with a Zeiss OPMI 19-FC stereomicroscope; magnification ×6.)

Fig 49 Intracrevicular positioning in the labial area of the margin of the telescopic abutment.

Fig 50 Equigingival positioning of the palatal and interproximal margins of the telescopic abutment.

the cast and finished with rubber points until it fit perfectly on the separate implant analog and transmucosal area of the cast (Fig 44). Only then can the geometric design of the telescopic abutment be milled using diamond-tipped burs[51] and water (Fig 45). Some areas of the transmucosal zone could not be produced by the CAD/CAM Procera system (Nobel Biocare, Göteborg, Sweden) because it cannot reproduce angles of more than 30 degrees. Instead, these areas were produced by hand using a specific ceramic for zirco-

nium (Fig 46). After sandblasting and applying the bonding agent to the abutment, the modified shoulder ceramic was added and fired. The shoulder ceramic was refined and perfectly adapted to the transmucosal zone of the implant cast. It was then polished and fired for autoglazing (Figs 47 to 50).

The implant antirotational transfer and positioning key[7] was made using heat-hardening acrylic resin with a modified composition and heating modality to make it more stable and rigid (Fig 51).

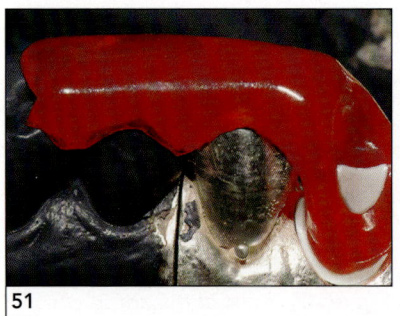

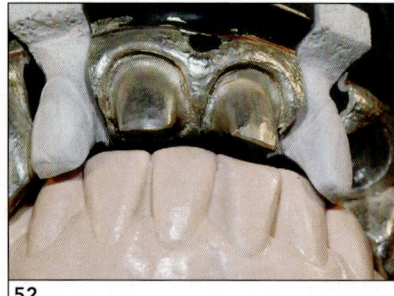

Fig 51 Implant jig, which permits the exact transfer and positioning of the telescopic abutments from the working cast to the oral cavity and vice versa.

Fig 52 Duplicate dies of the lateral incisors made in refractory material.

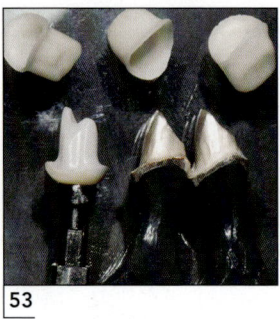

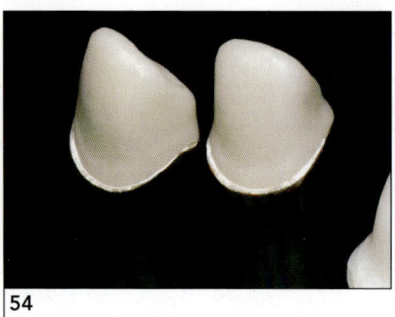

Fig 53 Densely sintered aluminum oxide copings *(top)*. Implant abutments in densely sintered zirconia *(bottom)*.

Fig 54 Surface of the copings treated to receive the ceramic. Note the marginal reduction to allow a sufficient quantity of translucent orange and fluorescent ceramic to be applied.

Scans of the central incisors and left canine were sent to the Nobel Biocare production facility, which produced three copings in aluminum oxide.

Duplicate dies of the lateral incisors were made in refractory material and used to make the veneers. The refractory material was degassed by heating it in a vacuum at 1,000°C for 11 minutes. The dies were then held in normal atmospheric pressure at 1,052°C for 7 minutes (Fig 52). The T-Glass feldspathic ceramic (Vintage Halo, Shofu, San Marcos, CA, USA) was applied and heated at 1,000°C for 2 minutes. The waxups of the central incisor and left canine crowns were replaced on their respective dies to provide reference points and aid in the fabrication of the veneers. The intensified dentinal and translucent ceramics were layered and heated at 940°C for 1 minute. The various enamels were heated at 930°C for 1 minute. An additional heating was done for autoglazing, which included some additional ceramics and stains, at 920°C for 1 minute. Finally, the veneers were refined.

To match the color of the cervical zone of the natural teeth, the entire margin of the Procera copings was reduced horizontally by 0.2 to 0.4 mm (Figs 53 and 54). The copings were fitted not only on the segmented dies, but also on the dies of the implant cast, where the ceramic layering was performed later. The copings were treated with diamond-tipped ceramic burs and sanded with highly pure, reddish-brown, 50-Ì aluminum oxide from Brazil (Perio-R-Blast, Talladium, Valencia, CA, USA) at 2.5 atm. They were then placed in a container with carbon tetrachloride and immersed in an ultrasonic bath at 80°C for 5 minutes, followed by steam cleaning and boiling in purified water for 10 minutes in a ceramic pan.

The all-ceramic crowns for the central incisors and left canine were then fabricated via layering with Nobel Rondo Alumina ceramic (Nobel Biocare). First, an initial application of the shoulder ceramic was made and fired, followed by a second application and corrective firing (Fig 55). Next, the dentinal ceramics were applied, with intense chroma (chromatizer) at high values, along with the translucent ceramics, from clear to colored, to create a very irregular and uneven surface (Fig 56). This distributes the light inside the restorations, as in natural teeth. The alternation of the various ceramics and the absorption, reflection, and refraction of the diffused light allow the light to circulate

Fig 55 All-ceramic crown after firing of the shoulder ceramic. Note the degree of precision achieved at this stage. (Photographed with a Zeiss OPMI 19-FC stereomicroscope; magnification ×6.)

Fig 56 Application of dentinal and translucent ceramics, from pure to colored, forming an irregular and uneven surface that will react positively to light. (Photographed with a Zeiss OPMI 19-FC stereomicroscope; magnification ×6.)

Fig 57 Layering of the dentinal ceramics and dentinal cuts.

Fig 58 Packed and condensed ceramics[52] of the left central incisor before sintering.

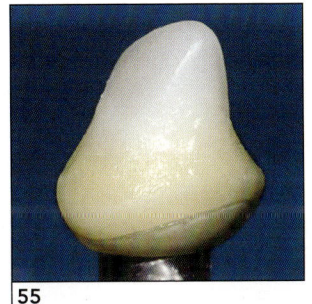
55

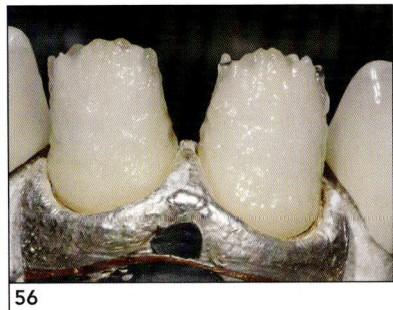
56

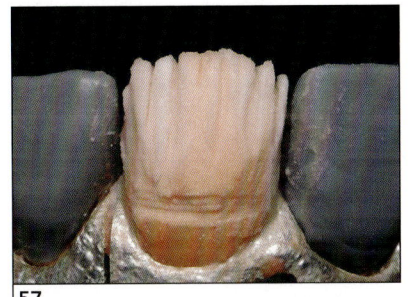
57

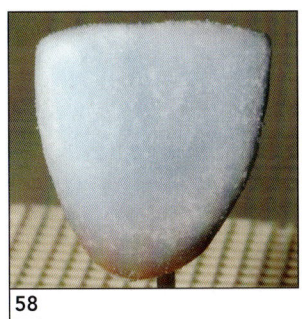
58

inside the restorations, thanks in part to the irregularity and unevenness of the layers of ceramic. This creates a live, natural appearance for the prosthetic teeth. In the same way, the dentin of the teeth was stratified, and a dentinal cut was made for the application of the successive ceramic, based on the color stratification found in the natural teeth (Fig 57). The translucent ceramics were applied, from clear to colored, depending on the values found in the natural teeth, followed by the various enamels, alternated with the opalescent and fluorescent ceramics in both vertical and horizontal layers with the mother-of-pearl modifiers. The teeth were made with a slightly larger total volume to (1) eliminate the effect of the contraction of the ceramic when fired; (2) define the anatomy of the teeth by firing the dentin and enamel only once and using only the nucleus of the ceramic, which offers superior quality; and (3) finish the teeth with just three firings, including the autoglaze, stains, and final corrections of the shoulder ceramic (Fig 58).

This way, the physical properties of the ceramics remain unaltered and the restorations have a more natural look, because the various ceramic layers have been sintered, not vitrified, and are

less stressed because they have been fired fewer times. In fact, the more ceramic is fired, the more its coefficients of thermal expansion and contraction will vary.[52] This can generate radial tension instead of radial compression, which can lead to failure. In addition, a limited number of firings will help produce an optimal match between the restoration and the patient's natural teeth in terms of opalescence, iridescence, and fluorescence.

Finally, the ceramic teeth were refinished, defined, and polished using specific rubber tips (Fig 59).

At this point, the clinician should schedule an appointment for a trial fitting of the restorations before they are completed to assess the precision (Figs 60 and 61), function (Fig 62), physiology (Figs 63 and 64), and esthetics (Figs 65 to 68).

In order to achieve excellent results, each prosthesis must be unique, just like the individual who will wear it. There are no hard and fast rules for making restorations that have a truly natural appearance. Knowledge, skill, experience, and the ability to relate to others must combine synergistically to produce the optimal outcome. To this end, the clinician and the dental technician must scrupulously collect all the data, along with the expectations of the patient, so that they can work

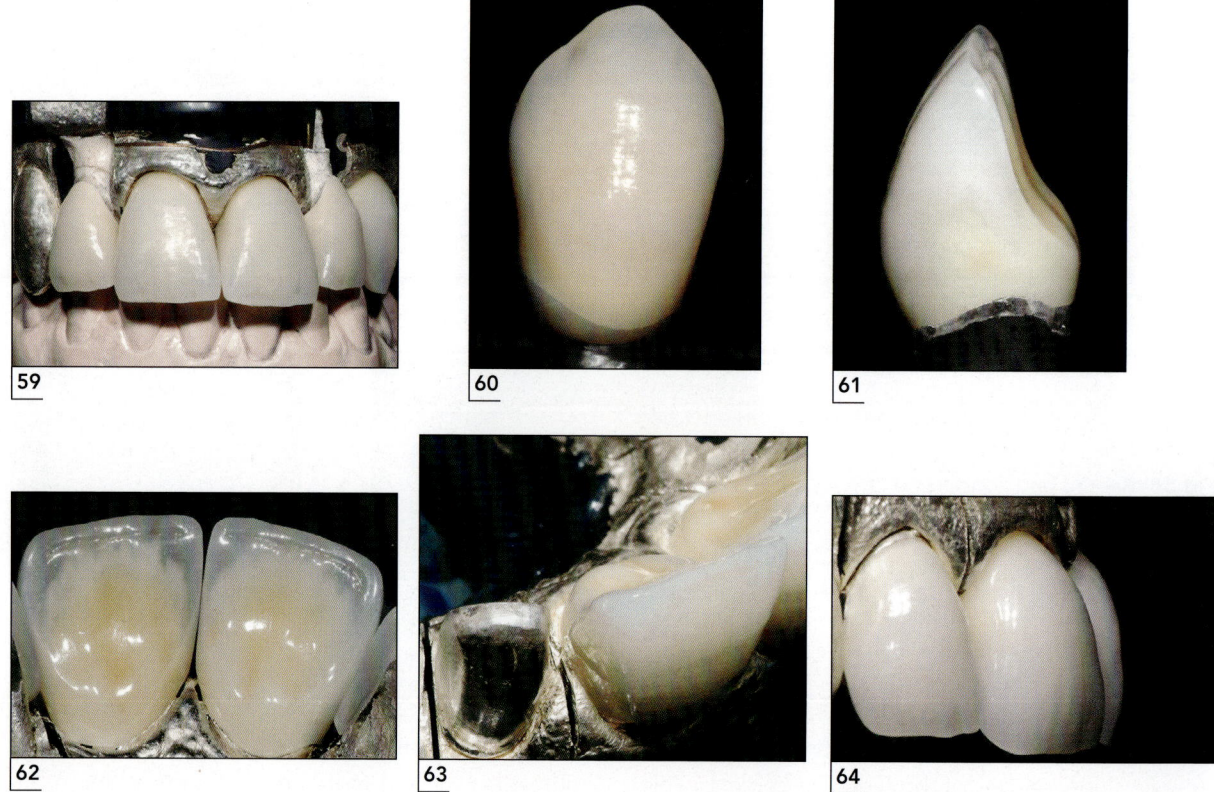

Fig 59 Physiology and functional anatomy of the definitive restorations, created with carbon-silicon and diamond-tipped burs on a water turbine and abrasive and polishing rubber tips on an electric handpiece.

Fig 60 Finished canine. Note the precision of the margin and the continuity between the contour of the crown and the transmucosal contour of the abutment. (Photographed with a Zeiss OPMI 19-FC stereomicroscope; magnification ×9.)

Fig 61 Distal view of the right central incisor. Note the anatomy of the labial and palatal contours of the crown, the gradual inclination of the functional area, and the precision of the margin. It was decided to eliminate the ceramic in the two areas of the preparation margin where there were imperfections, because they might have damaged the ceramic during cementation. (Photographed with a Zeiss OPMI 19-FC stereomicroscope; magnification ×6.)

Fig 62 Palatal view of the central incisors showing the perfectly polished functional surface. The margins of the two crowns were closed perfectly on the individual dies and then transferred and fitted to the dies of the implant cast with the aid of a microscope, in order to perform an accurate static and dynamic functioning check. (Photographed with a Zeiss OPMI 19-FC stereomicroscope; magnification ×9.)

Fig 63 Distal portion of the left central incisor. Note (1) the perfectly polished, extremely compact surface, which is easier for the patient to keep clean; (2) the three-dimensional anatomy of the incisopalatal and incisolabial thirds, which characterize and personalize the tooth; (3) the gradual inclination of the functional area, which ensures freedom of movement and comfort; and (4) the special shape of the distal side, from the middle third to the cervical third, with the excess ceramic used to close the papillary space.

Fig 64 Contour and labial surface of the restorations of the right lateral incisor and central incisors.

together to realize a custom-designed prosthetic device—perfect in anatomy, function, precision, and esthetics—that reflects the personality of the patient[53] and is perfectly integrated over the long term in the biologic environment of the oral cavity.

Cementing the Definitive Restorations

Once the definitive restorations were completed, the provisional restorations were removed. After removing the interim telescopic abutment,[7] it was ev-

Fig 65 Labial view of right lateral and central incisors.

Fig 66 The definitive restorations.

Fig 67 Labial view of left central incisor, lateral incisor, and canine. Note the harmonious relationship between the shapes and the precise polishing of the cervical surface of the ceramic, which reflects the electroplated areas of the cast.

Fig 68 Along with the definitive restorations and implant jig, the clinician should receive a new abutment screw and a locking, antirotational, titanium insert to connect the zirconium abutment to the implant. These have never been subjected to stress and are used only for the final attachment of the zirconium telescopic abutment.

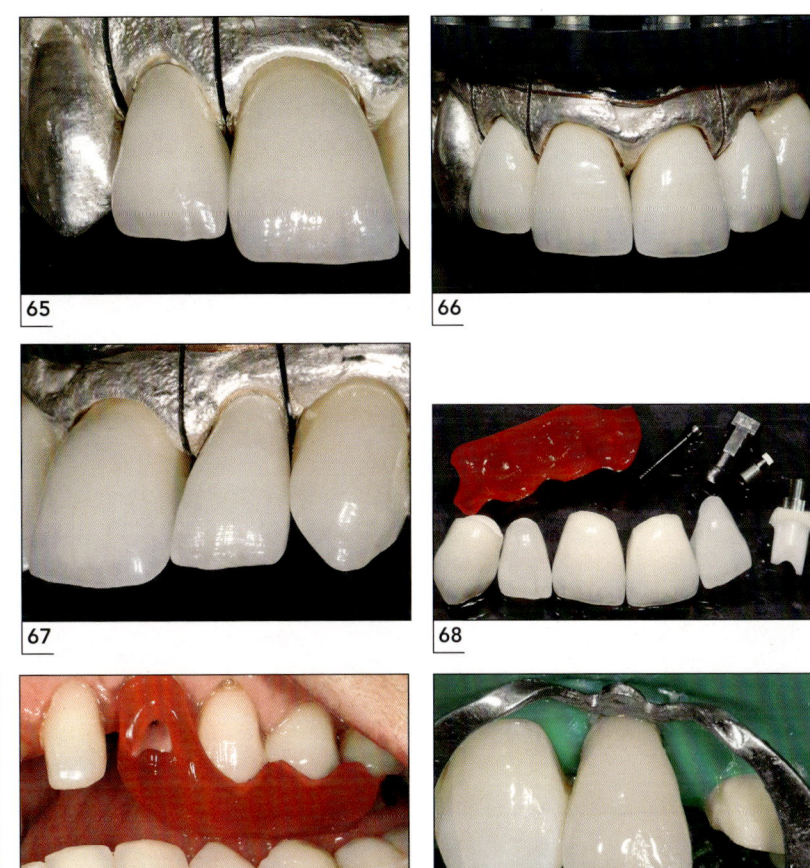

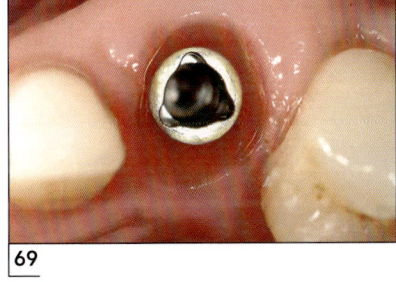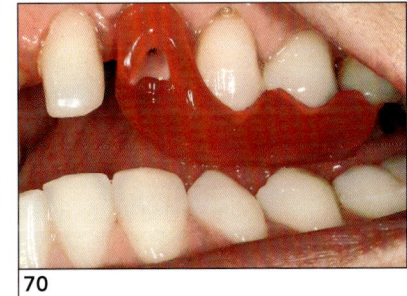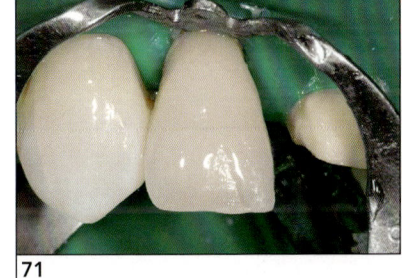

Fig 69 Implant and peri-implant tissues of the left canine. The tissues have perfectly matured around the contour of the crown and interim abutment. The tissues did not collapse, despite the removal of the provisional crown and the interim telescopic abutment.

Fig 70 Telescopic abutment in zirconium being attached to the implant head. The implant jig accurately engages the specific geometric profile of the telescopic abutment, allowing for exact positional transfer from the cast to the mouth. The jig also provides resistance to rotation and acts as a countertorque when fastening the screw.

Fig 71 Cementation of the ceramic veneer under rubber dam.

ident that the transmucosal zone had been properly modified and was now healthy and mature (Fig 69). The definitive zirconium telescopic abutment was torqued into place with the implant jig (Fig 70).[7] The jig accurately engaged the specific geometric profile of the abutment, thereby creating resistance to rotation and acting as a countertorque.

The two ceramic veneers were cemented under rubber dam using a light-cured resin cement (Rely X veneer cement, 3M ESPE, St Paul, MN, USA) (Fig 71). The three aluminium oxide crowns (Procera, Nobel Biocare) were cemented into place with a chemically cured resin cement (Panavia 21, Kuraray, Osaka, Japan).

Comparing the before and after photographs shows the importance of individualizing the tooth morphology according to the patient's unique facial features (Figs 72 to 81).

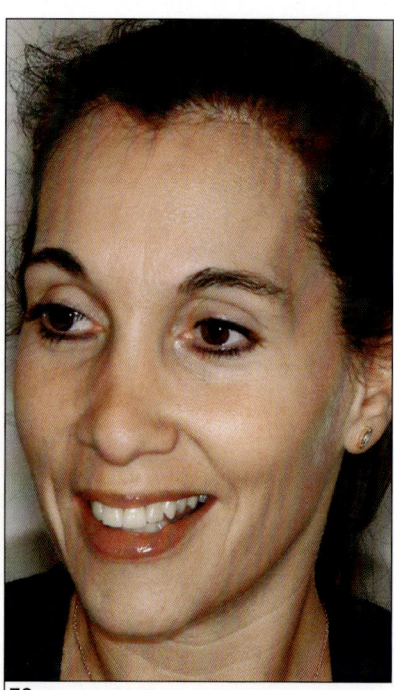

Fig 72 Left dentofacial view 1 week after cementation. Note the presence of a perspective progression, natural appearance of the incisal embrasures, specific anatomic character of each tooth, and improved relationship between the restorations and the lower lip.

Fig 73 A satisfied smile 1 week after cementation. Note the individual nature of the single restorations and their harmonious relationship to the facial composition.

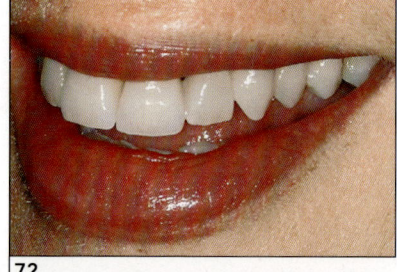

72

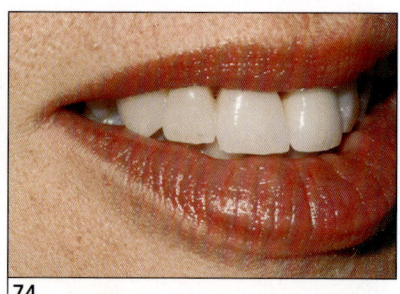

74

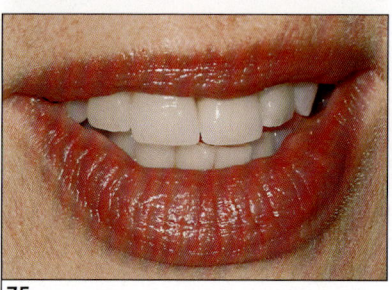

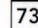

75

Fig 74 Right dentofacial view 1 month after cementation. Note the altered form of the lips caused by the reestablishment of natural support from the teeth, the improvement of the teeth-lips relationship, and the specific individual dominance of each tooth.

Fig 75 Frontal dentofacial view 1 month after cementation. Dominance of the individual teeth is an indispensable element in achieving a harmonious dentofacial composition.

Fig 76 Right intraoral view 1 month after cementation. The tissues around the restorations of lateral incisor and central incisors are beginning to recover their physiologic equilibrium. Note the anatomic details, such as the angular-axial transition lines, surface texture, and three-dimensional anatomy of the incisopalatal third and incisolabial third, which characterize and personalize the teeth. The contour of the crowns was shifted labially to stimulate and support the lips, and is in harmony with the gingival contour.

Fig 77 Left intraoral view 1 month after cementation. The tissues around the restoration of the canine are reacting to the stimulus provided by the correct anatomy of the coronal and transmucosal contours.

Fig 78 Frontal intraoral view. Note the radiant symmetry produced by the balance between the forces of separation and forces of cohesion, which give dynamism and vitality to the dental composition. Also note the dynamism of the light generated by the contrast between the various colors, between the opacity and translucence, and between the lines and structures, which combine to produce a pleasant visual effect.

Fig 79 Frontal dentofacial view 7 months after cementation. The curvature of the lower lip follows the arc of the maxillary teeth, and the smile has a defined, balanced appearance.

Fig 80 Left dentofacial view 8 months after cementation. The tissues around the restorations of the central incisors and left lateral incisor and canine continue to adapt and integrate with the restorations. Note that the papilla between the left central and lateral incisors has occupied most of the physiologic space available.

Fig 81 Before beginning the esthetic treatment, the patient was dissatisfied and discouraged by the unnatural appearance of her prosthesis (see Fig 1). Eight months after the insertion of the definitive restorations, the patient is relaxed and confident.

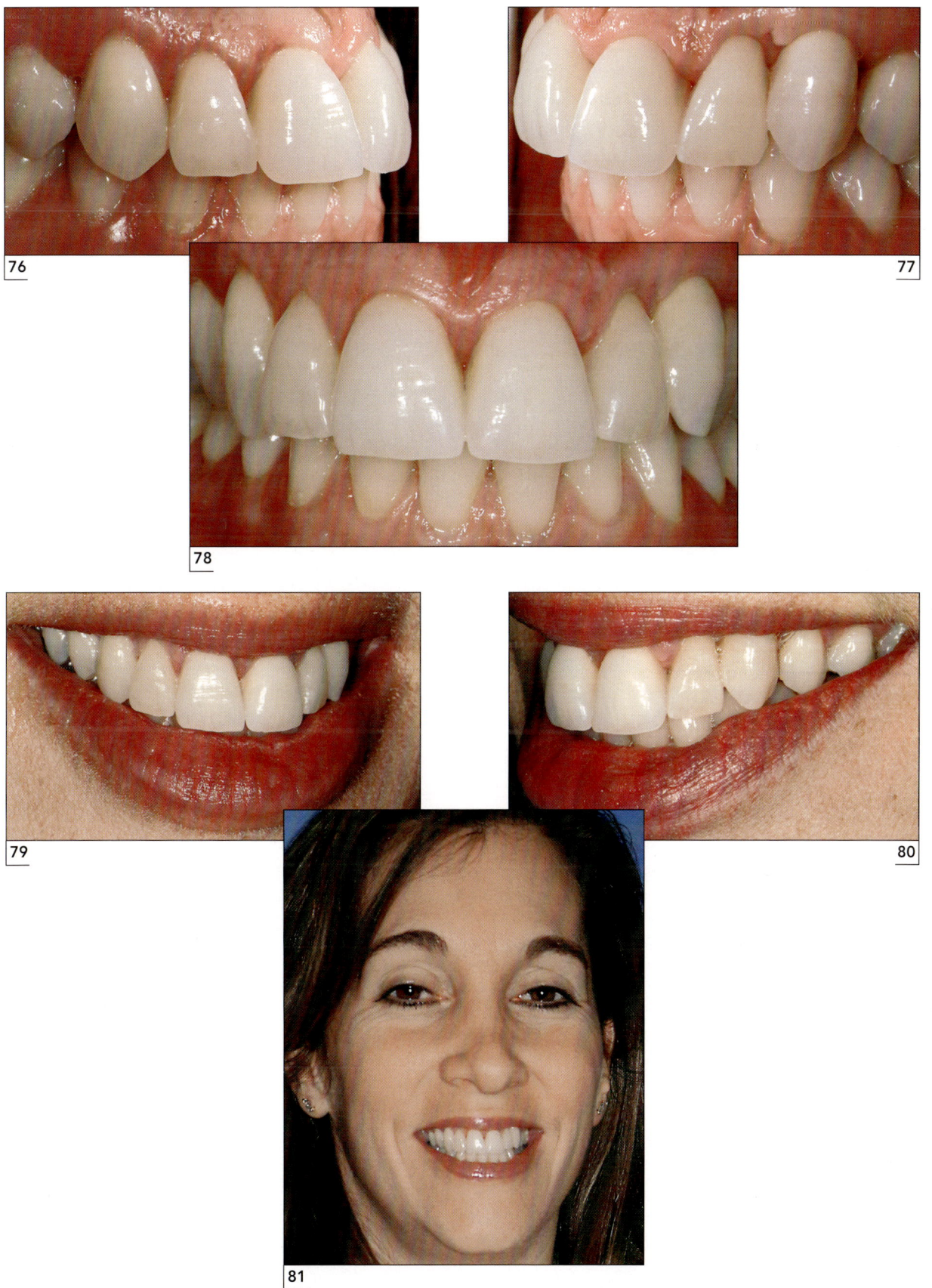

76

77

78

79

80

81

CONCLUSIONS

Every face has individual features and characteristics, and this individuality should be imparted to the restorations and smile design. Applying generic smile design recipes without understanding and modifying the unique tooth morphology will create characterless and unnatural restorations. In cases such as the one presented in this article, the clinician can be easily misled into thinking that the treatment will be simple and can be completed in a short period of time. However, because of the patient's specific features, generically shaped teeth would have yielded a compromised result. Only through a continuous dialogue between the clinician, dental technician, and patient, and by properly evaluating and modifying the provisional restorations, can excellent, individualized results be achieved.

ACKNOWLEDGMENTS

The authors wish to thank Dr Ines Capobianco for her precious collaboration in reviewing this article.

REFERENCES

1. Magne P, Belser U. Bonded Porcelain Restorations in the Anterior Dentition: A Biomimetic Approach. Chicago: Quintessence, 2002.

2. Chiche GJ, Pinault A. Esthetics of Anterior Fixed Prosthodontics. Chicago: Quintessence, 1994.

3. Scharer P, Rinn LA, Kopp FR. Aesthetic Guidelines for Restorative Dentistry. Chicago: Quintessence, 1982.

4. Caradonna C, Caruso C, Lotti M. Ortognatodonzia come arte. Ortognatodonzia Italiana 1998;7:69–96.

5. Owen CP, Goolam R. Disinfection of impression materials to prevent viral cross contamination: A review and a protocol. Int J Prosthodont 1993;6:480–494.

6. Sgrò S, Eliseo M. Galvanoplastica in argento. Ottimizzazione del metodo. Dental Labor 1998;5:449–456.

7. Sgrò S. Accurate positional impression, accurate positional cast, and antirotational transfer and positioning key in the fabrication of implant-supported prostheses. Quintessence Dent Technol 2005;28:27–48.

8. Pedroli G. Il modello di studio ortodontico. La Quintessenza Odontotecnica 1992;4:383–394.

9. Köhler H. Utilizzo della dima angolare di Leleux secondo Köhler e Döring. La Quintessenza Odontotecnica 1994;8:783–793.

10. Yamamoto M, Miyoshi Y, Kataoka S. Basi fondamentali di estetica: Tecniche di modellazione per i restauri metallo-ceramici. Quintessenza Odontotecnica 1991;15:10–81.

11. Boyarsky HP, Loos LG, Leknius C. Occlusal refinement of mounted casts before crown fabrication to decrease clinical time required to adjust occlusion. J Prosthet Dent 1999;82:591–594.

12. Loos LG, Boyarsky HP, Quiring DJ. Procedure for occlusal refinement of mounted definitive casts to reduce clinical time required for adjustment of occlusion. J Prosthet Dent 2001;85:246–251.

13. Carossa S, Lojacono A, Schierano G, Pera P. Evaluation of occlusal contacts in the dental laboratory: Influence of strip thickness and operator experience. Int J Prosthodont. 2000;13:201–204.

14. DeLong R, Ko CC, Anderson GC, Hodges JS, Douglas WH. Comparing maximum intercuspal contacts of virtual dental patients and mounted dental casts. J Prosthet Dent 2002;88:622–630.

15. Davies S, Al-Ani Z, Jeremiah H, Winston D, Smith P. Reliability of recording static and dynamic occlusal contact marks using transparent acetate sheet. J Prosthet Dent 2005;94:458–461.

16. Millstein P, Maya A. An evaluation of occlusal contact marking indicators. A descriptive quantitative method. J Am Dent Assoc 2001;132:1280–1286.

17. Schelb E, Kaiser DA, Bruckl CE. Thickness and marking characteristics of occlusal registration strips. J Prosthet Dent 1985;54:122–126.

18. Proschel PA, Maul T, Morneburg T. Predicted incidence of excursive occlusal errors in common modes of articulator adjustment. Int J Prosthodont 2000;13:303–310.

19. Morneburg TR, Proschel PA. Predicted incidence of occlusal errors in centric closing around arbitrary axes. Int J Prosthodont 2002;15:358–364.

20. Wang RL, Moore BK, Goodacre CJ, Swartz ML, Andres CJ. A comparison of resins for fabricating provisional fixed restorations. Int J Prosthodont 1989;2:173–184.

21. Mojon P, Oberholzer JP, Meyer JM, Belser UC. Polymerization shrinkage of index and pattern acrylic resins. J Prosthet Dent 1990;64:684–688.

22. Ness EM, Nicholls JI, Rubenstein JE, Smith DE. Accuracy of the acrylic resin pattern for the implant-retained prosthesis. Int J Prosthodont 1992;5:542–549.

23. Moulding MB, Loney RW, Ritsco RG. Marginal accuracy of indirect provisional restorations fabricated on polyvinyl siloxane models. Int J Prosthodont 1994;7:554–548.

24. Takahashi J, Kitahara K, Teraoka F, Kubo F. Resin pattern material with low polymerization shrinkage. Int J Prosthodont 1999;12:325–329.

25. Burns DR, Beck DA, Nelson SK. A review of selected dental literature on contemporary provisional fixed prosthodontic treatment: Report of the Committee on Research in Fixed Prosthodontics of the Academy of Fixed Prosthodontics. J Prosthet Dent 2003;90:474–497.

26. Nejatidanesh F, Lotfi HR, Savabi O. Marginal accuracy of interim restorations fabricated from four interim autopolymerizing resins. J Prosthet Dent 2006;95:364–367.

27. Sato Y, Koretake K, Hosokawa R. An alternative procedure for discrimination of contacts in centric occlusion and lateral excursion. J Prosthet Dent 2002;88:644–645.

28. Harper KA, Setchell DJ. The use of shimstock to assess occlusal contacts: A laboratory study. Int J Prosthodont 2002;15:347–352.

29. Noveri F. Elementi Storici Critici Filosofici Pratici di Gnatologia. Milan: Edi-Ermes, 1982.

30. Bruni A, Luzit R. Maggiore estetica nel settore cervicale. L'impianto-abutment individuale. Dental Labor 1998;1:19–29.

31. Hinds KF. Custom impression coping for an exact registration of the healed tissue in the esthetic implant restoration. Int J Periodontics Restorative Dent 1997;17:584–591.

32. Hochwald DA. Surgical template impression during stage 1 surgery for fabrication of a provisional restoration to be placed at stage 2 surgery. J Prosthet Dent 1991;66:796–798.

33. Dieterich J. Corona naturescente su monoimpianto con emergence profile. Dental Dialogue 2002;6:640–647.

34. Bengazi F, Wennstrom JL, Lekholm U. Recession of the soft tissue margin at oral implants: A 2-year longitudinal prospective study. Clin Oral Implants Res 1996;7:303–310.

35. Ekfeldt A, Eriksson A, Johansson LA. Peri-implant mucosal level on patients with implant-supported fixed prostheses: A 1-year follow-up study. Int J Prosthodont 2003;16:529–532.

36. Pagniano RP, Scheid RC, Clowson RL, Dagefoerde RO, Zardiackas LD. Linear dimensional change of acrylic resins used in the fabrication of custom trays. J Prosthet Dent 1982;47:279–283.

37. Valderhaug J, Floystrand F. Dimensional stability of elastomeric impression materials in custom-made and stock trays. J Prosthet Dent 1984;52:514–517.

38. Baker PS, Frazier KB. Water immersion procedure for making light-cured custom trays with wax spacers. J Prosthet Dent 1999;82:714–715.

39. Wirz J. L'importanza del portaimpronta individuale. La Quintessenza Odontotecnica 1999;16:489–497.

40. Takahashi Y, Chai J, Kawaguchi M. Equilibrium strengths of denture polymers subjected to long-term water immersion. Int J Prosthodont 1999;12:348–352.

41. Dixon DL, Breeding LC, Brown JS. The effect of custom tray material type and adhesive drying time on the tensile bond strength of an impression material/adhesive system. Int J Prosthodont 1994;7:129–133.

42. Peregrina A, Land MF, Wandling C, Johnston WM. The effect of different adhesives on vinyl polysiloxane bond strength to two tray materials. J Prosthet Dent 2005;94:209–213.

43. Huang FM, Tai KW, Hu CC, Chang YC. Cytotoxic effects of denture base materials on a permanent human oral epithelial cell line and on primary human oral fibroblasts in vitro. Int J Prosthodont 2001;14:439–443.

44. Campanha NH, Pavarina AC, Giampaolo ET, Machado AL, Carlos IZ, Vergani CE. Cytotoxicity of hard chairside reline resins: Effect of microwave irradiation and water bath postpolymerization treatments. Int J Prosthodont 2006;19:195–201.

45. Silva MM, Vergani CE, Giampaolo ET, Neppelenbroek KH, Spolidorio DM, Machado AL. Effectiveness of microwave irradiation on the disinfection of complete dentures. Int J Prosthodont 2006;19:288–293.

46. Vergani CE, Seo RS, Pavarina AC, dos Santos Nunes Reis JM. Flexural strength of autopolymerizing denture reline resins with microwave postpolymerization treatment. J Prosthet Dent 2005;93:577–583.

47. Witkowski S. (CAD-)/CAM in dental technology. Quintessence Dent Technol 2005;28:169–184.

48. Hegenbarth EA. Pilastri implantari individuali e sovrastrutture realizzati con tecniche di design computerizzato. Quintessence International 2000;11/12:377–387.

49. Andersson B, Taylor A, Lang BR, et al. Alumina ceramic implant abutments used for single-tooth replacement: A prospective 1- to 3-year multicenter study. Int J Prosthodont 2001;14:432–438.

50. Glauser R, Sailer I, Wohlwend A, Studer S, Schibli M, Scharer P. Experimental zirconia abutments for implant-supported single-tooth restorations in esthetically demanding regions: 4-year results of a prospective clinical study. Int J Prosthodont 2004;17:285–90.

51. Park SW, Driscoll CF, Romberg EE, Siegel S, Thompson G. Ceramic implant abutments: Cutting efficiency and resultant surface finish by diamond rotary cutting instruments. J Prosthet Dent 2006;95:444–449.

52. Sgrò S. Principles of the metal framework design in metal-ceramic reconstructions. Quintessence Dent Technol 2002;25:21–52.

53. Rufenacht CR. Principi di Estetica. Milan: Scienza e Tecnica Dentistica Edizioni Internazionali, 1992.

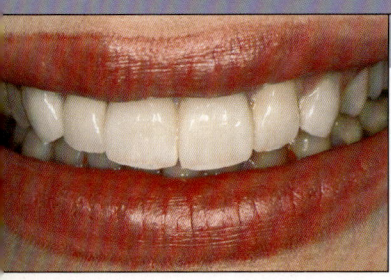

ESTHETIC RESTORATION OF THE ANTERIOR TEETH USING ALL-CERAMIC CROWNS

Lior Angelovici, DDS[1]
Maurizio Gualandri[1]

A 26-year-old female model presented with a disharmonic smile. The esthetics were unacceptable for her age and profession.

The treatment plan was to replace the porcelain-fused-to-metal crowns with all-ceramic crowns in order to create a more pleasing smile.

[1]Private practice, Rome, Italy.

Correspondence to: Dr Lior Angelovici, Via Frattina 35, Rome 00187, Italy. E-mail: drlior@yahoo.it

CASE PRESENTATION

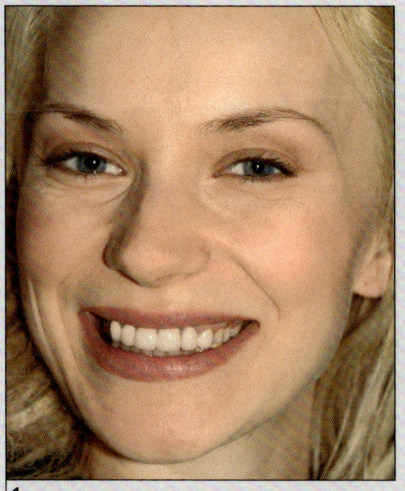

1a

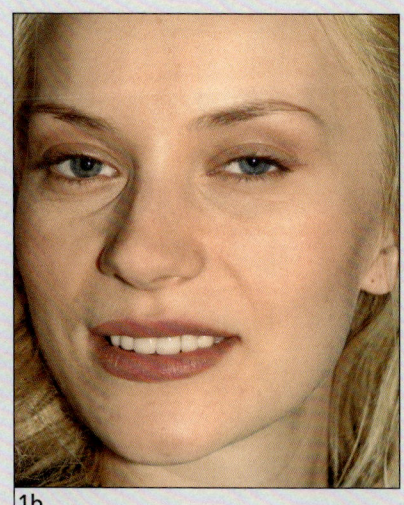

1b

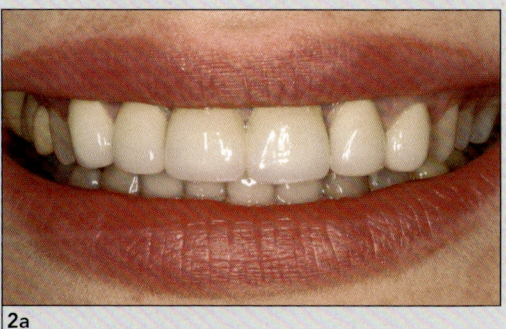

2a

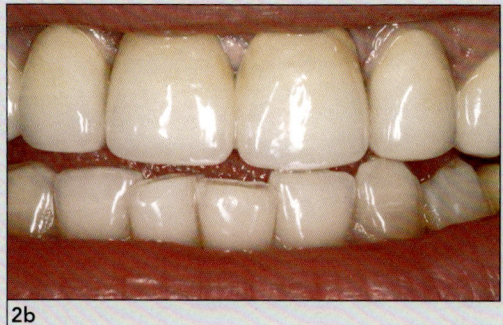

2b

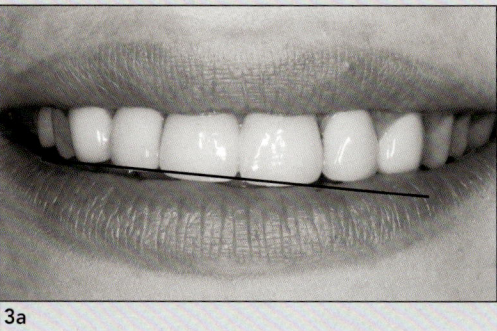

3a

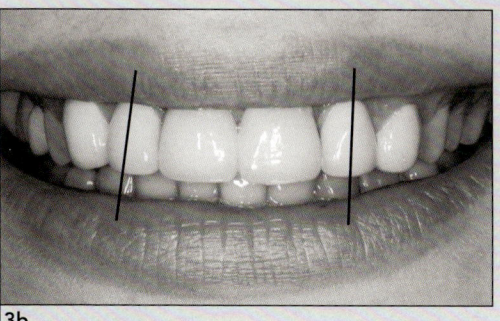

3b

Figs 1a and 1b Preoperative views. Note the disharmonic smile caused by the unsuitable color and shape of the porcelain-fused-to-metal crowns.

Figs 2a and 2b With the lips in the normal position, the gingiva showed a grayish appearance created by the color of the existing porcelain-fused-to-metal crowns.

Figs 3a and 3b The horizontal and sagittal lines show the disharmony of the shape and alignment of the teeth.

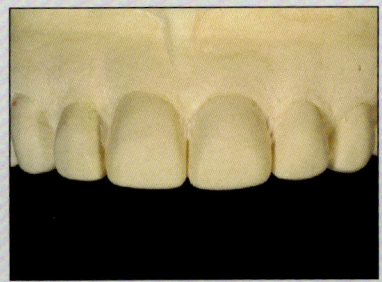

Fig 4 Study cast.

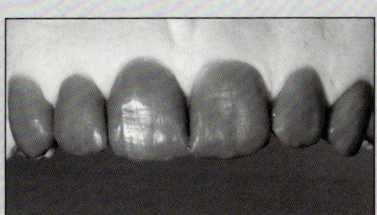

Figs 5a and 5b The diagnostic waxup demonstrates improved tooth form and texture.

Figs 6a and 6b Occlusal view of the existing restorations *(left)* versus the provisional restorations *(right)*. Note the difference in thickness.

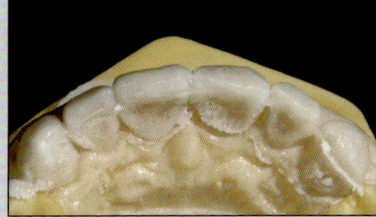

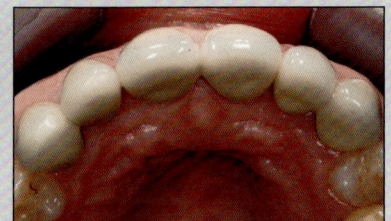

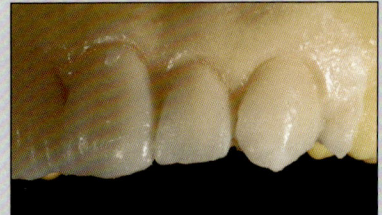

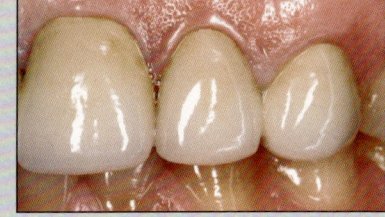

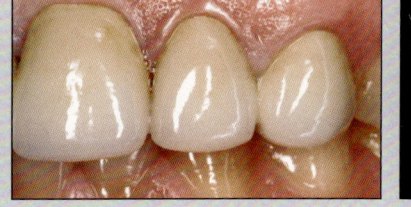

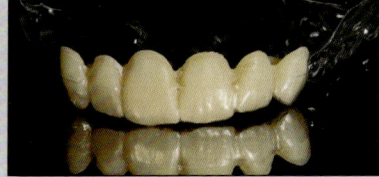

Figs 7a and 7b Lateral view of the preoperative situation *(left)* versus the provisional restorations *(right)*.

Fig 8 The provisionals with the vacuum-formed matrix.

Fig 9a to 9c After removing the porcelain-fused-to-metal crowns and placement of retraction cords, the preparations were completed.

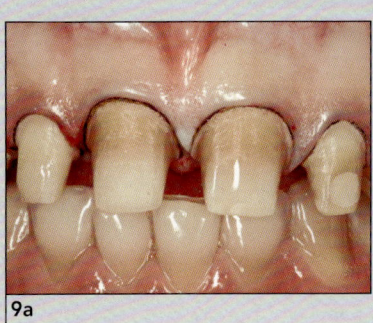

9a

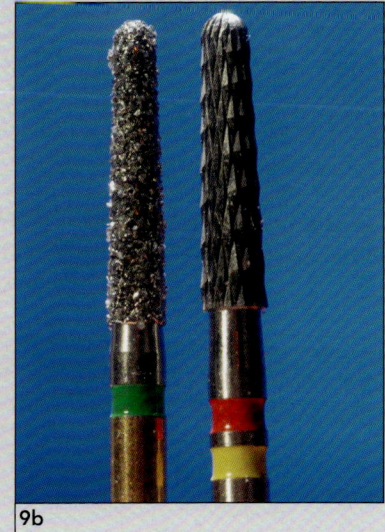

9b

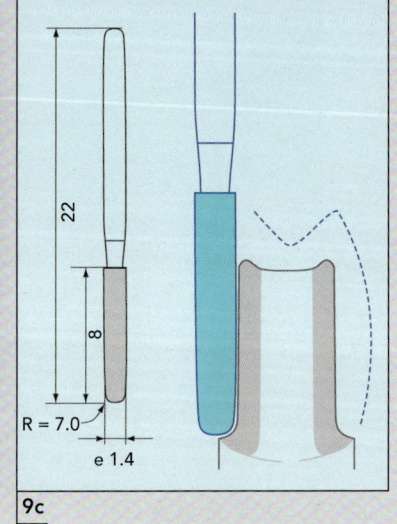

9c

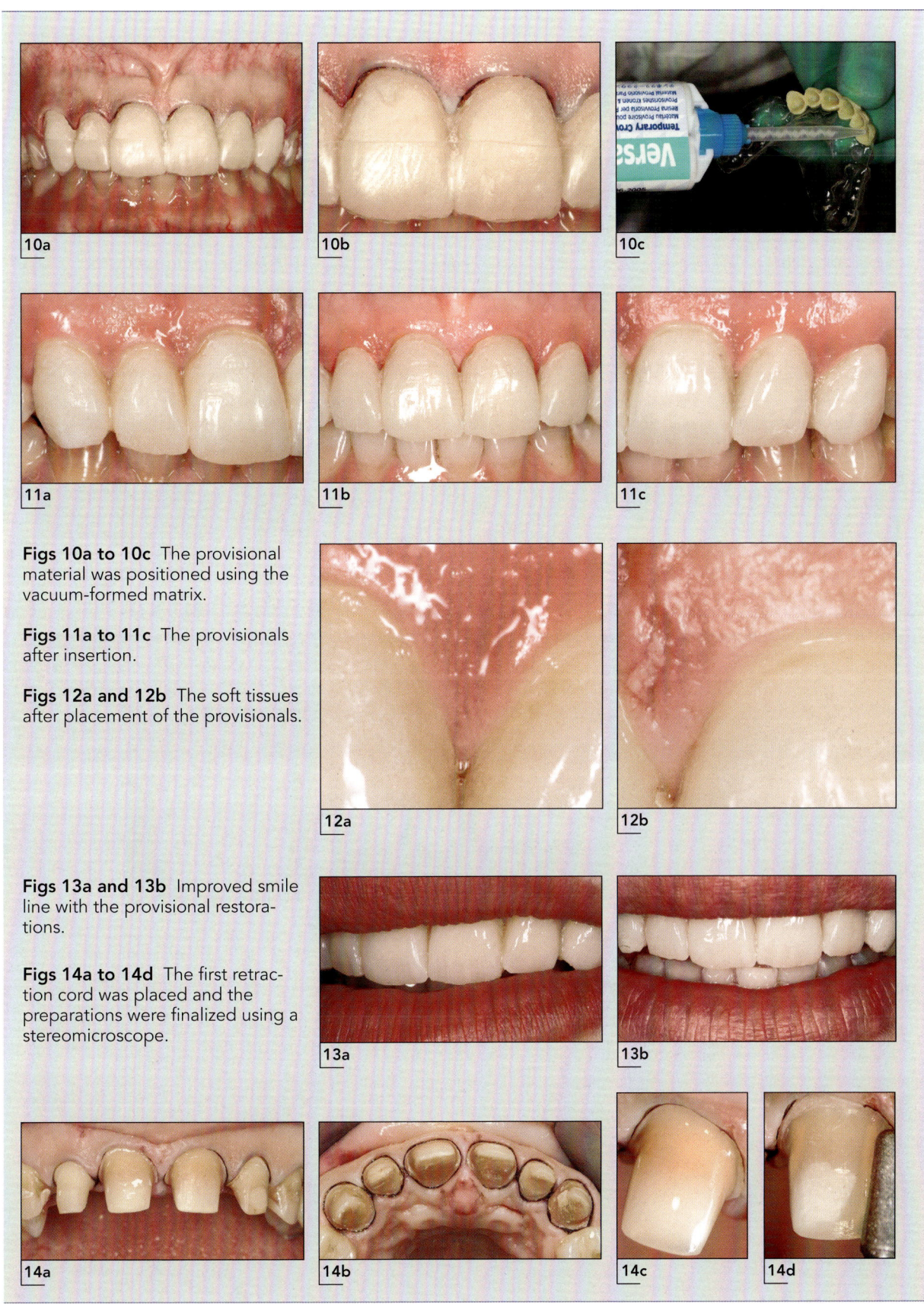

Figs 10a to 10c The provisional material was positioned using the vacuum-formed matrix.

Figs 11a to 11c The provisionals after insertion.

Figs 12a and 12b The soft tissues after placement of the provisionals.

Figs 13a and 13b Improved smile line with the provisional restorations.

Figs 14a to 14d The first retraction cord was placed and the preparations were finalized using a stereomicroscope.

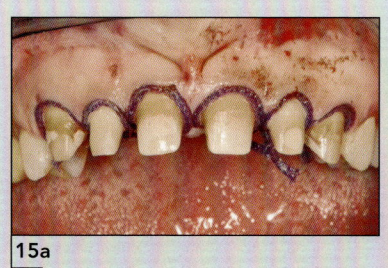
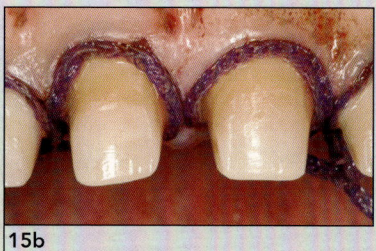
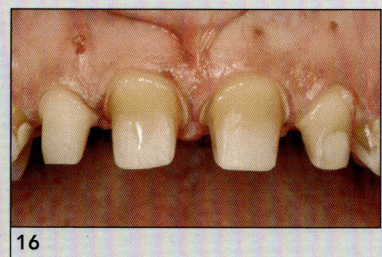

15a | 15b | 16

Figs 15a and 15b A second retraction cord was placed to facilitate fabrication of the final impression.

Fig 16 After removal of the impression material and first retraction cord, the harmonious shape of the gingiva could be observed because of the absence of bleeding.

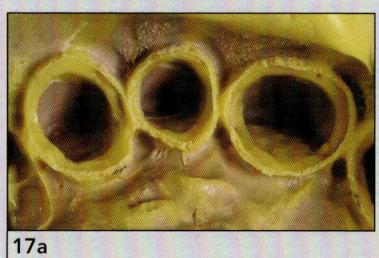
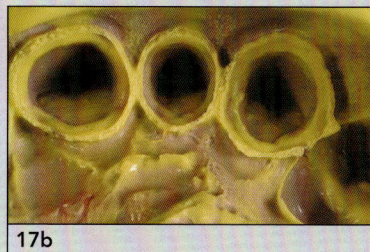
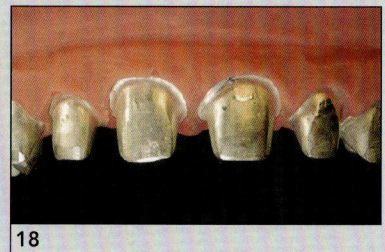

17a | 17b | 18

Figs 17a and 17b Closeup views of the final impressions.

Fig 18 The galvanic technique was used to fabricate a silver master cast, which offers good mechanical properties, stability, and hardness.

Figs 19a and 19b Try-in of ceramic copings. The shade of the coping should mask the color of the underlying tooth.

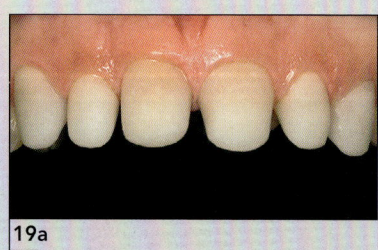
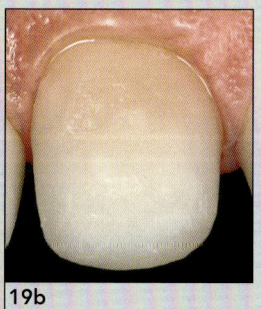

19a | 19b

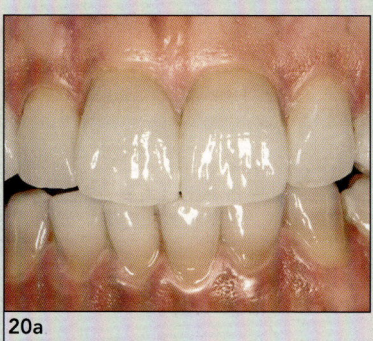
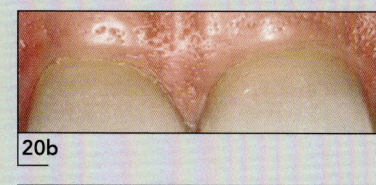
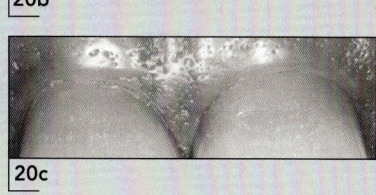
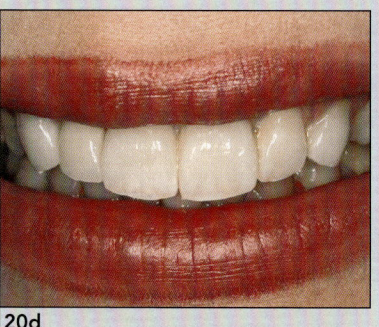

20a | 20b | 20c | 20d

Figs 20a to 20d The restored smile showed an improved smile line and no discoloration of the soft tissues.

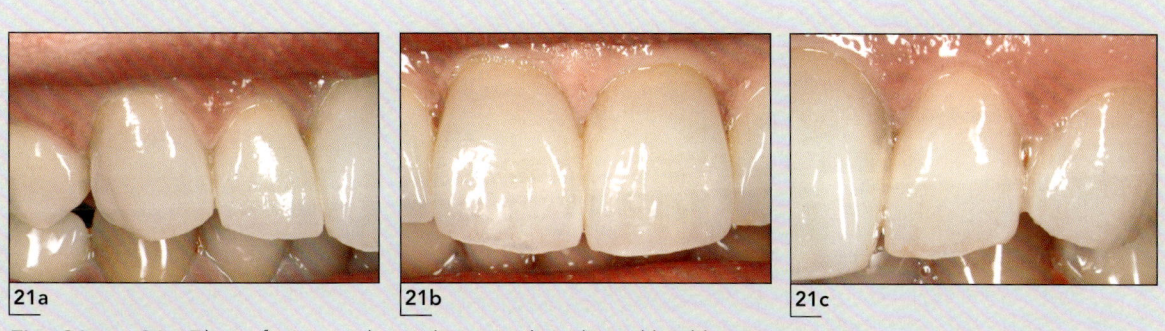

Figs 21a to 21c The soft tissues showed a natural, pink, and healthy appearance.

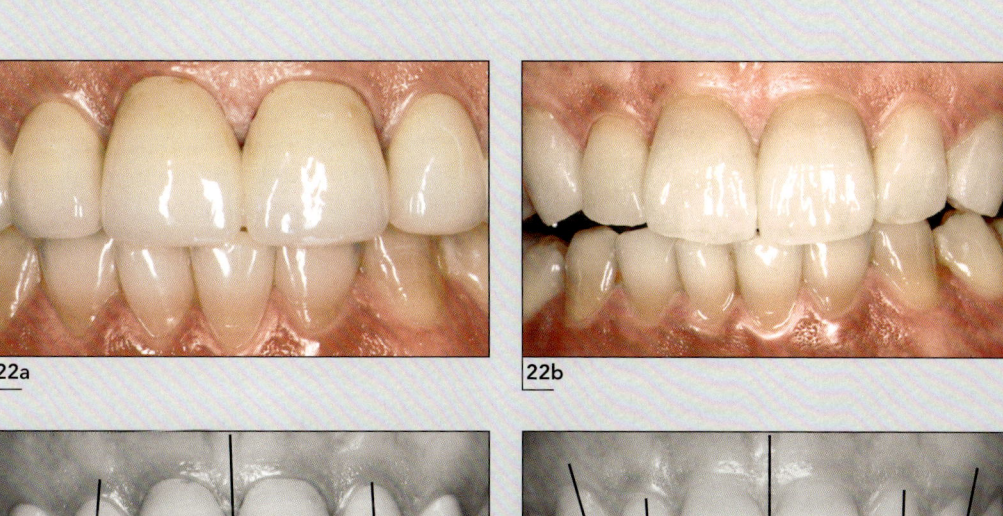

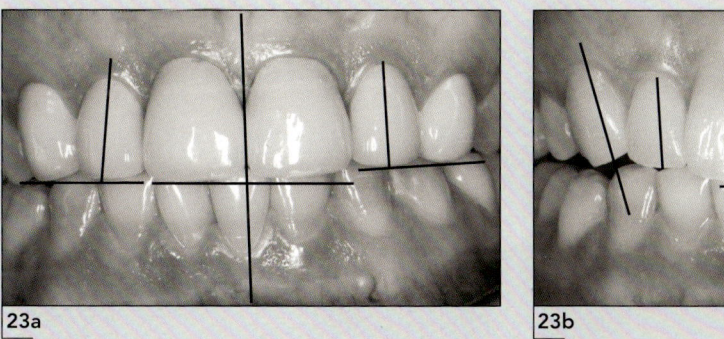
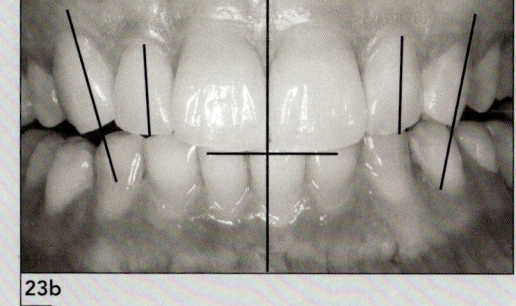

Figs 22a and 22b Preoperative (left) and postoperative (right) views.

Figs 23a and 23b Preoperative (left) and postoperative (right) views with the guidelines in place show the restored shape and alignment of the teeth.

Fig 24 Postoperative facial view.

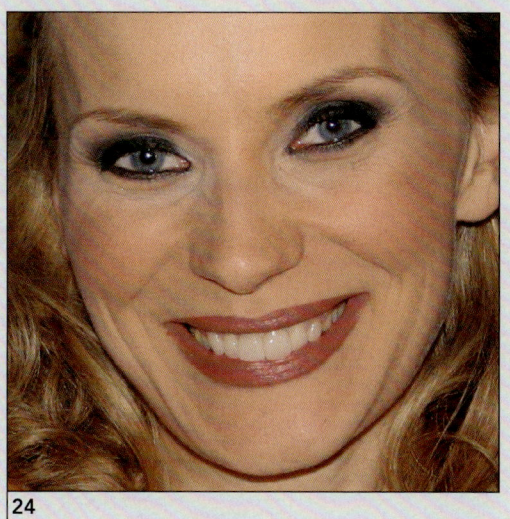

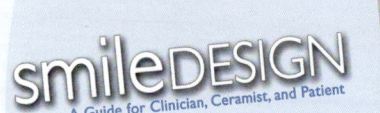
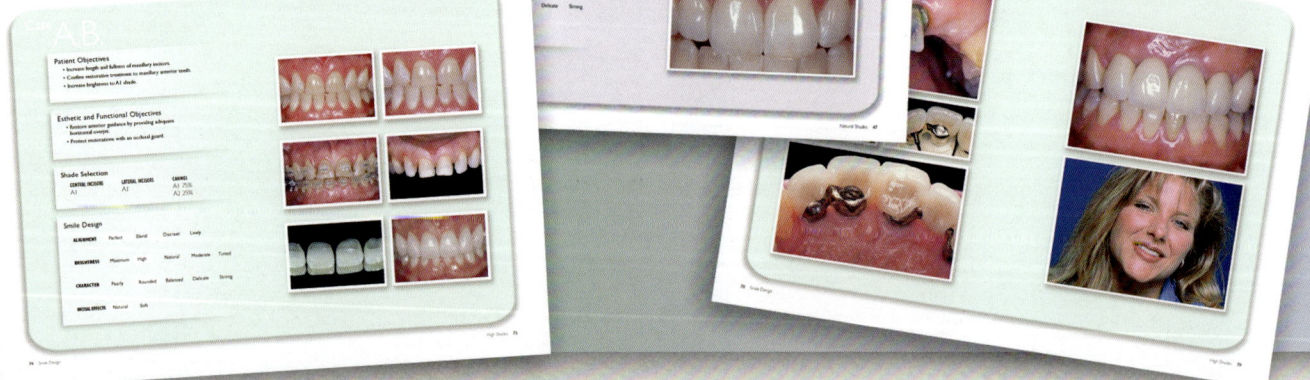
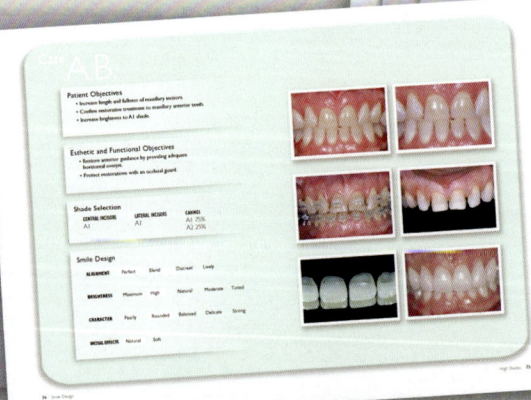
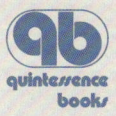

ESTHETICS COMPROMISED BY TOOTH WEAR: ETIOLOGY, DIAGNOSIS, MANAGEMENT, AND RESTORATION

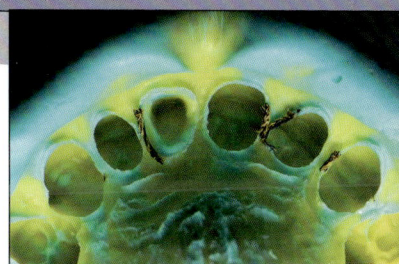

Irfan Ahmad, BDS[1]

In developed countries, infectious diseases such as caries and periodontitis are easily recognized and universally managed by established clinical protocols. However, at the dawn of a new century, the prevalence of an insidious, noninfectious dental "disease" is looming: tooth wear. *Tooth wear* is defined as a noncarious, irreversible loss of dentin and enamel, caused not by bacteria, but by a combination of factors. Tooth wear is a lesion in the waiting, presenting a twenty-first century clinical challenge[1] to a healthy and long-lasting dentition (Fig 1).

[1]Private practice, Middlesex, United Kingdom.

Correspondence to: Dr Irfan Ahmad, 173 The Ridgeway, North Harrow, Middlesex, HA2 7DF, United Kingdom. Fax: +44 020 8861 6181. E-mail: iahmadbds@aol.com

Unlike caries and periodontal disease, which compromise the survival of a tooth via a third party (bacteria), tooth wear is primarily the result of personal choices and habits, similar to smoking or alcohol abuse. The manifestations of wear are varied, ranging from innocuous cervical lesions to profound changes in tooth morphology, discoloration, fractures, cracks, sensitivity, and loss of vertical dimension of occlusion (VDO). In the anterior regions of the mouth, disfiguration and discoloration are esthetically unacceptable, and require intervention to restore the appearance of the smile and halt further degradation of the dentition (Fig 2). The purpose of this paper is to review the literature, demystify the terminology, and present the current thinking about tooth wear, including its etiology, diagnosis, and management. Finally, a case study will be presented, showing how lost tooth tissues can be treated to restore anterior esthetics (Fig 3).

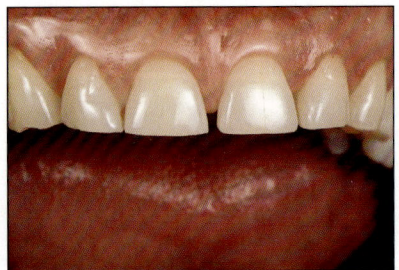

Fig 1 Tooth wear of the maxillary anterior sextant caused by noncarious enamel and dentin loss.

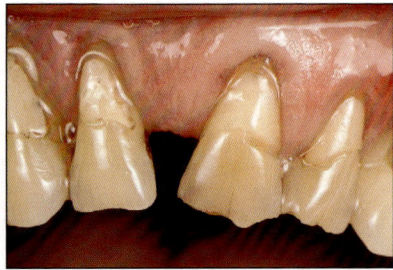

Fig 2 Severe tooth wear of maxillary anterior teeth, resulting in discoloration, disfigurement, and compromised esthetics.

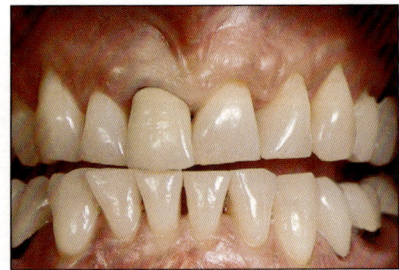

Fig 3 Three primary questions should be answered when handling cases of tooth wear: What is the cause? How should it be managed? Which treatment modality should be used?

ETIOLOGY

There are three ways that tooth substrate can be damaged or lost: caries, acute trauma, and wear. Noninfectious and nontraumatic tooth loss is attributed to four factors: erosion, abrasion, attrition, and abfraction. Before discussing pathogenesis, it is important to define the various terms used for describing different types of tooth wear. The commonly accepted terms are those just mentioned—*erosion*, *abrasion*, *attrition*, and *abfraction*—but obscure terminology, such as *tribology*, is perhaps more apt for describing the method of wear.[2] Tribology is the science of wear, lubrication, and friction, and is more descriptive of the mechanism of tooth loss.

Erosion is the loss of dental hard tissues by chemical means, eg, acidic drinks. *Abrasion* is the interaction between teeth and extraneous materials, eg, dentifrice. *Attrition* is tooth loss caused by tooth-to-tooth contact, eg, bruxism. *Abfraction* is a condition in which wedge-shaped lesions are formed at the buccocervical margins of the teeth. The etiology of tooth wear is multifactorial and rarely isolated to one specific cause. Usually, one factor dominates, and secondary factors interact to alter the clinical appearance. Furthermore, most of the evidence is derived from in vitro and in situ studies, since in vivo models are complicated by a myriad of variables. Thus, the etiology of tooth wear is circumstantial, rather than factual scientific evidence.

Erosion

The most common form of tooth wear is erosion, ie, the dissolution of enamel by intrinsic or extrinsic acids. Intrinsic acids are derived from the digestive tract, namely the stomach via the esophagus. Esophageal reflux is characterized by gastric acid emanating from the stomach and entering the esophagus (ie, heartburn), a relatively common occurrence after consumption of spicy and hot foods that is inconsequential to dental erosion.[3] However, with conditions such as acidic projectile vomiting, gastric contents pass beyond the upper esophageal sphincter and enter the oral cavity. This can be either spontaneous or deliberate, presenting in conditions such as rumination, anorexia nervosa, and bulimia.[4] Whatever the cause, the risk of erosion in the mouth is profound (Fig 4).

The second form of erosion is caused by extrinsic acids resulting from particular dietary preferences (effervescent drinks, acidic fruits, wine, vinegar, and pickles), or occupational hazards (industrial toxic fumes). It is important to note that the mode of ingestion is probably more destructive that the quantity of the offending agent.[5] Habits such as retaining carbonated drinks in the oral cavity before swallowing or mulling fruit between the posterior teeth are highly damaging. In addition, the erosive potential of titratable acid is also influenced by the frequency of intake.

Below the critical threshold of pH 5.5, decalcification of all dental hard tissues (enamel, dentin,

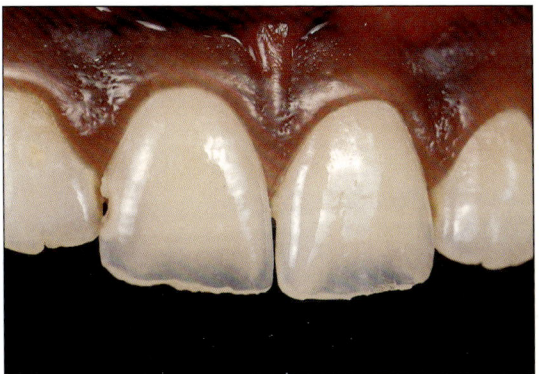

Fig 4 Thinning of the enamel at the incisal edges resulting from palatal erosion caused by gastric regurgitation.

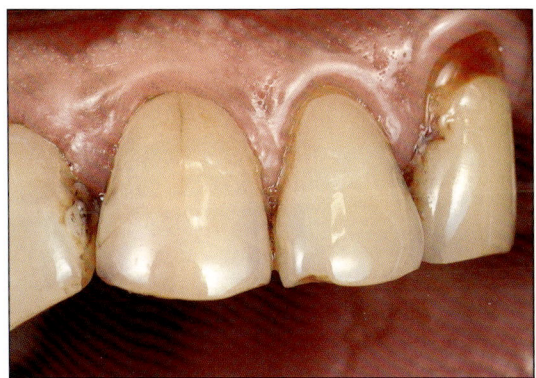

Fig 5 Enamel loss at the buccocervical region of the maxillary left canine, exposing underlying dentin.

and cementum) is evident.[6] Saliva modulates the erosive process through its buffering and clearing capacity and formation of a salivary pellicle, but is unable to prevent demineralization in the presence of continual acidic assaults.[7] Following acidic exposure, saliva has the potential to remineralize softened enamel after 4 to 6 hours,[8] but has little ability to protect dentin. Subsequent to enamel erosion, exposed dentin becomes vulnerable to acidic attack, forming a demineralized collagenous matrix, similar to a smear layer after cavity preparation with rotary instruments (Fig 5). The smear layer offers limited protection from further destruction and is readily lost by tooth brushing (even without dentifrice), leaving the exposed dentin susceptible to further attack.[9]

Abrasion

Refined contemporary diets are less fibrous and therefore have less abrasive potential than medieval diets, which caused extensive wear. Consequently, in developed countries, wear caused by abrasion is pathologic, requiring clinical intervention for prevention. Although tooth brushing is beneficial to oral health, it is also the major culprit of dental abrasion. Brushing alone, using a toothbrush with rounded bristles, causes little or no abrasion of enamel, and will result in only 1 mm

of tooth loss over 100 years.[10] But tooth wear is substantial in combination with abrasive dentifrices, especially those claiming to whiten teeth.[11] Tooth loss from toothbrush abrasion is dependent on frequency, duration, and the force of brushing strokes. In severe situations, patients who develop discoloration caused by toothbrush abrasion may enter into a viscious circle of events, with the belief that overzealous brushing will remove the stains, when in fact the opposite is true, as the worn enamel exposes the darker dentin layer.

Another serious concern regarding abrasion is tribochemical wear.[12] Tribochemical wear is erosion of 3 to 5 μm of the superficial enamel layer, termed *softening*,[13] making it more susceptible to mechanical forces of tooth brushing, food particles, and even tongue movements.

Attrition

Attrition is the physiologic wear of tooth structure as a result of tooth-to-tooth contact, as in mastication. Attrition may be nonphysiologic when caused by parafunctional activity, primarily bruxism. This is distinguished from physiologic bruxism, which is prevalent in the entire population. However, with parafunctional activity, the degree of bruxism becomes pathologic, resulting

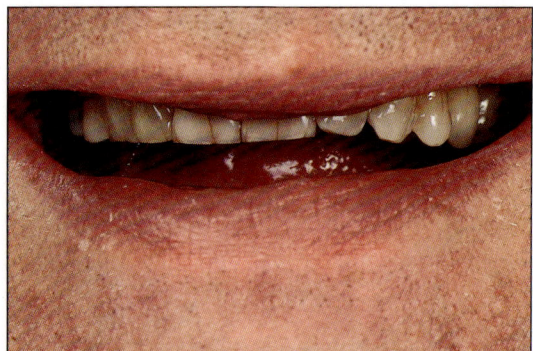

Fig 6 Shortened maxillary anterior teeth caused by pathologic bruxism.

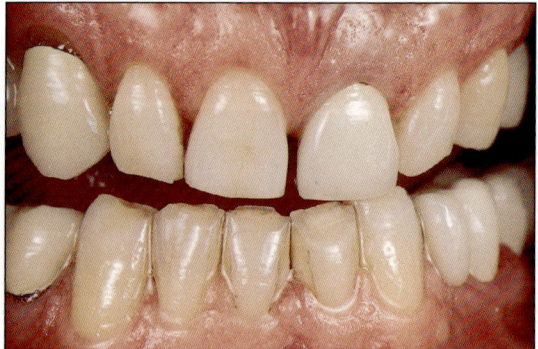

Fig 7 Pronounced incisal wear of the mandibular incisor caused by the porcelain palatal surface of the metal-ceramic crown on the maxillary left central incisor.

in abnormal amounts of tooth loss, which compromises esthetics if anterior teeth are involved (Fig 6). This is exacerbated if the opposing dentition has porcelain restorations, which may be highly abrasive and cause rapid loss of antagonist natural teeth (Fig 7). The etiology of bruxism is predominantly psychologic and stress related.[14] Generally, bruxists are high-strung, tense individuals, who concurrently perform heavy-handed brushing procedures that further accelerate tooth loss.

Abfraction

Abfraction is a theoretic fatigue concept defined as nonaxial tensile forces flexing the cusps at the dentinoenamel junction, resulting in bucco-cervical notches or wedges.[15] The reason for these lesions is that enamel is less capable of absorbing tensile forces compared to dentin. This means that under stress, enamel is more susceptible to abrasion and erosion, thus leaving the sensitive dentin exposed. Credence for this concept has been provided via finite element analysis,[16] with the observation that abfractions may be subgingival, thus eliminating causes such as toothbrush abrasion or acidic insult. However, recent documentation has questioned the existence and mechanism of abfraction lesions.[17]

Miscellaneous

Other esoteric causes of tooth loss are attributed to pipe smoking, playing musical wind instruments, snuff dipping, beetle nut chewing, occupational practices (eg, holding sewing needles between anterior teeth), pica[18] (eating nonfood substances, eg, soil, glass, paper clips, fingernails) and clandestine oral habits.

DIAGNOSIS

Accurate diagnosis requires taking a painstaking history and performing a detailed oral examination. In addition, study casts and photographs are essential to assess, monitor, and review tooth wear. The initial consultation should gauge the patient's symptoms (if any), oral hygiene procedures, lifestyle, and psychologic makeup. Most patients only seek dental advice when tooth wear is relatively advanced, with symptoms such as hypersensitivity, discoloration, or altered tooth morphology, particularly of the anterior teeth.

Tooth loss can potentially affect any tooth and any site on a tooth. A meticulous examination is crucial to note the location, quantity, and quality of wear, which provide clues to the predominant pathogenic agent. Plaster casts and photographs are essential documentation and diagnostic tools to assess findings and for differential diagnosis. A

Table 1 Differential Diagnosis of Tooth Wear[19]

| | Clinical findings | | | | Diagnosis | |
Affected teeth	Site of wear	Morphology of wear	Interdigitation of worn teeth	Loss of VDO	Primary factor	Secondary factor(s)
Maxillary anterior and posterior	Palatal surfaces	Amorphous and smooth, elevated amalgam restorations, cupping and cratering*	No	Possible†	Acidic regurgitation	—
Posterior, especially mandibular first molars	Occlusal surfaces	Sharp enamel edges	No	Possible	Effervescent drinks	—
Maxillary and mandibular posterior	Occlusal surfaces	Abraded enamel edges, cupping and cratering	Yes	Possible	Acidic fruits	—
Anterior and posterior	Buccal surfaces of mandibular canines and premolars	Faded anatomic detail, smooth and polished dental restorations	No	Possible†	Abrasion	—
Anterior and posterior	Buccal surfaces of mandibular canines and premolars	Faded anatomical detail, smooth and polished dental restorations, cupping and cratering	No	Possible†	Dentifrice abuse	Erosion
Anterior and posterior	Buccocervical	Smooth saucer shaped	No	No	Toothbrush abrasion	Gingival recession‡
Anterior and posterior	Buccocervical	Wedge shaped	No	No	Abfraction	Gingival recession‡
Anterior and posterior	Incisal edges and occlusal surfaces	Flat	Yes	Yes¶	Bruxism#	—
Anterior and posterior	Incisal edges and occlusal surfaces§	Cupping and cratering	Yes	Yes¶	Bruxism#	Abrasion/erosion
Specific tooth	Unique wear	Any	Possible	Possible†	Miscellaneous	Miscellaneous

*Stained surfaces indicate a previous episode of regurgitation, while stain-free surfaces indicate an active condition.
†If occlusal surfaces are involved.
‡Sensitivity is a common symptom.
§In Angle Class III occlusion, wear may be evident on facial surfaces of maxillary teeth. With an anterior open bite, the wear is limited to the posterior teeth.
¶Check for alveolar compensation by the location of the cementoenamel junction of worn teeth.
#Masseteric hypertrophy is possible.

useful method of differential diagnosis of wear has been proposed using pathognomonic wear patterns on plaster casts of worn dentitions. As previously stated, tooth wear is multifactorial and often presents as an interaction of various causes. Further, patients are usually oblivious to wear until symptoms appear or discoloration and morphologic changes are bought to their attention. Thus, the clinical manifestation is likely to be the result of combined causes, often masking the initial causative agent or habit. Nevertheless, as a starting point, and to ascertain the predominant causative factor, pathognomonic wear patterns are helpful for clinical diagnosis (Table 1).[19]

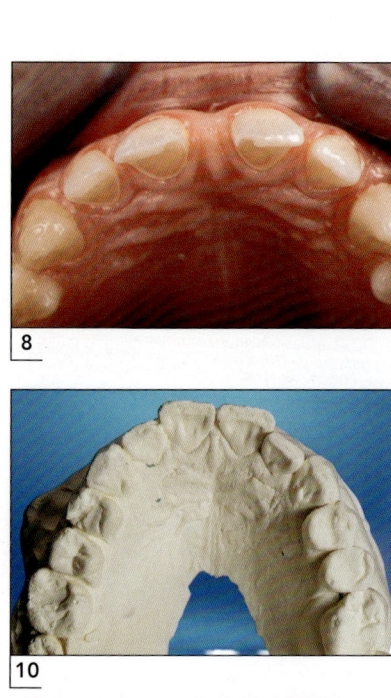

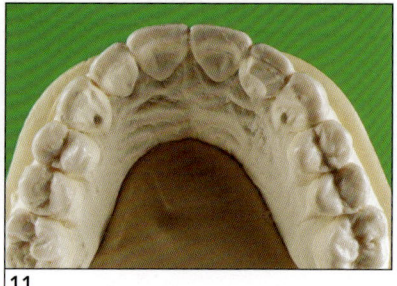

Fig 8 Erosion of the palatal surfaces of maxillary anterior teeth caused by intrinsic acidic erosion.

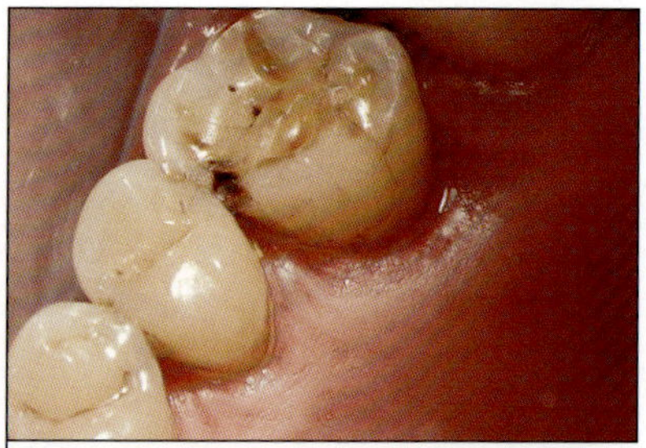

Fig 9 Cupping and cratering on the occlusal and palatal surfaces of the maxillary first molar caused by acidic erosion.

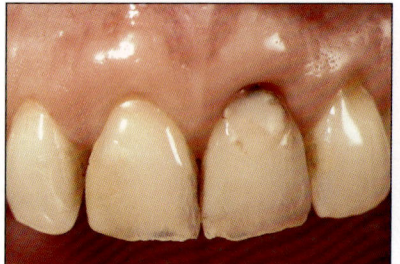

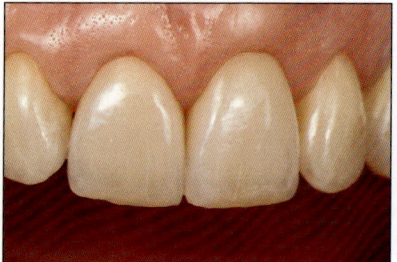

Fig 10 Pretreatment cast showing abraded, smooth occlusal wear patterns of the maxillary arch. The patient reported a history of fruit mulling.

Fig 11 Diagnostic waxup showing the amount of occlusal buildup necessary to restore function.

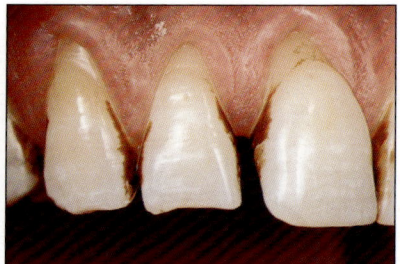

Fig 12 Dentifrice abuse has caused wear on the facial surfaces of the maxillary incisors.

Fig 13 Esthetics are restored with all-ceramic crowns and porcelain laminate veneers. (Ceramics by Willi Geller, Zurich, Switzerland.)

Fig 14 Gingival recession caused by toothbrush abrasion, exposing vulnerable dentin to dentifrice abuse and acidic erosion.

Erosion

Intrinsic acidic erosion caused by gastric regurgitation presents as dissolution of the palatal surfaces (predominantly) of the maxillary teeth (Figs 8 and 9), combined with elevated amalgam restorations. The mandibular teeth escape wear because of the protection of the tongue. Extrinsic erosion patterns depend on the type of acidic foodstuff, ie, effervescent drinks, wines, salad dressings, vinegar, or acidic fruits (lemons, limes, oranges, or tomatoes).[20] With acidic drinks, wear is limited to the posterior teeth, especially the mandibular molars, which display sharp enamel edges, while the anterior mandibular teeth remain unaffected. With acidic fruits, the pattern of loss is equally evident on the posterior maxillary and mandibular teeth because of the horizontal grinding of fruit pulp, similar to herbivores (Figs 10 and 11). Unlike acidic drinks, the enamel edges are not sharp, but are abraded by the grinding action, which differentiates this type of erosion from those mentioned above.

Abrasion

The main culprit of abrasion is dentifrice abuse. Clinically, this presents as faded anatomy of the buccal surfaces, which may or may not include the

Fig 15 Cupping and cratering on the incisal surfaces of the mandibular incisors and canines.

Fig 16 Interdigitation of worn anterior teeth, with a loss of VDO.

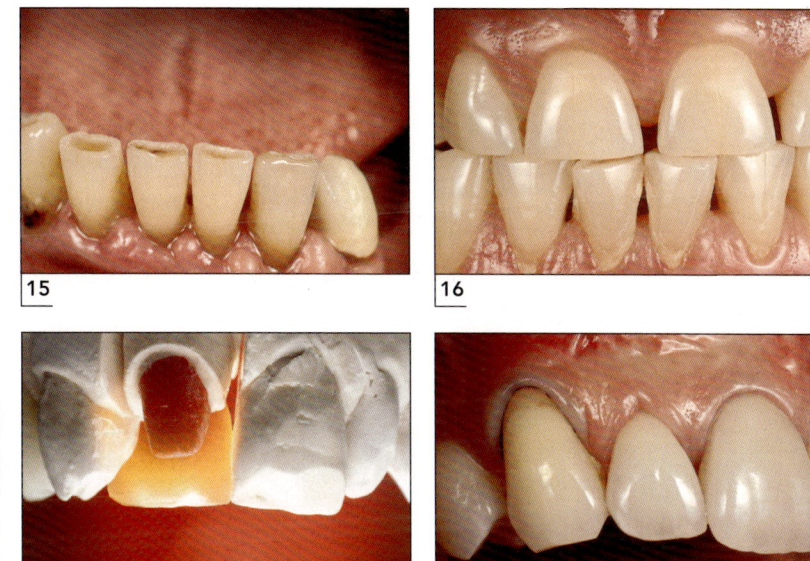

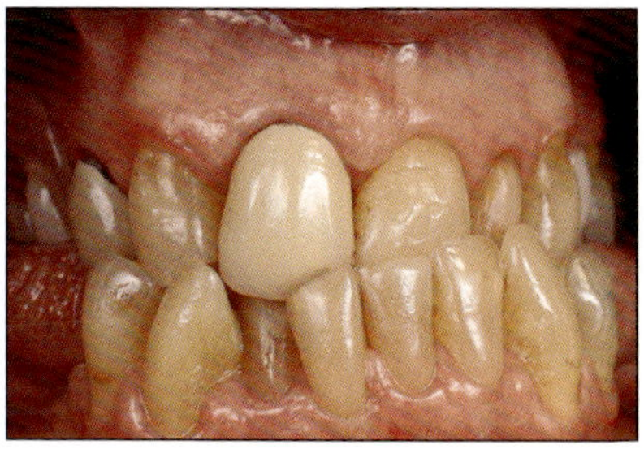

Figs 17 and 18 Angle Class III occlusion showing wear on the facial surfaces of the maxillary anterior teeth. The defective metal-ceramic crown on the right maxillary central incisor was replaced with an all-ceramic crown using low-abrasive veneering porcelain.

Fig 19 Buccocervical abfraction lesion on the maxillary canine, which clicks against the fingernail.

cervical areas. Dental restorations, especially amalgam, appear polished and shiny, and if occlusal surfaces are involved, loss of VDO is evident. In the presence of secondary erosive factors, cupping and cratering are also visible.

It is important to distinguish between toothbrush abrasion and dentifrice abuse, which are usually grouped together as toothbrush abrasion. Dentifrice abuse can affect any tooth surface regardless of the type of toothbrush (Figs 12 and 13). Conversely, toothbrush abrasion results from brushes with firm nonrounded bristles, leading to gingival recession and exposed dentin, which is subsequently susceptible to dentifrice abuse or acidic erosion (Fig 14).[21]

Attrition

Pathologic bruxism is usually associated with incisal wear of the maxillary and mandibular anterior teeth. The latter is often overlaid with cupping and cratering caused by secondary factors such as dentifrice abuse. Cups and craters are formed as a result of initial enamel loss that exposes the softer

dentin, which wears faster than the peripheral enamel because of subsequent abrasion or erosion (Fig 15). The wear facets of opposing teeth coincide, and there may be a reduction in VDO (Fig 16). Furthermore, because of adaptive alveolar compensation by overeruption,[22] worn teeth interdigitate, leaving no space for restorative materials to replace the lost tooth substrate. In Angle Class III occlusion, wear may be evident on the facial surfaces of maxillary teeth (Figs 17 and 18), and with an anterior open bite, wear is limited to the posterior teeth.

Abfraction

The typically recognized abfraction lesion is a wedge-shaped cervical enamel notch with sharp line angles. A readily distinguishing characteristic is that the buccocervical lesion clicks against the fingernail (Fig 19). In isolation, abfraction is readily differentiated from the smooth cervical saucer-shaped lesions of abrasion and/or gingival recession. In addition, abfraction lesions may also occur without gingival recession.

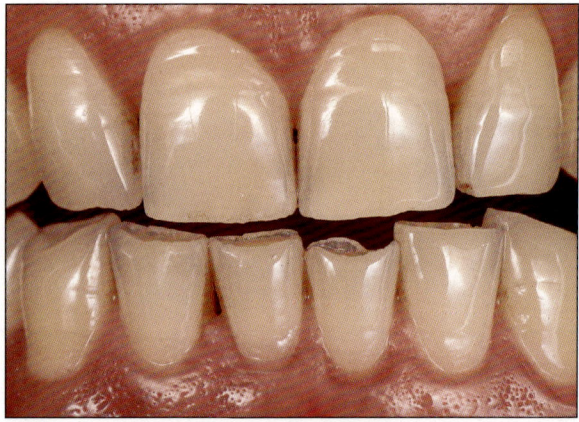

Fig 20 A history of retaining and sucking lemons with the anterior teeth resulted in incisal wear of the mandibular teeth.

MANAGEMENT

The three main strategies of management are counseling for prevention, periodic recalls for monitoring, and clinical intervention for replacing or repairing lost tooth structure.

Prevention depends on the cause of wear. The clinical picture is usually unclear regarding the particular type of wear. Consequently, combined with clinical findings, differential diagnosis is heavily dependent on an accurate history to elucidate the primary cause. If the primary etiologic factor is determined, preventive advice is straightforward. However, in certain circumstances, the patient is reticent to disclose his or her medical history or specific habits. For example, bulimia is perceived as a social stigma, and the individual may avoid admitting this medical condition. In these situations, the clinician is completely reliant on intraoral findings and a sympathetic approach to gain a confession. In extreme cases, referral to a psychologist may be the only option.

If the cause of erosion is from an extrinsic source, providing dietary advice involves a pragmatic, rather than a dogmatic, approach. Dietary advice should be aimed at modifying, as opposed to stopping, a given habit, because a judgmental approach is frequently ignored and ineffective. It is best to provide a simple explanation that focuses on the benefits of modifying a given lifestyle. These modifications include reducing the quantity, timing, and method of ingestion of an offending food or drink. Since the rate of salivary flow is reduced during sleep (thus reducing its buffering capabilities), consuming acidic products before sleeping is particularly damaging. Chilled rather than frozen acidic drinks are the least harmful, while warm or hot formulations elevate enamel dissolution.[23] Similarly, acidic fruits, which are part of a balanced healthy diet, should not be discouraged, but should be consumed rapidly to minimize contact with the dentition (Fig 20). In addition, eating alkaline foods, such as cheese or chewing gum, to encourage saliva production after an acidic meal helps neutralize acidity. Since recent research has revealed that acid softens the surface enamel, brushing immediately after a meal should be discouraged. Instead, brushing should be performed before a meal or several hours afterward, to allow the buffering capacity of saliva to take effect. In cases of xerostomia caused by antidepressants and tranquilizers or Sjogren disease, measurement of salivary flow rate is indicated with a prescription for saliva-stimulating lozenges. For erosion from an intrinsic source, appropriate steps include referral for social counseling or to a gastroenterologist for further tests and antireflux and antacid medication.

Abrasion lesions dictate the use of a round-ended soft-bristle toothbrush with a low-abrasive dentifrice. High fluoride–content dentifrices may also be effective against erosion and abrasion via hardening, rather than by remineralizing the surface enamel.[24] With continual use, a new dentifrice, Sensodyne Pronamel (GSK, Middlesex, United Kingdom), claims to microharden softened surface enamel, thereby making it resistant to further acidic attack.[25]

Bruxism is stress related and therefore requires patients to consider lifestyles changes, which may or may not be feasible. Nocturnal guards or splints are useful for protecting worn dentitions (from abraded natural or porcelain surface antagonists), and help to break parafunctional habits. However, if erosion is the suspected cause, splints have no therapeutic value.

Looking to the future, a recent breakthrough has used nanotechnology, via a hydrothermal method, to create synthetic enamel for coating engineering components subjected to excessive wear and tear. The researchers are now developing thicker apatite blocks, which could one day be used as veneers to replace lost enamel caused by tooth wear, caries, or traumatic injuries.[26]

RESTORATION

Whatever the etiology, if clinical intervention is necessary it should be implemented at the earliest possible stages of wear to prevent future esthetic or functional deterioration, and preventative advice must be given and followed.

The type of restorative therapy may be minimal or extensive. The complexity of treatment is determined by the extent of tooth loss. For innocuous wear such as buccocervical lesions, use of a dentin-bonding agent may suffice to stop hypersensitivity by hybridization. While the alleviating properties of dentin-bonding agents are ephemeral, requiring periodic applications, this treatment modality is desirable for its minimal intervention approach.[27]

If restorations are necessary, minimally invasive protocols are mandatory to preserve an already compromised dentition. The durability of a restoration is determined by the choice of material, type of tooth, site on the tooth, amount of tooth loss, and occlusal and esthetic considerations. The materials available are glass ionomers, resin composites, indirect ceramic laminates or onlays, and full-coverage crowns. Since tooth wear is a chemicomechanical process, a restorative material should exhibit properties to resist both chemical and mechanical challenges, particularly in circumstances in which preventative measures are ineffective and wear is continuing.

Glass ionomers are an ideal choice for wear lesions, particularly buccocervical lesions, because of their adhesive and noninvasive potential. However, glass ionomers are mechanically weak and hydrophilic, which makes them vulnerable in an acidic or load-bearing environment compared to composites.[28] Therefore, glass ionomers are suited for areas of minimal load and in which acidic erosion is controlled by preventative measures. Resin composites, in combination with dentin-bonding agents, also offer a minimal approach, but are technique sensitive. Although mechanically superior to glass ionomers, resin composites suffer from polymerization shrinkage, and are also prone to degradation than can lead to microleakage and discoloration.

In situations in which substantial tooth loss has caused profound discoloration, anatomic deformity, and diminished VDO, ceramics are indicated for superior esthetics and mechanical resilience. Nevertheless, caution is still necessary in cases of ongoing bruxism, which can result in catastrophic fractures of the brittle porcelain on incisal and occlusal surfaces. For extensive oral rehabilitation involving alveolar compensation, space for ceramics is created by orthodontic means using Dahl appliances. This avoids extensive provision of crowns on posterior teeth (if unaffected) to raise the VDO for creating adequate clearance for anterior restorations.

The type of ceramic coverage depends on the amount of tooth to be replaced, occlusal load, and structural integrity of the remaining tooth. Porcelain laminate veneers and onlays are the preferred choice, as they require minimal or no tooth removal and are highly esthetic; however, they are also clinically demanding. If structural or pulpal integrity is in question, the only option is full-coverage crowns, possibly preceded by endodontic therapy. Full-coverage crowns may be either all-ceramic or metal-ceramic. All-ceramic units show superior esthetics, and the newer systems using alumina and zirconia as a substructure offer enhanced mechanical properties. For unabated bruxism, prescribing porcelain on occlusal or incisal surfaces usually predisposes to fractures and may accelerate wear of opposing natural teeth. To mitigate this scenario, the use of metal-ceramic units with gold occlusal or incisal surfaces is a prudent alternative. Table 2 summarized the advantages and limitations of various restorative materials.

Table 2 Restorative Options for Restoring the Worn Dentition

Treatment	Advantage	Disadvantage
Splint	Minimally invasive, allow assessment without restorative intervention	Poor patient compliance
Dentin-bonding agent	Minimally invasive, alleviate sensitivity	Ephemeral
Glass ionomer	Minimally invasive, adhesion to dentin	Poor mechanical and physical properties, crack formation, poor esthetics
Resin composite	Superior esthetic and mechanical properties	Microleakage, technique sensitive, degradation over time
Ceramic onlay	Esthetic, conservative compared to full coverage	Poor bonding potential in presence of sclerotic dentin, invasive, technique sensitive, vulnerable to high occlusal loads
Porcelain laminate veneer	Esthetic, conservative compared to full coverage	Poor bonding potential in presence of sclerotic dentin, invasive, technique sensitive, vulnerable to high occlusal loads, requires fabrication by skilled ceramist, increased cost
All-ceramic crowns	Esthetic, increased strength with alumina or zirconia substructures	Invasive, vulnerable to high occlusal loads (bruxism), requires fabrication by skilled ceramist, increased cost
Metal-ceramic crowns	Mechanically resilient	Invasive, reduced esthetics, vulnerable to high occlusal loads with porcelain coverage on incisal/occlusal surfaces, increased cost
Full-metal crowns	Useful for palatal surfaces in Angle Class II occlusion or continuing bruxism, minimal wear of antagonist natural teeth	Poor esthetics, invasive

CASE REPORT

The following clinical study depicts a woman in her late thirties with multifactorial tooth wear. The desire of the patient was to improve the anterior esthetics compromised by tooth loss. In addition, she requested elimination of sensitivity, whiter and brighter teeth, and the prevention of any further deterioration of her dentition (Figs 21 and 22).

The dental history revealed the etiology of tooth wear caused by anorexia nervosa, bruxism, and toothbrush abrasion (Figs 23 and 24). Besides the obvious incisal wear of the anterior teeth, defective metal-ceramic crowns were evident posteriorly. The maxillary right central incisor had a defective metal-ceramic crown, supported by a cast metal post and core. In addition, the patient was

highly strung with a vigorous tooth-brushing habit using abrasive whitening dentifrice, which caused buccocervical lesions on numerous teeth. This resulted in hypersensitivity, exacerbated by a home bleaching regime with hydrogen peroxide.

Diagnosis was confirmed following an oral examination, photographs, and study casts. Attrition was evident on the anterior teeth, while the buccocervical enamel loss was attributed to toothbrush abrasion and dentifrice abuse.

The first therapeutic phase of tooth wear is management by counseling and preventive advice to stop further damage. In this case, the patient's oral hygiene regime was modified by recommending the use of a soft toothbrush with a low-abrasive, high fluoride–content dentifrice. The medical history confirmed cessation of anorexia nervosa, but a night

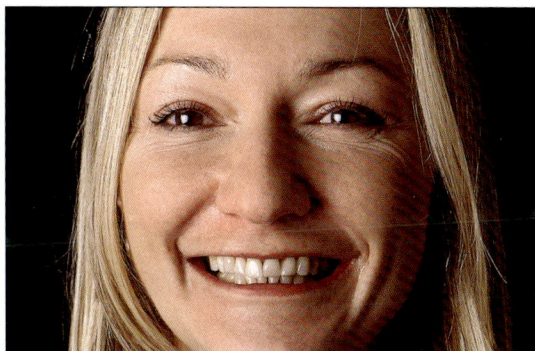

Fig 21 Preoperative facial view of the patient showing compromised anterior esthetics caused by tooth wear.

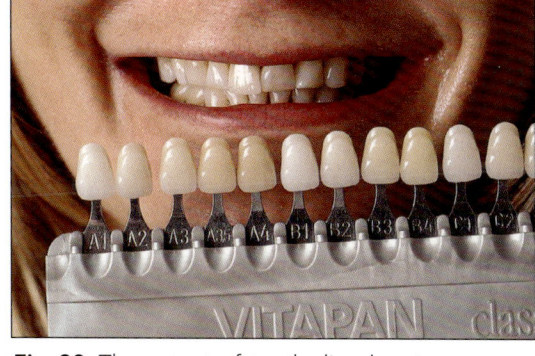

Fig 22 The extent of tooth discoloration was assessed using the Classic Vita shade guide as a reference.

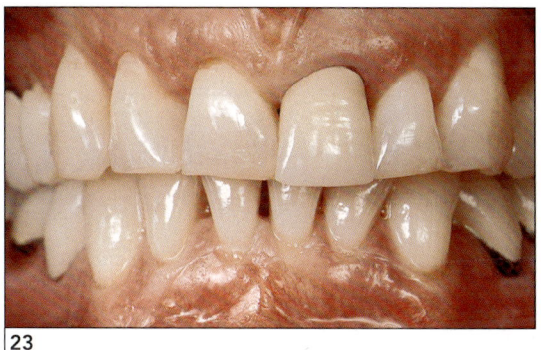

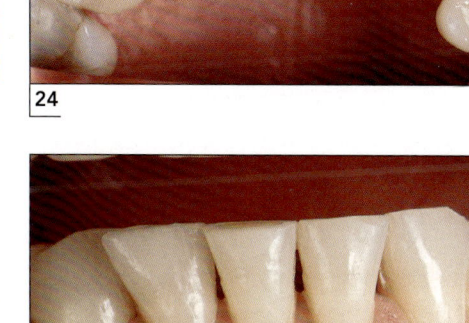

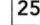

Fig 23 Multifactorial tooth wear caused by bruxism, toothbrush abrasion, and dentifrice abuse (facial view).

Fig 24 Multifactorial tooth wear caused by bruxism, toothbrush abrasion, and dentifrice abuse (occlusal view).

Fig 25 Restoration of the buccocervical abrasion lesions of the mandibular anterior teeth with resin composite fillings.

guard was advised following restorative therapy to protect the artificial prostheses. Finally, home bleaching was discouraged to mitigate sensitivity.

The next step was deciding on the type of restoration for improving the color and form of the worn dentition. Although incisal wear had contributed to loss of VDO, the amount was inconsequential and did not require extensive rehabilitation beyond replacing the posterior defective crowns. In addition, during smiling, the mandibular lip concealed attrition of the mandibular anterior teeth, and therefore monitoring was suggested at this stage rather than rebuilding the worn incisal edges. The only treatment necessary for the mandibular anterior teeth was restoration of the buccocervical lesions. A resin composite (HFO Enamel Plus, Optident, West Yorkshire, United Kingdom) was chosen for superior esthetic, optical (especially fluorescence), and mechanical properties compared to glass ionomer (Fig 25). Furthermore, if compliance with the recommended oral hygiene procedures was poor, resin composite fillings are more resilient and less likely to be abraded by toothbrush abrasion or dentifrice abuse.

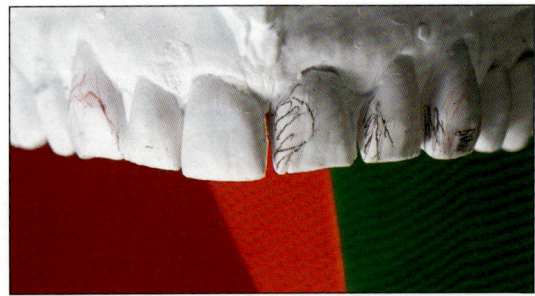

Fig 26 Preoperative plaster cast for fabricating an indirect resin composite mockup of the maxillary anterior sextant.

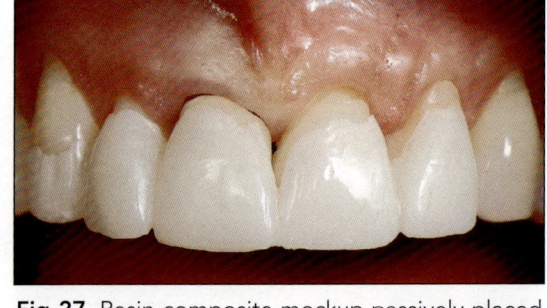

Fig 27 Resin composite mockup passively placed on the anterior maxillary teeth. Although the shape and alignment were satisfactory, the color was excessively bright (facial view).

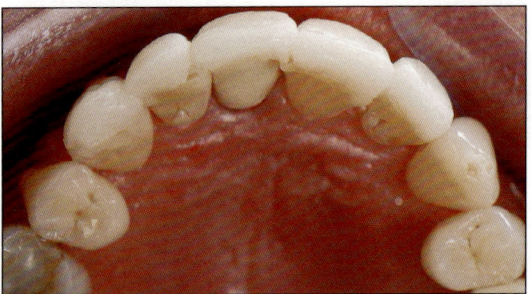

Fig 28 Resin composite mockup passively placed on anterior maxillary teeth (occlusal view).

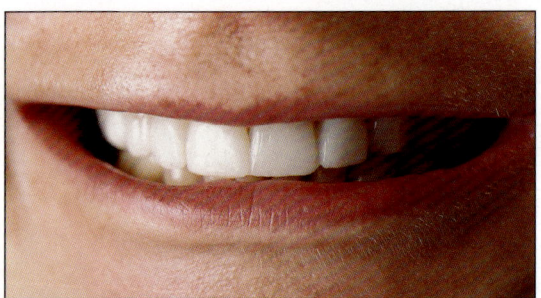

Fig 29 Dentofacial view with resin composite mockup to assess the incisal edge position (and degree of tooth exposure) of the maxillary incisors during smiling.

The primary factor contributing to the poor maxillary anterior esthetics was incisal edge wear of the anterior sextant and premolars, resulting in an erratic incisal plane, discoloration, flat incisal embrasures, and large width/length ratios. In addition, enamel loss was also evident at the buccocervical regions of the maxillary anterior teeth. The choice of materials for replacing the lost tooth substrate was either resin composite or porcelain laminate veneers.

The least invasive approach is resin composite fillings for the buccocervical lesions, followed by bleaching to improve color and resin composite fillings to improve incisal morphology. The disadvantage of this approach is that, although resin composite fillings are satisfactory cervically, they are clinically challenging and offer less latitude when restoring tooth morphology, especially at the incisal edges. Furthermore, fillings are prone to staining, discoloration, and periodic replacement. Another concern with fillings at the incisal

edges is that they may be prone to occlusal stress during protrusive excursions. The second, more extensive treatment option is porcelain laminate veneers, which are also technique sensitive, but offer superior esthetics and longevity, obviate the need for buccocervical resin composite fillings, and offer greater latitude for restoring tooth morphology. In addition, a replacement crown on the right central incisor will eliminate the buccomesial imbrication.

The two options were presented to the patient, and she opted for the porcelain laminate veneers with a crown on the right central incisor. Before commencing tooth preparation, it is essential to either carry out a diagnostic waxup or a composite mockup to assess shape, color, alignment, and tooth exposure (incisal edge position) in relation to the maxillary lip at rest and during smiling (Figs 26 to 29). Both of these approaches allow patient interaction and can be used for fabricating a silicone guide for intraoral tooth preparation.

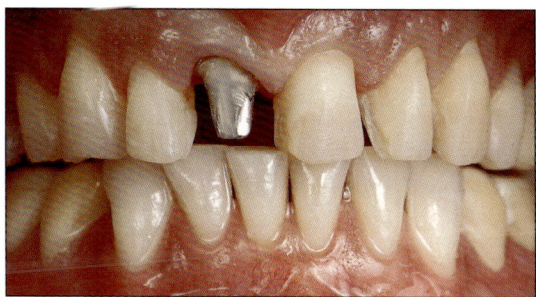

Fig 30 When possible, tooth preparations for the porcelain laminate veneers on the maxillary teeth were confined to enamel.

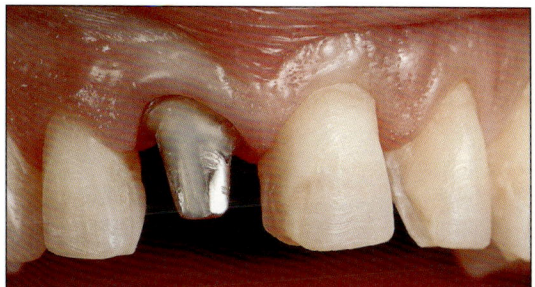

Fig 31 The full-coverage preparation for the crown on the right central incisor was refined.

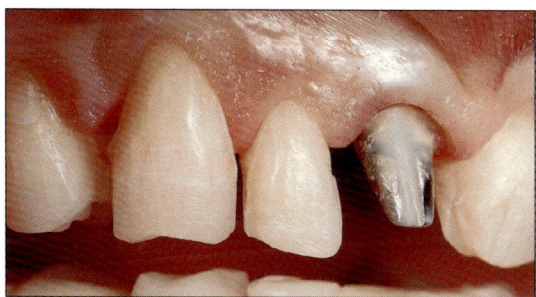

Fig 32 The interproximal contact points were broken for ease of fabrication and cementation of the porcelain laminate veneers.

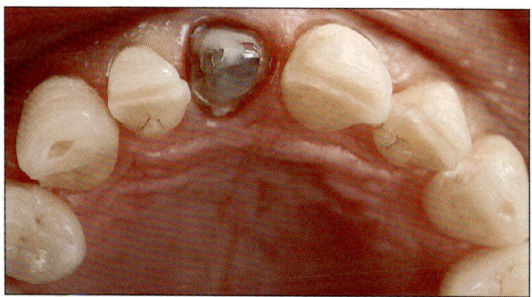

Fig 33 The incisal finish line was located palatally to increase the length of the porcelain laminate veneers to restore proper esthetics.

Tooth preparations for the porcelain laminate veneers, when feasible, were within enamel to maximize tooth structural integrity and provide superior bonding with resin cements. The preparations on the right first premolar, canine, and lateral incisor and left central incisor, lateral incisor, and canine were 0.3-mm cervical reductions, increasing to 0.7 mm incisally (Figs 30 to 33). Interproximal contacts were broken for ease of fabricating the porcelain laminate veneers on a refractory die and subsequent seating onto the abutments, and for concealing the cement lines. The right central incisor was prepared for a full-coverage metal-ceramic crown to mask the underlying cast metal core. The incisal finish line was located palatally for improved esthetics by incisal coverage, while avoiding centric contacts. A highly accurate addition-silicone impression material (Panasil, Kettenbach, Hesse, Germany), with a low contact angle, was used to capture the intracrevicular preparation margins and the minimal

facial enamel reductions (Fig 34). The plaster casts showed faithful reproduction of finish lines and roughened bur stokes, which increase micromechanical retention with a resin-luting agent (Figs 35 to 37).

The porcelain laminate veneers were fabricated using a low-abrasive porcelain and bonded with a resin cement after pretreatment of the intaglio surfaces with hydrofluoric acid and silane. The postoperative results showed impeccable integration of the metal-ceramic crown and porcelain laminate veneers with the surrounding healthy and stippled gingiva (Figs 38 to 41). The preoperative imbrication of the crown on the right central incisor was eliminated and was in line with the surrounding porcelain laminate veneers. A slight shadowing was noticeable on the free gingival margin around the right central incisor caused by root discoloration (Fig 42). However, because the patient had a low lip line, this was not detrimental to the final esthetic outcome (Figs 43 and 44).

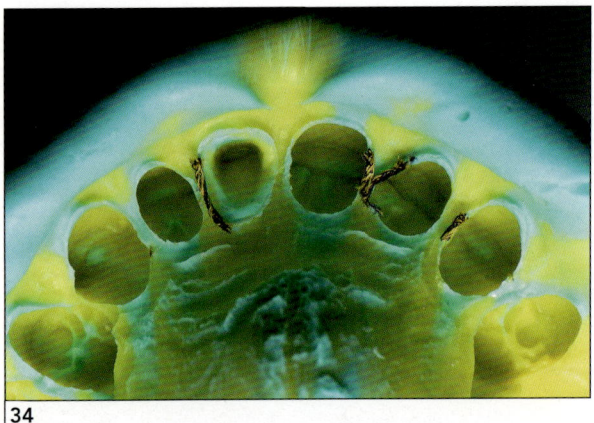

34

Fig 34 Addition-silicone impression of tooth preparations. Note that any tenaciously embedded retraction cord is left in situ and removed after pouring the plaster cast to avoid tearing the delicate finish lines.

Fig 35 Plaster cast showing detailed reproduction of tooth preparations.

Fig 36 An area apical to the finish line was faithfully reproduced, allowing the ceramist to obtain the correct emergence profiles of the prostheses.

Fig 37 Occlusal view of plaster cast showing the location of the palatal finish lines for the porcelain laminate veneers.

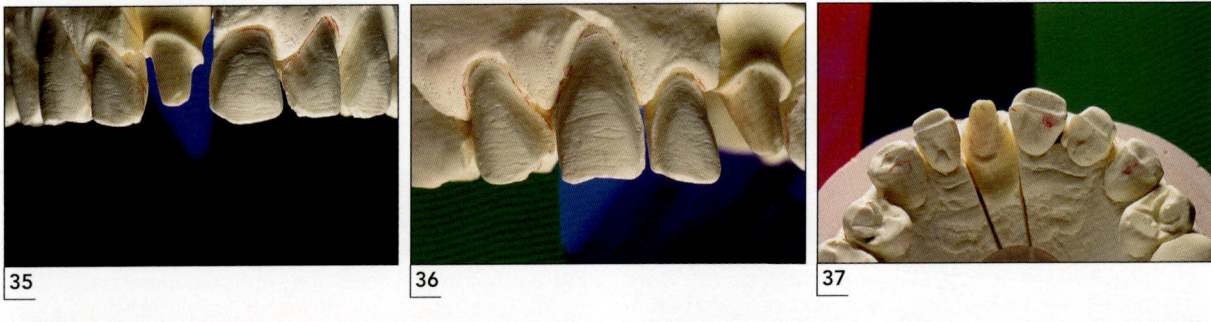

35   36   37

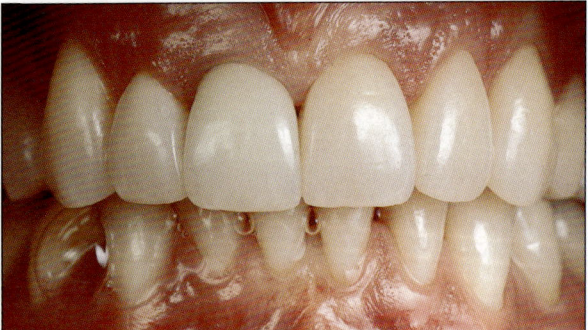

Fig 38 Postoperative facial view in centric occlusion.

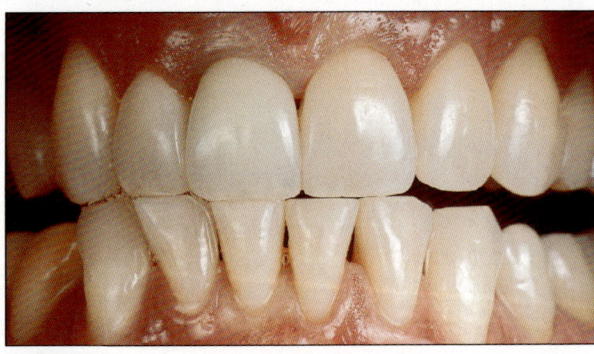

Fig 39 Postoperative facial view in protrusive excursion.

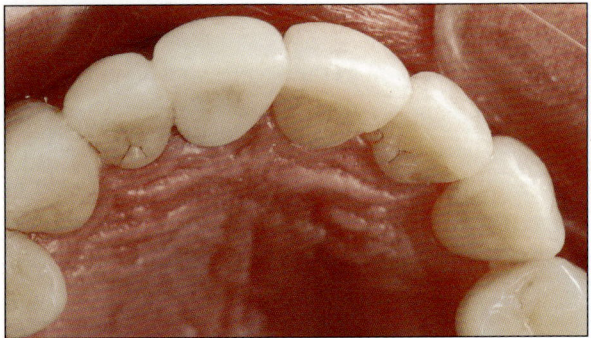

Fig 40 Postoperative occlusal view.

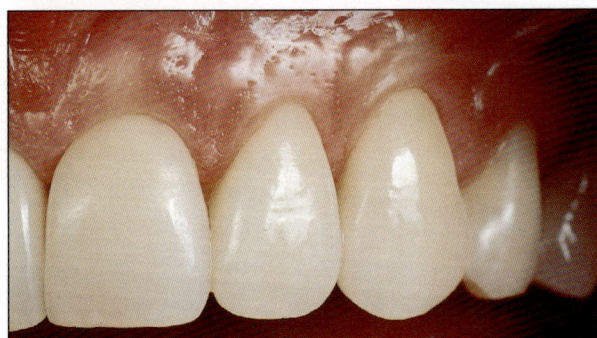

Fig 41 Postoperative detail view showing improved color and restoration of the width/length ratio and incisal embrasures, with healthy surrounding soft tissues. (Ceramics by Gerald Ubassy, Avignon, France.)

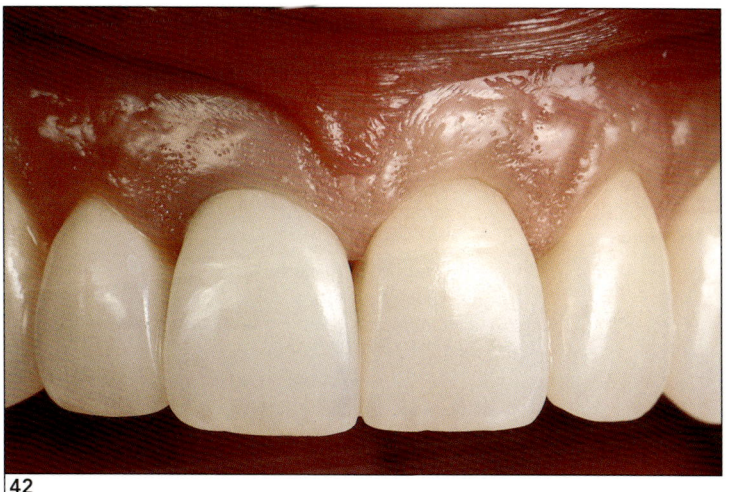

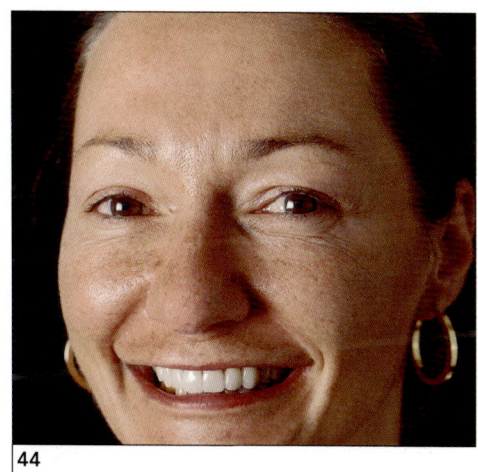

Fig 42 Postoperative detail view showing acceptable color harmony of the metal-ceramic crown on the right central incisor with adjacent porcelain laminate veneers. Note the slight shadowing of the gingival margin around the metal-ceramic crown; however, this did not detract from the final esthetics because of the patient's low lip line.

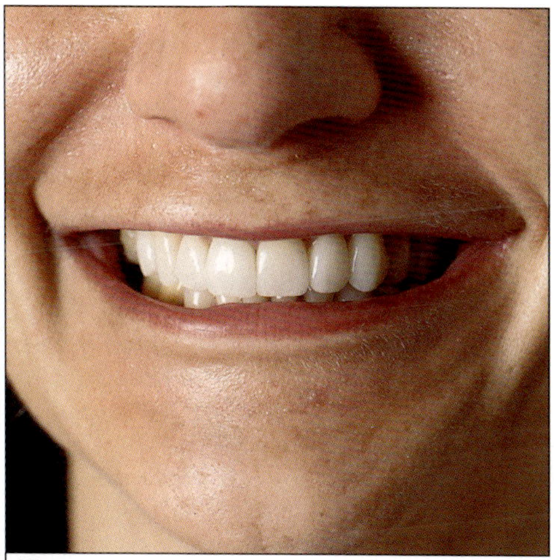

Fig 43 Postoperative dentofacial view.

Fig 44 Postoperative facial view.

CONCLUSION

Tooth wear is a ubiquitous condition, affecting the majority of the population at some stage of their lives. Because of its innocuous nature and slow progression, it often remains unnoticed until symptoms such as sensitivity, discoloration, or changes in tooth morphology become apparent. The etiology largely results from lifestyle choices and is preventable by appropriate counseling and periodic monitoring. If treatment is required, it should be provided immediately to halt further tooth loss. The treatment modality should be minimally invasive to preserve the maximum tooth structure of an already compromised dentition. Finally, it must achieve the objectives of function and esthetics, and satisfy the patient's wishes.

REFERENCES

1. Hancocks S. Tooth wear—A condition in the waiting. Int Dent J 2005;55:260.

2. Addy M, Shellis RP. Interaction between attrition, abrasion and erosion in tooth wear. Monogr Oral Sci 2006;20: 17–31.

3. Jones R, Lydeard S. Prevalence of symptoms of dyspepsia in the community. Br Med J 1989;298:30–32.

4. Jarvinen V, Meurman JH, Hyvarinen H. Dental erosion and upper gastrointestinal disorders. Oral Surg Oral Med Oral Pathol 1988;65:298–303.

5. Moazzez R, Smith BGN, Bartlett DW. Oral pH and drinking habit during ingestion of a carbonated drink in a group of adolescents with dental erosion. J Dent 2000; 28:395–397.

6. Eccles JD, Jenkins WG. Dental erosion and diet. J Dent 1974;2:153–159.

7. Amaechi BT, Higham SM. Eroded enamel lesion remineralisation by saliva as a possible factor in the site-specificity of human dental erosion. Arch Oral Biol 2001;46:697–703.

8. Eisenburger M, Addy M, Hughes JA, Shellis RP. Effect of time on the remineralization of enamel after citric acid erosion. Caries Res 2001;35:211–215.

9. Kinney JH, Balooch M, Haupt DL, Marshall SJ, Marshall GW. Mineral distribution and dimensional changes in human dentine demineralization. J Dent Res 1995;74:1179–1184.

10. Hunter ML, Addy M, Pickles MJ, Joiner A. Role of toothpastes and toothbrushes in the aetiology of toothwear. Int Dent J 2002;52:399–405.

11. Fischman S. Oral hygiene: How far have we come in 6000 years? Periodontol 2000 1997:15:7–14.

12. Mair LH. Wear in the mouth: The tribological dimension. In: Addy M, Embery G, Edgar WM, Orchardson R (eds). Tooth Wear and Sensitivity. London: Martin Dunitz, 2000.

13. Attin T, Zirkel C, Hellwig E. Brushing abrasion of eroded dentine after application of sodium fluoride solutions. Caries Res 1998;32:344–350.

14. Rugh JD, Harlan J. Nocturnal bruxism and temporomandibular disorders. Adv Neurol 1988;49:329–341.

15. Grippo JO. Abfractions: A new classification of hard tissue lesions of teeth. J Esthet Dent 1991;3:14–19.

16. Rees JS, Hammadeh M, Jagger DC. Abfraction lesion formation in maxillary incisors, canines and premolars: A finite element study. Eur J Oral Sci 2003;111:149–154.

17. Litonjua LA, Andreana S, Bush PJ, et al. Non-carious cervical lesions and abfractions: A re-evaluation. J Am Dent Assoc 2003;134:845–850.

18. Barker D. Tooth wear as a result of pica. Br Dent J 2005;199:271–273.

19. Abrahamsen TC. The worn dentition—Pathognomonic patterns of abrasion and erosion. Int Dent J 2005;55:268–276.

20. Oral health care epidemic causing irreversible damage to teeth. IPU Rev 2006;7:25.

21. Sangnes G. Traumatization of teeth and gingiva related to habitual tooth cleaning procedures. J Clin Periodontol 1975;3:94–103.

22. Dahl BL, Krogstad O. The effect of partial bite raising splint on the occlusal face height. An x-ray cephalometric study in human adults. Acta Odontol Scand 1982;40:17–24.

23. West NX, Hughes JA, Addy M. Erosion of dentine and enamel in vitro by dietary acids: The effect of temperature, acid character, concentration and exposure time. J Oral Rehabil 2000;27:875–880.

24. Bartlett DW, Smith BG, Wilson RF. Comparison of the effect of fluoride and non-fluoride toothpaste on tooth wear in vitro and the influence of enamel fluoride concentration and hardness of enamel. Br Dent J 1994;174:346–348.

25. Rees GD. Enamel protection and repair by a new desensitising anti-erosion toothpaste. Presented at the International Association for Dental Research Pan European Federation, Dublin, 14 Sept 2006.

26. Clarkson BH. Acellular synthesis of a human enamel-like microstructure. Adv Mater 2006;18:1846–1851.

27. Azzopardi A, Bartlett DW, Watson TF, Sherriff M. The surface effects or erosion and abrasion on dentine with and without a protective layer. Br Dent J 2004;196:351–354.

28. Shabanian M, Richards LC. In vitro wear rates of materials under different loads and varying pH. J Prosthet Dent 2002;87:650–656.

MICRO-OPERATIVE DENTISTRY: WHY DO IT?

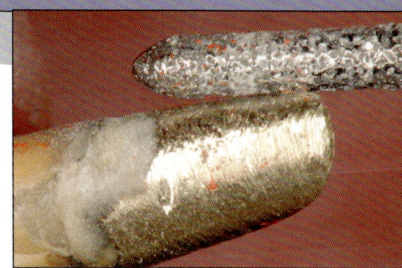

Claudia Cia Worschech, DDS, MS, PhD[1]
José Roberto Moura, Jr, DDS, MS[1]
Dickson Fonseca, DDS, MS[2]

When the profession of dentistry was established in the nineteenth century, operative dentistry was considered an entirely mechanical practice with almost no relation to the techniques or physical and biological properties of dental materials. At that time, there were only a few restorative materials available, such as gold and amalgam, to meet patients' needs for the restoration of damaged anterior and posterior teeth.

As the science of dentistry progressed into the twentieth century, new materials were developed by dental manufacturers, and so more complex restorative techniques became available.[1] Significant advancements were achieved in operative dentistry, such as the adhesion of composites to enamel and dentin, which allowed more conservative restorative procedures to preserve sound dental structure during the process of caries removal.[1] Knowledge of the physical, chemical, and mechanical properties of recent dental materials, as well as their correct applications, is essential to achieve successful long-term clinical performance.

To enhance clinical diagnostics, cavity preparations, and restorative procedures, an increasing number of dental practitioners are using magnification in their practices. Although this concept is not new to dentistry—loupes have been used for many years—the use of operating microscopes is gaining acceptance among clinicians. Operating microscopes optimize the viewing of images, amplify details, and provide the best lighting of the working field.[2]

Dental professionals have also begun to recognize that the amount and quality of light in the working field is just as important as magnification.[2] Under an operating microscope, the structures of the oral cavity can be seen with greater clarity. The illumination of the operating field along the optical axis eliminates shadows and optical illusions. The anatomy of the oral cavity appears in an impressive and vibrant manner, which is difficult or impossible to reproduce in a photograph.[3]

[1]Private practice, São Paulo, Brazil.
[2]Private practice, Rio Grande do Norte, Brazil.

Correspondence to: Dr Claudia Cia Worschech, Rua Florindo Cibin, 313 Americana, São Paulo, CEP 13465-000, Brazil. E-mail: claudiacw@terra.com.br

Margins of restorations that feel rough or seem to be open when checked with an explorer will appear as blatantly ragged or open under an operating microscope.[3]

The operating microscope not only provides a variety of magnification options, it also offers control of coaxial illumination for a shadow-free visual field. In addition, it allows the dental practitioner and the auxiliary staff to work in precise concert with one another, because they share the same visual access to the procedure being performed via the use of accessory binoculars.[4]

For several decades, many dental technicians have used stereomicroscopes for trimming dies, refining castings, and performing other procedures that require a high degree of precision. Now, clinicians may benefit from magnification as well.

Improved lighting, coupled with magnification, provides a clear distinction between surfaces that may look similar in color or texture under traditional working conditions. The clarity and detail are so vivid and revealing that the clinician will immediately recognize the potential for improved precision in both diagnostic and treatment procedures.[2]

LEARNING TO USE AN OPERATING MICROSCOPE

The first consideration is setup of this equipment in a given working environment. Often, clinicians buy an operating microscope before locating an adequate place to put it. The microscope must be placed in a position that allows maneuverability around the head of the patient without restricting the clinician's access to the oral cavity. The arms of the microscope must support the weight of the binocular head and any accessories (observer tube, inclinable binoculars, cameras, etc), and there must be enough space for all parts to move freely.

Another important aspect is the initial reduced productivity phase, in which the clinician must relearn the usual dental/restorative procedures. All manual and visual skills must be retrained to work with high magnification, as this usually marks the beginning of a complete change of working philosophies and paradigms. The brain will need time to adjust to the new visual information and to the magnified field of view.[2]

The patient's position should also be reviewed when using an operating microscope. The microscope can be placed in many different positions; however, the clinical procedure is most efficient when the patient's head, the mirror, or the chair are moved during treatment, rather than the microscope's head or arm.[4]

Use of the operating microscope allows for more ergonomic positions and minimal movement for the clinician and auxiliary staff, thus reducing the amount of pain and discomfort experienced after a procedure (Fig 1). Most general practitioners feel that an operating position that approximates the 12 o'clock position is the most convenient when working with the operating microscope. This position allows the auxiliary staff to work from an efficient and comfortable position as well (Fig 2).[4]

Documentation may also be improved, as operating microscopes allow the placement of accessories such as video and picture cameras to capture images of the treatment. These images can be stored in digital files, which are helpful for legal reasons and can be used as a source of patient education.[5]

Often, when clinicians understand how to work with magnification, they realize that the quality of past procedures needs to be reviewed. The increased vision and accuracy makes the professional more demanding over time, as most treatment elements can now be seen in much more detail, such as adaptation of porcelain, adhesion, caries lesions, or irregularities in a cavity restoration.

After the initial adaptation, the work in the dental office will return to normal, and the schedule can be followed as it was before introduction of the operating microscope. With each procedure, the microscope becomes easier to use. Eventually, clinicians can use it for all procedures.

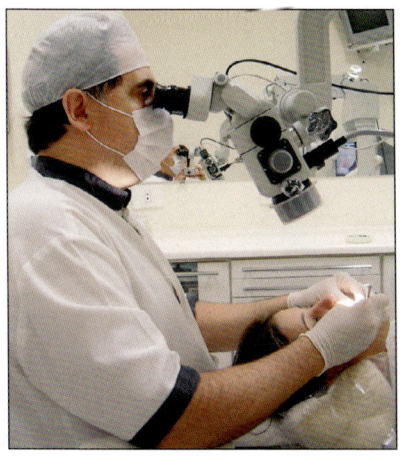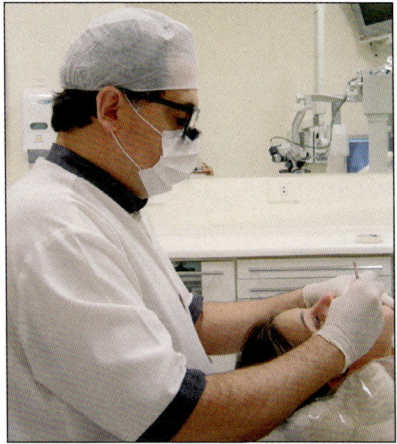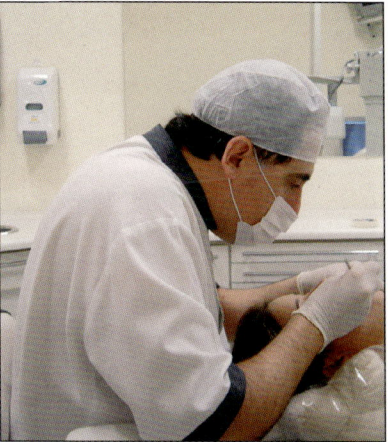

Figs 1a to 1c Ergonomics are improved when using the operating microscope **(a)**, compared to loupes **(b)**, and no magnification **(c)**.

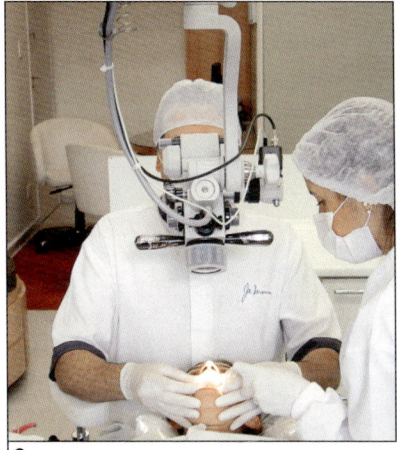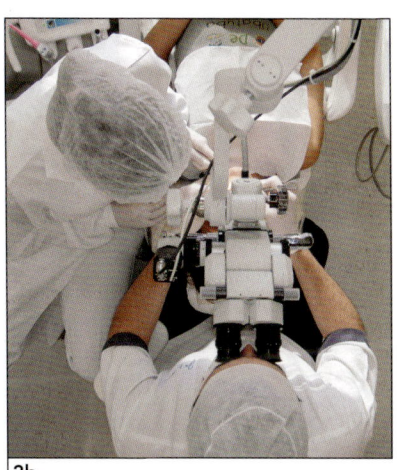

Figs 2a and 2b The best position when using an operating microscope is the 12 o'clock position, while sitting in a chair with an armrest.

An operating microscope can be expensive, requires time and effort to introduce in a dental office, and may also require the purchase of new instruments, mirrors, tips, etc. Nevertheless, the clinician will be rewarded by the beauty and superior adaptation of any new restorations, as well as the improved integration to the adjacent soft tissues. In turn, these enhancements will improve the clinician's credibility, satisfaction, and professional growth.[3]

WHY USE AN OPERATING MICROSCOPE?

The advantages of microscope-enhanced dentistry can be summarized as follows[6]:

- Better ergonomics
- Shadow-free illumination
- Intense lighting (80,000 lux)
- Clear visualization of details
- Better technical quality of clinical work
- Longer durability of clinical work
- Easy communication with patients and dental technicians
- Improved documentation

Although operating microscopes can greatly enhance a dental practice, there are some disadvantages, especially at the initial stages, which can be summarized as follows:

- High initial cost
- Need for rescheduling (increase in treatment costs and reduction in initial productivity)

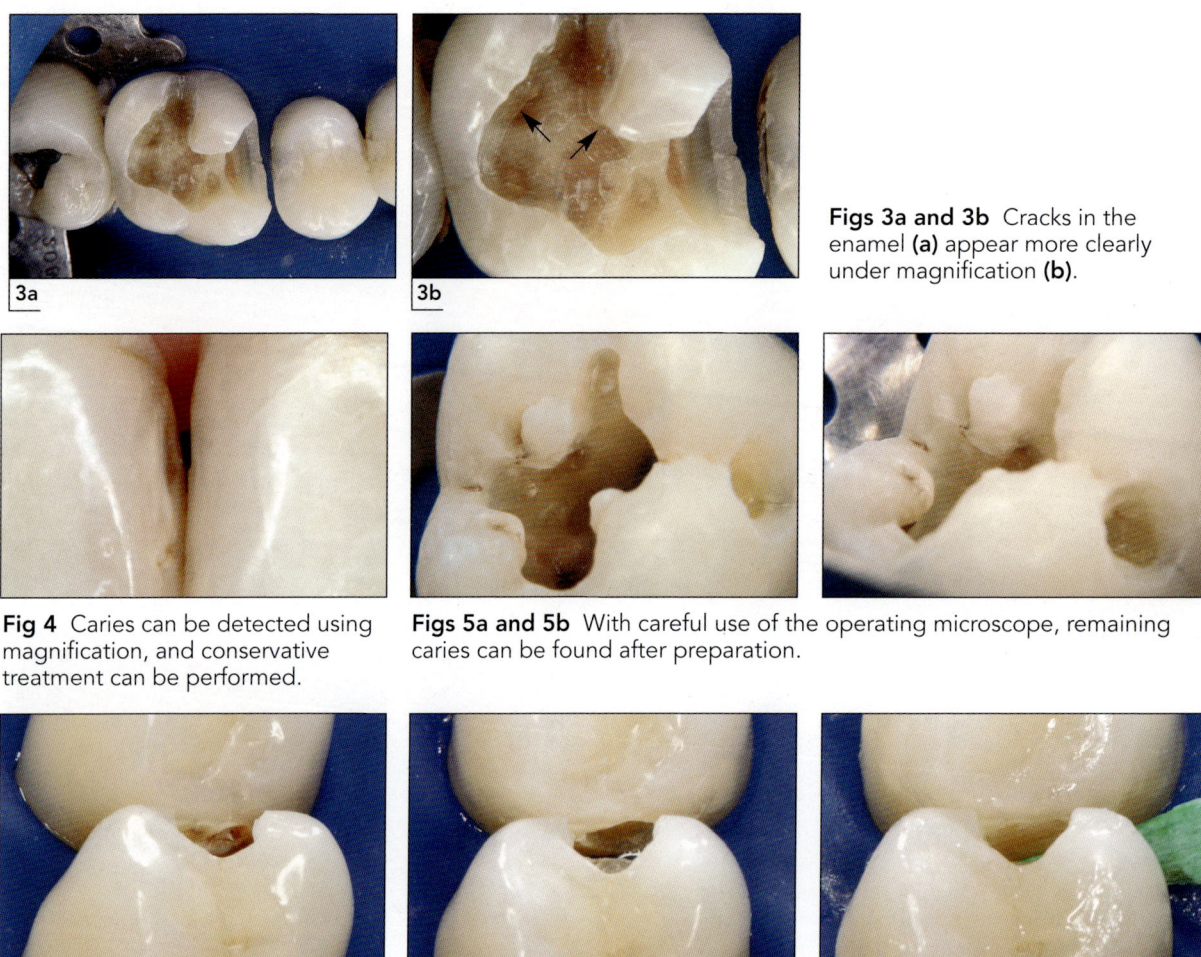

Figs 3a and 3b Cracks in the enamel (a) appear more clearly under magnification (b).

Fig 4 Caries can be detected using magnification, and conservative treatment can be performed.

Figs 5a and 5b With careful use of the operating microscope, remaining caries can be found after preparation.

Figs 6a to 6c Detecting and restoring caries proximally becomes more efficient under an operating microscope.

- Need for retraining of the auxiliary staff
- Need to rearrange office to find an adequate place for the equipment
- Adjustment period for the new treatment paradigms and postures

The diagnosis of early enamel cracks (cracked teeth and incomplete fracture) has historically been symptom based. The operating microscope at 16× magnification can fundamentally change a clinician's ability to diagnose such conditions. Thanks to microscope-enhanced dentistry, patterns have become clear that indicate treatment before the occurrence of symptoms or devastation of tooth structure (Fig 3).[7]

Use of an operating microscope also aids in the detection and restoration of caries, allowing for a conservative preparation (Fig 4). Further, the exact fit and adaptation of crowns and laminates can be checked in detail (Figs 5 to 11).

High accuracy is provided by 16× or 25× magnification to obtain superficial smoothness. The contour, shade, and superficial texture of composite restorations are easier to visualize and achieve (Figs 12 to 15).

An operating microscope may elicit a strong emotional response from the patient, because most likely he or she has never seen such a thing in a dental office. However, most patients approve of their clinician's use of the most up-to-

Fig 7 A gap can be seen between the coping and the preparation.

Figs 8a to 8e The preparation is cleaned and the fit is checked with the occlusion spray.

Fig 9 The contact points inside the coping are adjusted.

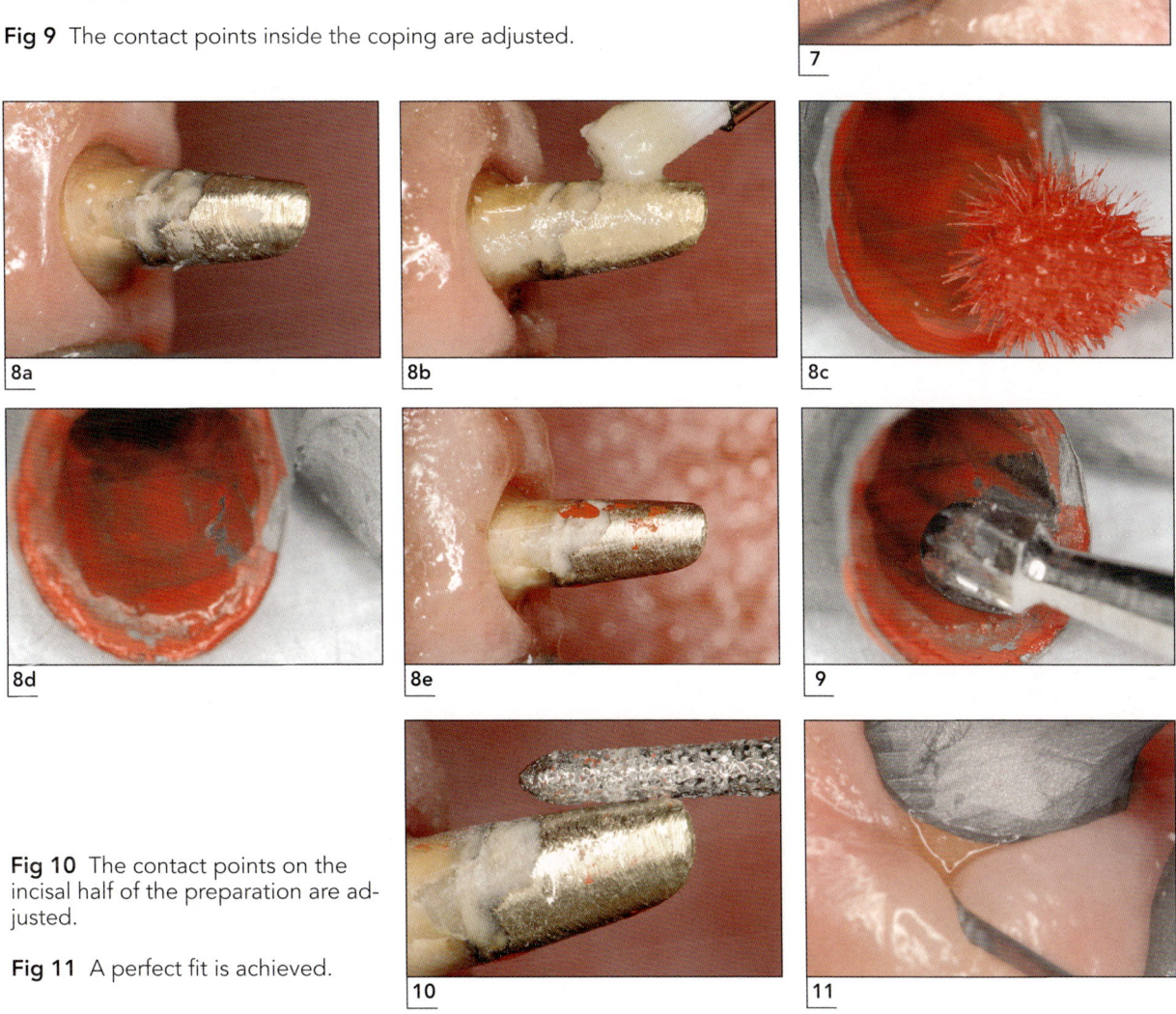

Fig 10 The contact points on the incisal half of the preparation are adjusted.

Fig 11 A perfect fit is achieved.

date technology. The clinician should explain how any procedures will be performed.

Many residents and students in the endodontic specialty are introduced to the operating microscope very early in their career. However, any general practitioner, with the proper equipment and training, can benefit from seeing the operative field magnified and clearly illuminated (Fig 16). Further, older professionals can rejuvenate their careers by learning this new technology and using different techniques.[5]

For tooth preparations, magnification can greatly enhance outcomes, particularly via more precise drilling procedures, which allow the clinician to avoid pulpal exposure and injury to the surrounding tissues.[3]

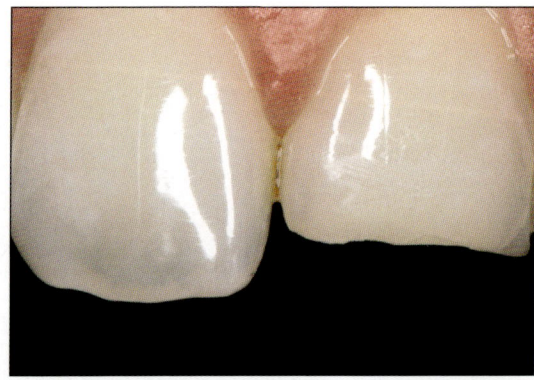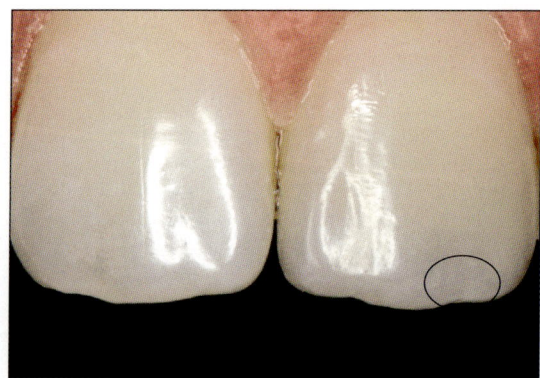

Figs 12a and 12b Magnification allows exact configuring and texturing of the restorations, and avoids the presence of bubbles inside the bulk of the resin composite.

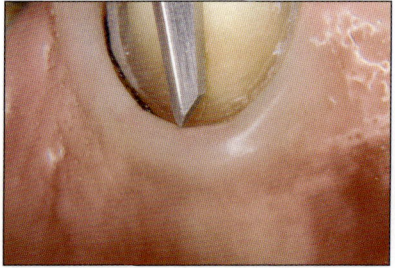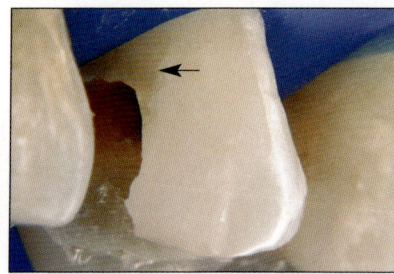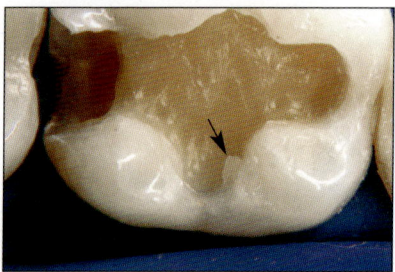

Fig 13 Hand instruments are used to remove unsupported enamel from the margin of the preparation.

Fig 14 Plaque is still visible on the surface of the tooth, which will prevent ideal bonding.

Fig 15 Old restorative material still remains on the enamel after preparation.

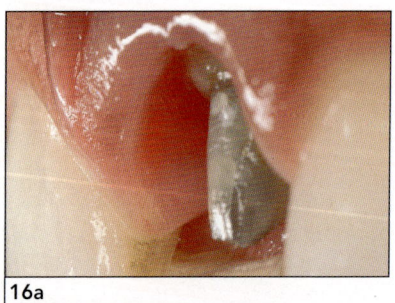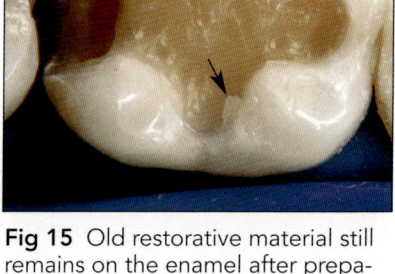

Figs 16a to 16e Excess resin cement can be easily identified and removed before polymerization, thus avoiding gingival retraction, periodontal inflammation, and other complications that may arise without magnification.

16a

16b

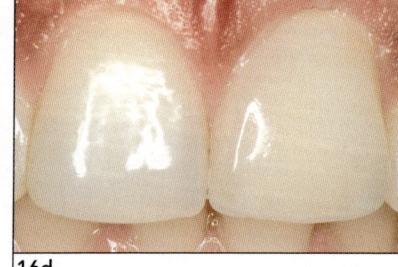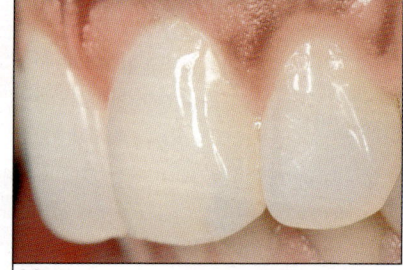

16c

16d

16e

CONCLUSIONS

There is no doubt that the use of operating microscopes can improve the quality of restorations, ceramic adaptation, precision of preparations, and removal of caries lesions, because the lighting is vibrant and shadow free, and the magnification provides excellent vision of the operating field.

Optical magnification has expanded the horizons of dentistry, not only in surgical endodontics, but in prosthodontics, operative dentistry, implant therapy, periodontic treatments, and every other aspect of the dental profession.

The improvement of visual acuity through optical magnification is part of modern dental practices. This article aimed to give clinicians a brief overview of magnification in dentistry and how they may benefit from the enhanced precision and quality in dental procedures.

The most important benefits when using an operating microscope are increased precision in cavity preparations, better vision of tiny details and imperfections, more precise execution of all dental techniques, better treatments for patients, less iatrogenic occurrences, less removal of sound tooth structure, better communication between clinicians and patients and laboratory technicians, and improved documentation of each treatment case.[6]

REFERENCES

1. Sheets CG, Paquette JM, Hatate K. The clinical microscope in an aesthetic restorative practice. J Esthet Restor Dent 2001;13:187–200.

2. Friedman M, Mora A, Schmidt R. Microscope-assisted precision dentistry. Compend Contin Educ Dent 1999; 20:723–735.

3. Baumann RR. How may the dentist benefit from the operating microscope? Quintessence Int 1977;5:17–18.

4. Friedman MJ, Landesman HM. Microscope-assisted precision (MAP) dentistry. A challenge for new knowledge. J Calif Dent Assoc 1998;26:900–905.

5. Koch K. The microscope. Its effect on your practice. Dent Clin North Am 1997;41:619–625.

6. Gondim E Jr, Murgel CAF, Sousa Filho FJ. Microscópio cirurgico: la nueva frontera de la Odontología clínica del siglo. Fola/Oral 1997;3:147–152.

7. Clark DJ, Sheets CG, Paquette JM. Definitive diagnosis of early enamel and dentinal cracks based on microscopic evaluation. J Esthet Restor Dent 2003;15:391–401.

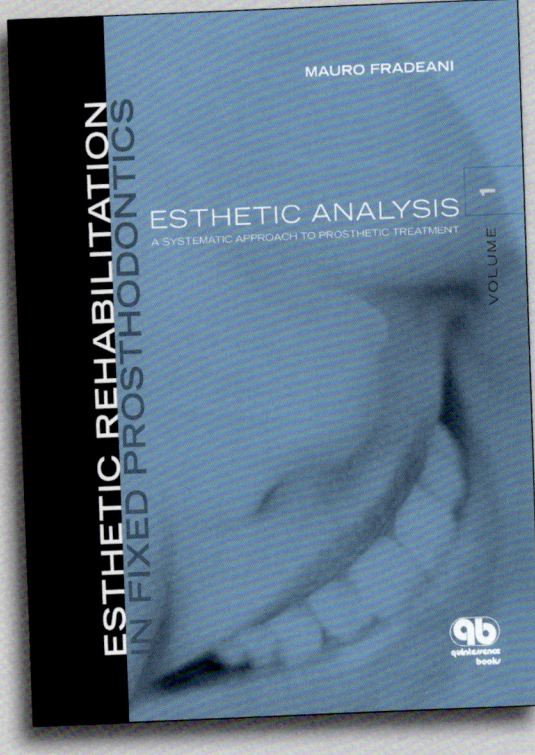
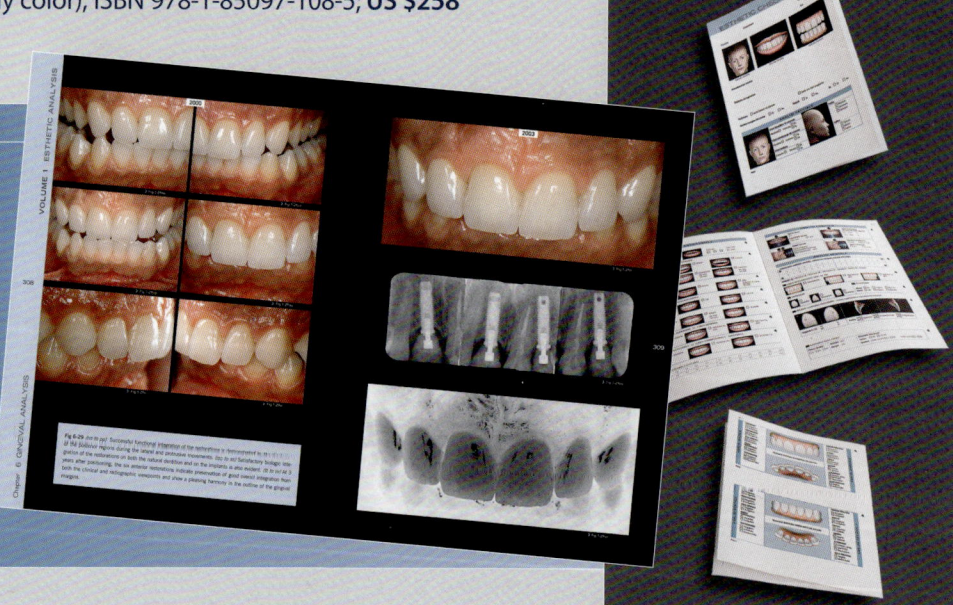
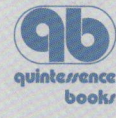

FUNCTIONAL AND ESTHETIC REHABILITATION USING ALL-CERAMIC CROWNS AND VENEERS: A CASE REPORT

Luigi Iannessi, DMD[1]

Anna Claudia Iannessi, DMD[1]

Angelo Canale, OT[2]

Angela Giordano, OT[2]

Barbara Bergantini, OT[2]

Daniela Bergantini, OT[1]

[1]Private practice, L'Aquila, Italy.

[2]Private dental laboratory, Rimini, Italy.

Correspondence to: Dr Luigi Iannessi, Via Fontesecco, 16 67100 L'Aquila, Italia. E-mail: studioiannessi@katamail.com

Recent advances in dental technology have led to the development of new restorative materials that provide excellent esthetics and affordability. These materials offer clinicians more options for selection of the best material for each specific case.[1] Therefore, it is crucial for clinicians to have a complete understanding of a patient's medical history and any special considerations when performing complex rehabilitations. This article describes a treatment approach using all-ceramic crowns and veneers in a patient who exhibited significant esthetic and functional compromise as a result of a previous medical condition.

The main goal of the restorative dentist is to recreate the physiologic occlusion using biocompatible materials that provide precise, esthetic, and durable restorations. Due to advances in dental technology, it is possible to use all-ceramic restorations for the posterior teeth.[2–4] All-ceramic restorations are physically and mechanically strong, highly biocompatible, and resist fracture, thermal shock, and erosion.[5–8] Further, ceramic is the material best tolerated by the gingiva.[9–12] The bulk of evidence suggests that all-ceramic restorations benefit from using adhesive cementation techniques. Therefore, all-ceramic restorations may offer a conservative treatment modality especially in patients with vital, worn teeth with healthy attachment apparatus.[13–15]

CASE PRESENTATION

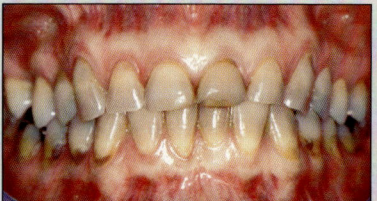

Fig 1 The initial situation.

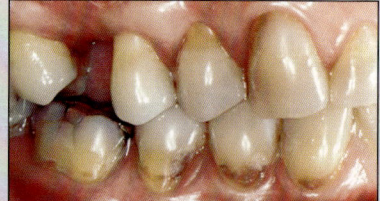

Fig 2 Pretreatment view showing the missing maxillary right first molar.

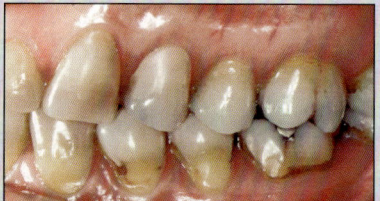

Fig 3 Pretreatment view of the maxillary left quadrant. The dentition exhibits significant esthetic problems.

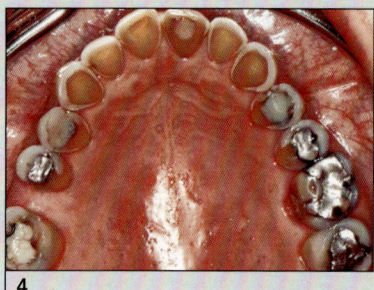

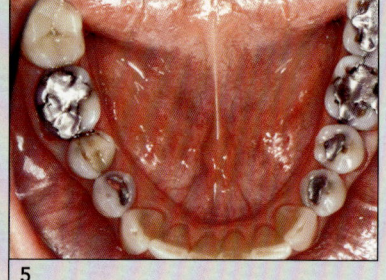

Fig 4 Occlusal view of the maxilla. Note the significant enamel erosion.

Fig 5 Occlusal view of the mandible.

The use of adhesive cementation provides improved resistance to the crowns that may preclude the need for endodontic treatment and surgical crown lengthening.[16–20] Since clinicians have several treatment options, careful and comprehensive treatment planning is even more important.[21] One of the most crucial steps is to collect all necessary information at the first appointment. It is also important to understand the patient's problems and treatment goals. Finally, a comprehensive occlusal analysis is essential for fabrication of functional provisional and definitive restorations.

CASE PRESENTATION

A 37-year-old woman presented with pulpitis of the mandibular left first molar. She also was worried about the erosion of her teeth, which resulted in hypersensitivity and esthetic problems (Figs 1 to 3).[22] The medical history included bulimia that was no longer active but had caused many dental problems, especially enamel erosion caused by self-induced acidic regurgitation (Figs 4 and 5). The patient reported high consumption of acidic beverages.[23–25] The extraoral examination was within normal limits; however, intraoral assessment revealed numerous large erosions, especially on the maxillary premolars and molars, where the supporting cusps were destroyed and the pulp was exposed. Significant erosion of the occlusal surfaces of the mandibular teeth was noted. In both arches caries lesions were evident, especially at the cervical areas, and many inadequate restorations were present. The maxillary right first molar was missing, and the second and third molars were mesioinclined. A full radiographic exam was performed (Fig 6). Diagnostic impressions were taken, and a diagnostic waxup was fabricated (Fig 7).

Initial Treatment Plan

The patient was shown the radiographs, waxups, and photographs taken at the first visit, and all dental problems were carefully explained to her. The initial treatment plan included endodontic

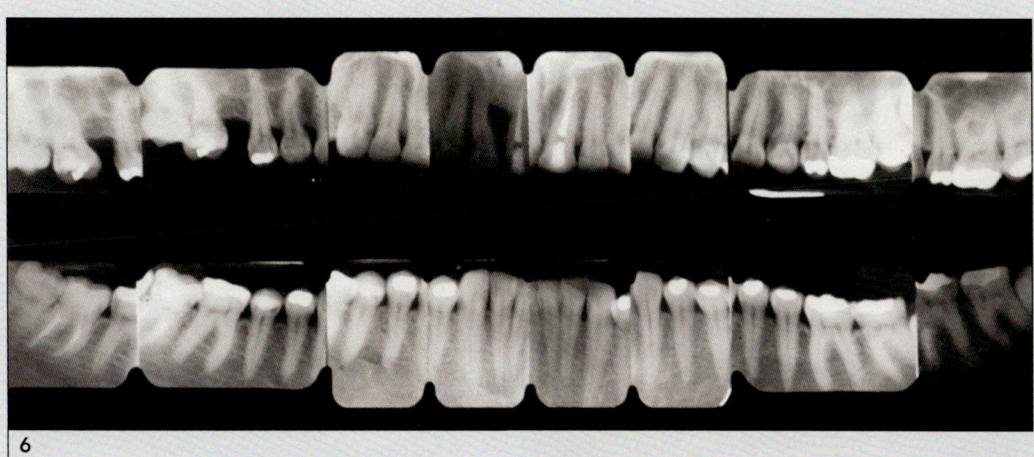

Fig 6 Pretreatment radiographs.

Fig 7 Diagnostic waxup.

Fig 8 Pretreatment occlusal view of the mandible with the old restorations removed, prior to the resin composite buildup.

Fig 9 Right posterior maxilla during orthodontic treatment.

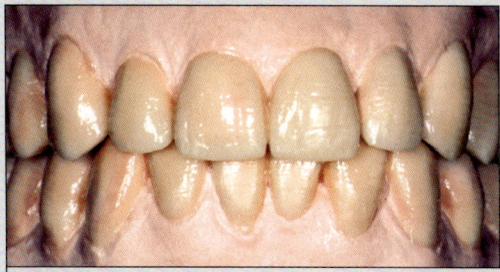

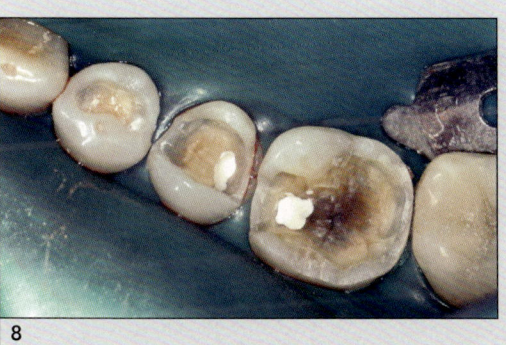

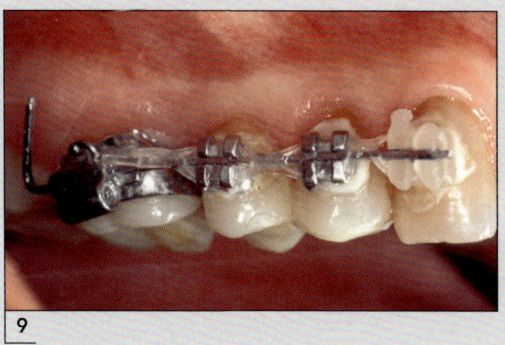

treatment of the molar with pulpitis, scaling, and extraction of the maxillary left and both mandibular third molars (Figs 8 and 9). The patient would then be reevaluated to assess her motivation and compliance.

Reevaluation

The patient improved her oral hygiene and a decrease in probing depth was found at the reevaluation appointment. She was motivated to correct her dental problems, and had stopped drinking acidic beverages. The patient's goals were to have whiter teeth, to prevent further erosion, and to receive fixed restorations. She also reported fear of surgery.

Definitive Treatment Plan

The treatment plan was to replace all amalgam restorations with resin composite buildups; refer the patient for orthodontic therapy to close the space from the missing maxillary right first molar by moving the third and second molars mesially[26,27]; and restore all teeth with single crowns, except

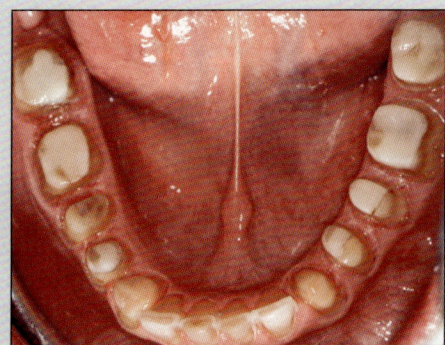

Fig 10 Occlusal view of tooth preparations in the mandible.

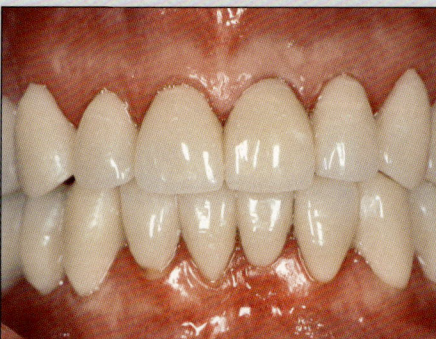

Fig 11 Frontal view of the provisional prostheses.

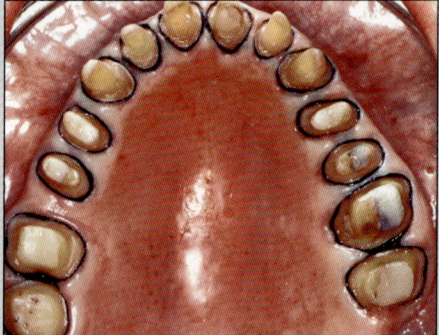

Fig 12 Occlusal view of the maxilla before final impressions were taken.

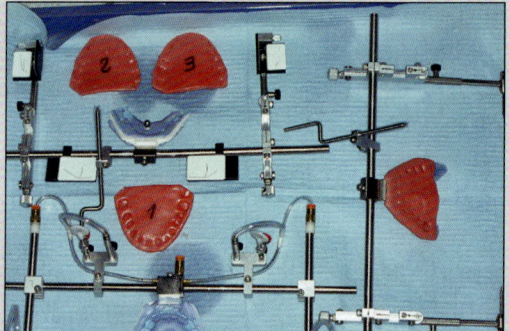

Fig 13 Pantographic registration.

the mandibular incisors which were to be restored with ceramic veneers.[28–36] The treatment sequence was described in detail to the patient.

Prosthetic Phase

The technician waxed up the mounted cast made from the impressions taken after orthodontic treatment and fabricated provisional crowns. The patient was satisfied using an occlusal appliance that increased the vertical dimension of occlusion (VDO) by 1.5 mm. Therefore, the provisional restorations were designed to increase the VDO by the same amount to provide space for the definitive restorations (Figs 10 and 11). In centric relation, a 3-mm space was noted between the arches.

The treatment goal was to restore adequate function and to improve esthetics.[37] The significant erosion had caused phonetic problems because

anterior guidance was lost, as well as esthetic problems because the smile was inverted. A tooth-to-tooth occlusal scheme was selected for the posterior teeth. Single-unit provisional prostheses were placed in both arches following preparation of all teeth. Because the plan was to use all-ceramic materials, a round chamfer was prepared at the gingival level.[38]

The patient wore the provisional restorations for 6 months to evaluate the restored vertical dimension.[4,39–42] During this period she was recalled regularly for oral hygiene maintenance and to check for marginal adaptation and seal, resin erosion, sensitivity, and muscular or articular pain. The esthetics and phonetics also were evaluated.

At the end of the 6-month period the patient was satisfied with the esthetics and function, and additional impressions were taken (Fig 12). Pantographs were taken to register the condylar pathway and posterior determinants of occlusion

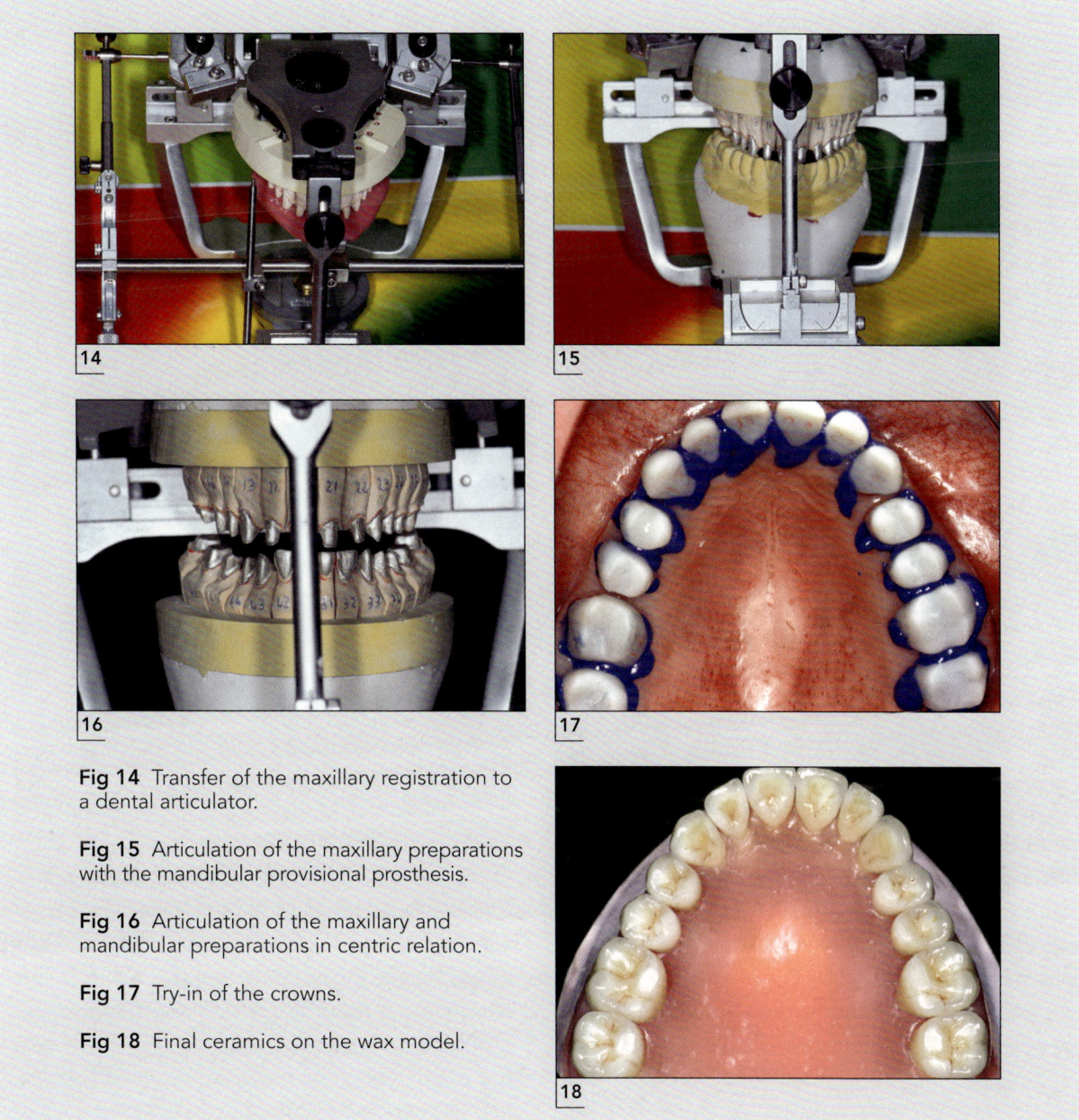

Fig 14 Transfer of the maxillary registration to a dental articulator.

Fig 15 Articulation of the maxillary preparations with the mandibular provisional prosthesis.

Fig 16 Articulation of the maxillary and mandibular preparations in centric relation.

Fig 17 Try-in of the crowns.

Fig 18 Final ceramics on the wax model.

(Fig 13) so the technician could fabricate more functionally adequate restorations. Anterior guidance was duplicated from the provisional restorations. The wax models were fabricated by mounting the mandibular provisional restorations opposing the maxillary preparations and the master casts of preparations opposing each other (Figs 14 and 15). The facebow record served to mount the maxillary cast using the pantographic registration (Fig 16). Final impressions of both arches were made with a polyether material and a triple-zero retraction cord.[43–46]

The definitive restorations were tried in for esthetics. Four ceramic veneers were cemented with a light-polymerizing resin composite (Enamel Plus, Micerium, Rosbach, Germany) (Fig 17).[47–50] Another impression was taken with the crowns on the waxup models of the teeth to ensure optimal occlusion was achieved. (Fig 18). After try-in of the prostheses and patient approval of the esthetics,

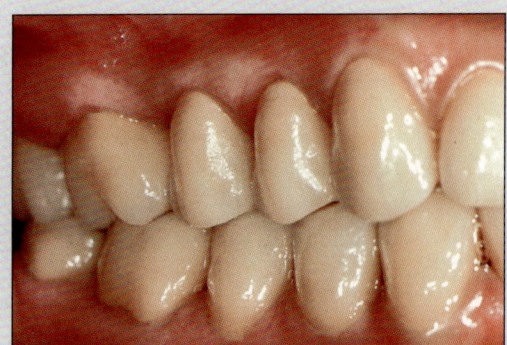

Fig 19 Final view of the right side.

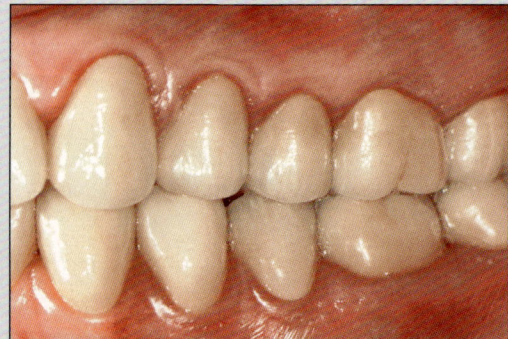

Fig 20 Final view of the left side.

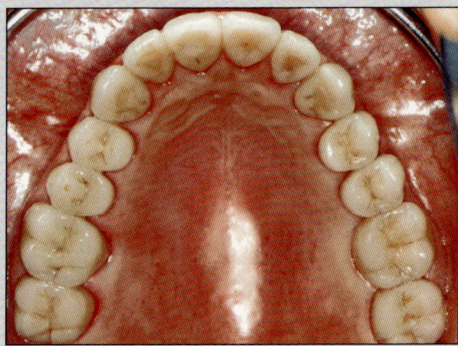

Fig 21 Final occlusal view of the maxilla.

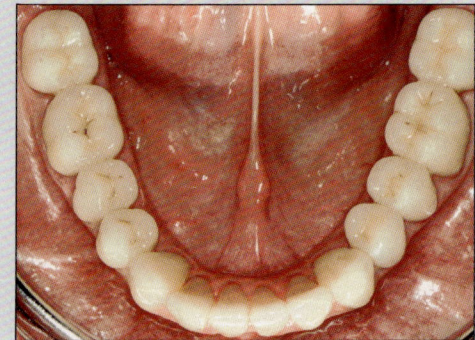

Fig 22 Final occlusal view of the mandible.

all crowns were cemented with an adhesive technique using a low-density dual-cured resin cement.[13,15,51–57] As in all restorative cases, the occlusion was carefully evaluated and final adjustments were performed intraorally. In this case the patient was very satisfied with the restorations and with her new smile (Figs 19 to 26).

DISCUSSION

It is important to determine patients' concerns about their teeth and their goals in terms of functional and esthetic outcomes. In complex cases it is not possible to prepare a definitive treatment plan after the first visit; an initial treatment should be performed, followed by a reevaluation to assess the patient's motivation and compliance. Then the clinician can present the definitive treatment plan and explain the changes that will be made, in-

cluding any modifications to the color, shape, tooth position, smile line, and occlusal plane.[58]

Continuous enamel erosion and dentin exposure can cause hypersensitivity and color alterations, leave the teeth at greater risk for caries, and limit the transmission of light. To solve these problems and recreate normal light transmission, the ceramic on a nonmetal crown should be stratified. All-ceramic restorations have good mechanical and physical characteristics and provide excellent esthetics.[59–62]

In the case presented, all treatment goals were achieved including good esthetics in terms of the color, shape, smile line, and preservation of function and tooth vitality. In fact, with adhesive cementation and resin composite buildups, sufficient retention was obtained without the need for endodontic therapy or periodontal surgery. Using a standardized protocol, occlusal precision and adequate function were achieved.

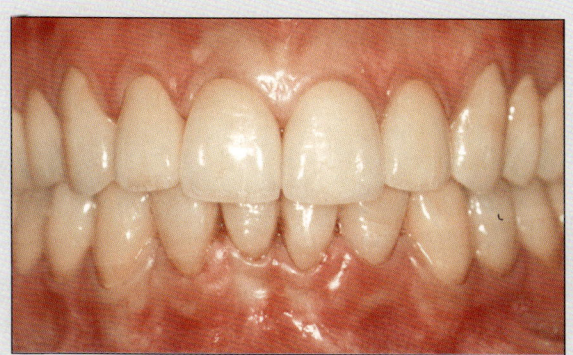

Fig 23 Final intraoral view.

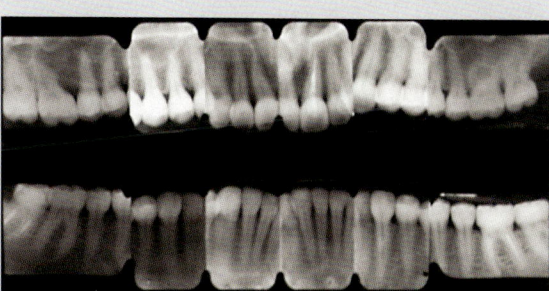

Fig 24 Final radiographs.

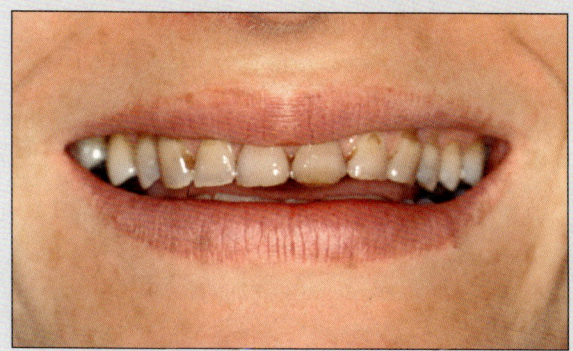

Fig 25 Initial smile.

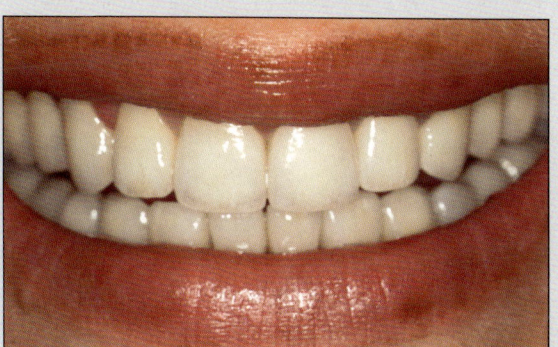

Fig 26 Final smile.

REFERENCES

1. Goodacre CJ, Bernal G, Rungcharassaeng K, Kan JY. Clinical complications in fixed prosthodontics. J Prosthet Dent 2003;90:31–41.

2. Blatz MB. Long-term success of all-ceramic posterior restorations. Quintessence Int 2002;33:415–426.

3. Fradeani M. The application of all-ceramic restorations in the anterior and posterior regions. Pract Proced Aesthet Dent 2003;Supple:13–17.

4. Magne P, Dietschi D, Holz J. Esthetic restorations for posterior teeth: Practical and clinic considerations. Int J Periodontics Restorative Dent 1996;16:104–119.

5. Probster L. Compressive strength of two modern all-ceramic crowns. Int J Prosthodont 1992;5:409–414.

6. Seghi RR, Sorensen JA, Engelman MJ, Rumanas E, Torres TJ. Flexural strength of new ceramic materials [abstract 1521]. J Dent Res 1990;69(special issue):299.

7. Zeng K, Oden A, Rowcliffe O. Flexure tests on dental ceramics. Int J Prosthodont 1996;9:434–439.

8. Zeng K, Oden A, Rowcliffe O. Evaluation of mechanical properties of dental ceramic care materials in combination with porcelains. Int J Prosthodont 1998;11:183–189.

9. Chan C, Weber H. Plaque retention on teeth restored with full-ceramic crowns: A comparative study. J Prosthet Dent 1986;56:666–671.

10. Koidis PT, Schroeder K, Johnston W, Compagni W. Color consistency, plaque accumulation and external marginal surface characteristics of the collarless metal-ceramic restoration. J Prosthet Dent 1991;65:391–400.

11. Smales KJ. Plaque growth on dental restorative materials. J Dent 1981;9:133–140.

12. Tullberg A. An experimental study of the adhesion of bacterial layers to some restorative dental materials. Scand J Dent Res 1986;94:164–173.

13. Blatz MB. Cementation of porcelain restorations. Pract Proced Aesthet Dent 2002;14:616.

14. Blatz MB, Sadan A, Kern M. Cementazione adesiva di restauri in ceramica integrale a elevata resistenza. Quintessenze Int 2004;3:71–81.

15. El-Mowafy O. The use of resin cements in restorative dentistry to overcome retention problems. J Can Dent Assoc 2001;67:97–102.

16. Lang NP, Kiel RA, Anderhalden K. Clinical and microbiological effects of subgingival restorations with overhanging or clinically perfect margins. J Clin Periodontol 1983;10:563–578.

17. Loe H. Reactions of marginal periodontal tissues to restorative procedures. Int Dent J 1986;18:759–778.

18. Newcomb E. The relationship between the location of subgingival crown margins and inflammation. J Periodontol 1974;45:151–154.

19. Silness J. Fixed prosthodontics and periodontal health. Dent Clin North Am 1980;24:317–330.

20. Tarnow D, Stahl SS, Magner A, Zamzok J. Human gingival attachment responses to subgingival crown placement. Marginal remodelling. J Clin Periodontol 1986;13:563–569.

21. Carnevale G, Di Febo G, Trebbi L. A patient presentation: Planning a difficult case. Int J Periodontics Restorative Dent 1981;6:51–63.

22. Jarvinen VK, Rytomaa II, Heinonem OP. Risk factors in dental erosion. J Dent Res 1991;70:942–947.

23. Deery C, Wagner ML, Longbottom C, Simon R, Nugent ZJ. The prevalence of dental erosion in a United States and a United Kingdom sample of adolescents. Pediatr Dent 2000;22:505–510.

24. Hurst PS, Lacey LH, Crisp AH. Teeth, vomiting and diet: A study of the dental characteristic of seventeen anorexia nervosa patients. Postgrad Med J 1977;53:298–305.

25. Rytomaa I, Jarvinen V, Kanerva R, Heinonen OP. Bulimia and tooth erosion. Acta Odontol Scand 1998;56:38–40.

26. Goldberg D, Turley PK. Orthodontic space closure of the edentulous maxillary first molar area in adults. Int J Adult Orthodon Orthognath Surg 1989;4:255–266.

27. Shraff B, Siegel SM, Feldman S, Siegel SC. Combined orthodontic and prosthetic therapy. Special considerations. Dent Clin North Am 1996;40:911–943.

28. Belser UC, Magne P, Magne M. Ceramic laminate veneers: Continuous evolution of indications. J Esthet Dent 1997;9:197–207.

29. Calamia JR. Etched porcelain facial veneers: A new treatment modality based on scientific and clinical evidence. N Y J Dent 1983;53:255–259.

30. Calamia JR. Clinical evaluation of etched porcelain veneers. Am J Dent 1989;2:9–15.

31. Cortellini D, Parvizi A. Rehabilitation of severely eroded dentition utilizing all-ceramic restorations. Pract Proced Aesthet Dent 2003;15:275–282.

32. Dietschi D, Spreafico R. Adhesive Metal-Free Restorations. Chicago: Quintessence, 1997.

33. Friedman MJ. A 15 year review of porcelain veneer failure: A clinician's observation. Compend Contin Educ Dent 1998;19:625–636.

34. Horn HR. Porcelain laminate veneers bonded to etched enamel. Dent Clin North Am 1983;27:671–684.

35. Walls AVV. The use of intensively retained all-porcelain veneers during the management of fractured and worn anterior teeth: Part 2. Clinical results after 5 years of follow up. Br Dent J 1995;178:333–340.

36. Walls AVV. The use of adhesively retained all-porcelain veneers during the management of fractured and worn anterior teeth: Part 1. Clinical technique. Br Dent J 1995;178:333–336.

37. Kopp FR. Esthetic principles for full-crown restorations. Part II: Provisionalization. J Esthet Dent 1993;5:258–264.

38. Reeves WG. Restorative margin placement and periodontal health. J Prosthet Dent 1991;66:733–736.

39. Garber DA. Porcelain laminate veneers: Ten years later. Part I: Tooth preparation. J Esthet Dent 1993;5:57–61.

40. Magne P, Douglas WH. Design optimization and evolution of bonded ceramics for the anterior dentition: A finite element analysis. Quintessence Int 1999;30:661–672.

41. Touati B, Plissart-Vanackere A. Ceramic bonded veneers. Toward a minimal prosthesis [in French]. Real Clin 1990;1:51–66.

42. Touati B, Pissis P, Miara P. Bonded single restorations and the concept of pellicular preparations [in French]. Cah Prothese 1985;13:95–130.

43. Jokstad A. Clinical trial of gingival retraction cords. J Prosthet Dent 1999;81:258–261.

44. Benson BW, Bomberg TJ, Hatch RA, Hoffmann W. Tissue displacement methods in fixed prosthodontics. J Prosthet Dent 1986;55:175–181.

45. Loe H, Silness JS. Tissue reactions to string packs used in fixed restorations. J Prosthet Dent 1963;13:318–323.

46. Ruel J, Schnessler PJ, Malament K, Mori D. Effects of retraction procedures on the periodontium in humans. J Prosthet Dent 1980;44:508–515.

47. McComb D. Adhesive luting cement classes, criteria and usage. Compend Contin Educ Dent 1996;17:759–762.

48. Magne P, Versluis A, Douglas WH. Effect of luting composite shrinkage and thermal loads on the stress distribution in porcelain laminate veneers. J Prosthet Dent 1999;81:335–344.

49. Nicholls JI. Esthetic veneer cementation. J Prosthet Dent 1986;56:9–12.

50. Nicholls JI. Tensile bond of resin cements to porcelain veneers. J Prosthet Dent 1988;60:443–447.

51. Blatz MB, Sadan A, Kern M. Resin-ceramic bonding—A review of the literature. J Prosthet Dent 2003;89:268–274.

52. Frenzel E, Kern M. Tensile bond strength of new Panavia F to tooth structure [abstract 1439]. J Dent Res 2001;80(special issue).

53. Paul SJ. Adhesive Luting Procedures. Chicago: Quintessence, 1997.

54. Paul SJ, Scharer P. The dual bonding technique: A modified method to improve adhesive luting procedures. Int J Periodontics Restorative Dent 1997;17:536–545.

55. Jensen ME, Sheth JJ, Tolliver D. Etched porcelain resin-bonded full veneer crowns: In vitro fracture resistance. Compend Contin Educ Dent 1989;10:336–346.

56. Jacques LB, Ferrari M, Cardoso PE. Microleakage and resin cement film thickness of inted all-ceramic and gold electroformed porcelain. J Adhes Dent 2003;5:145–152.

57. Touati B, Quintas AF. Aesthetic and adhesive cementation for contemporary porcelain crowns. Pract Proced Aesthet Dent 2001;13:611–620.

58. Magne P, Magne M, Belser U. Natural and restorative oral esthetics. Part II: Esthetic treatment modalities. J Esthet Dent 1993;5:239–246.

59. Burke FJT. Fracture resistance of teeth restored with dentine-bonded crowns. Quintessence Int 1996;27:115–121.

60. Dumfahrt H, Schaffer H. Porcelain laminate veneers. A retrospective evaluation after 1 to 10 years of service: Part II—Clinical results. Int J Prosthodont 2000;13:9–18.

61. Fradeani M, Aquilano A. Clinical experience with Empress crowns. Int J Prosthodont 1997;10:241–247.

62. Fradeani M. Six years follow up with Empress veneers. Int J Periodontics Restorative Dent 1998;18:216–225.

CAD/CAM MULTIPLE-IMPLANT SCREW-RETAINED RESTORATIONS: ILLUSTRATION OF A TECHNIQUE

Thomas J. Salinas, DDS[1]
Valmont Desa, DDS, MD[2]
Momo Vasilic, MDT, CDT[3]

It is challenging for the clinician and laboratory technician to attain a passive fit between cast metal structures that serve as a stable platform and base for reconstructing occlusion and esthetics. Much of this difficulty may result from a combination of impression techniques used to transfer the position of the implants.[1–3] Another variable is the deficiencies inherent in the casting techniques. Alternative strategies and techniques to attain a passive framework fit have been investigated,[4–11] but many of these continue to fall short. Fortunately, biologic tolerance allows for misfit of the system without significant negative biologic consequences.[11,12]

Recent development of immediate implant loading protocols in the anterior mandible and maxilla offer a time-efficient alternative to traditional 2-stage surgical treatment.[13–16] Coupled with the development of computer-aided design/computer-assisted manufacture (CAD/CAM), computer numeric-controlled techniques of duplication have increased the accuracy of fit of these frameworks.[17–20] The recent trend to use computer technology has led to the development of subtractive techniques that reduce a solid block of material, such as commercially pure grade 2 titanium, to contours and fitting surfaces that approach predesigned configurations.[21] Combined with computer-assisted planning and mirrored implant placement, these techniques make immediate loading ideal and set the standard for the future of implant prosthodontics.

[1]Associate Professor, Department of Dental Specialties, Mayo Clinic, Rochester, Minnesota, USA.

[2]Oral and Maxillofacial Surgeon, Omaha, Nebraska, USA.

[3]Master Dental Technician, Yorba Linda, California, USA.

Correspondence to: Dr Thomas J. Salinas, Department of Dental Specialties, Mayo Clinic, 200 First St, Rochester, Minnesota 55905, USA.

CASE PRESENTATION

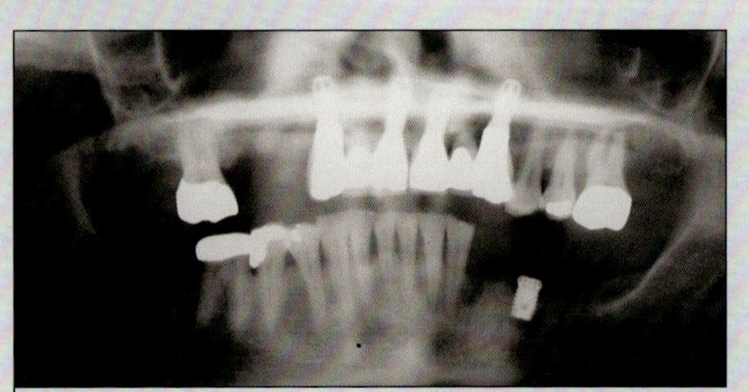

Fig 1 Preoperative panoramic radiograph.

Figs 2a to 2e Converting the complete denture to an implant fixed prosthesis. **(a and b)** Pick-up relation of titanium copings with acrylic resin. **(c and d)** Attachment of implant replicas to undersides of copings with guide pins. **(e)** Placement of assembly into dental-stone patty.

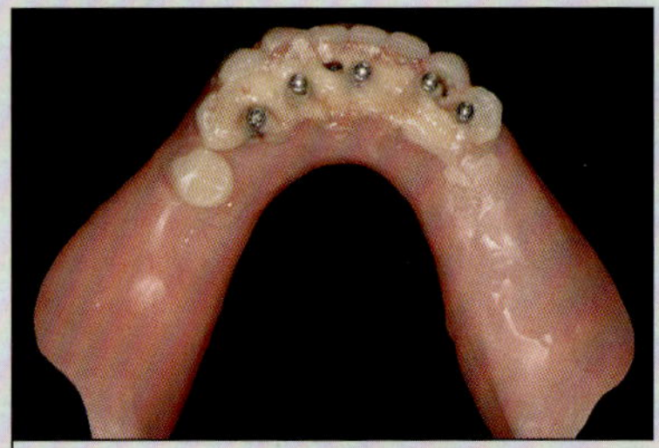

CASE PRESENTATION

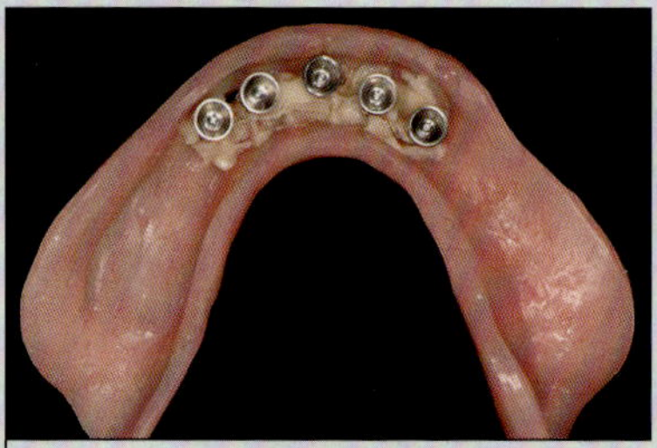

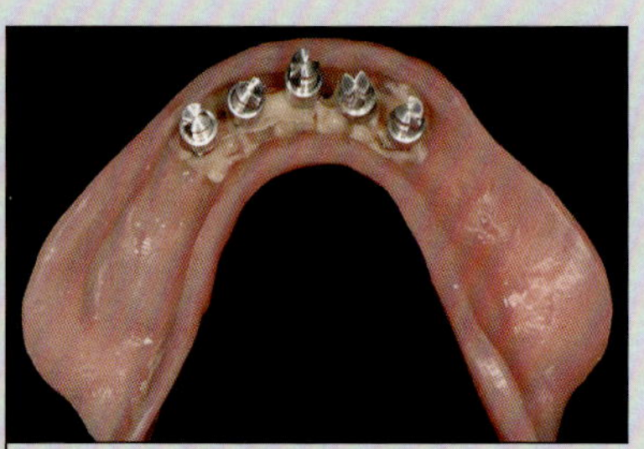

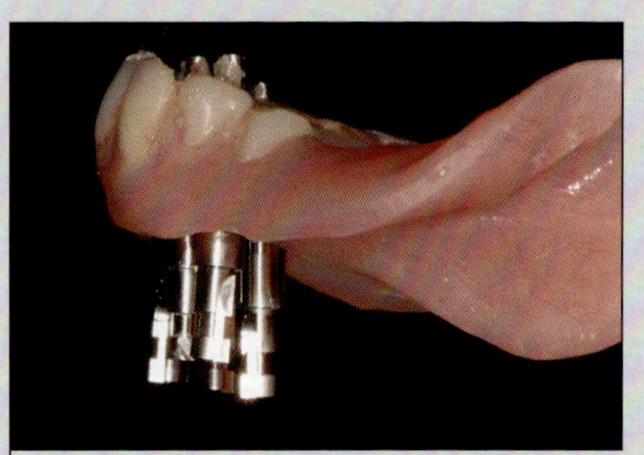

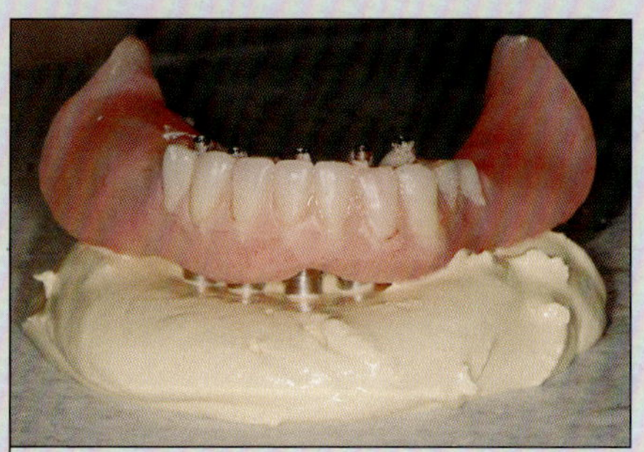

A 45-year-old white woman presented to the Oral and Maxillofacial Surgery Clinic at the University of Nebraska Medical Center for replacement of several missing teeth. The patient's medical history showed development of periodontal disease leading to loss of several teeth. Ten years earlier she received short implants in the anterior maxilla for placement of a fixed partial denture (Fig 1). After the failure of several of the implants, the patient was advised to have selected teeth removed for full-arch replacement. However, the bone in the posterior maxilla was deficient and would not sup-

port a full complement of implants. It was therefore decided to remove the mandibular anterior teeth and the remaining maxillary posterior teeth to create strategic anchorage for a full-arch rehabilitation.

Before surgery, the patient was prepared for an immediate mandibular denture with an immediate load restoration. During surgery, the nine remaining mandibular teeth were removed, and ostectomy of the apical sockets of the anterior teeth created about 15 mm of anterior restorative dimension. Five 3.75 × 15-mm Mark III implants (Nobel Biocare, Göteborg, Sweden) were placed between the mental foramina and torqued in excess of 45 Ncm. At that time, 4-mm multiunit abutments were in-

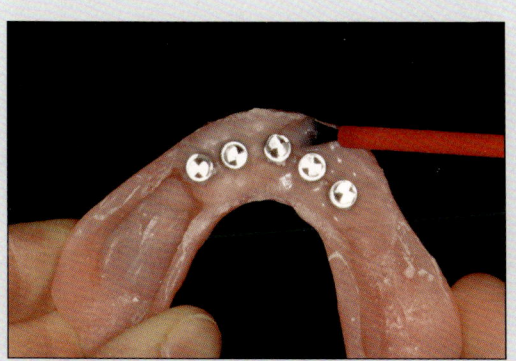

Fig 3a Incremental application of autopolymerizing acrylic resin.

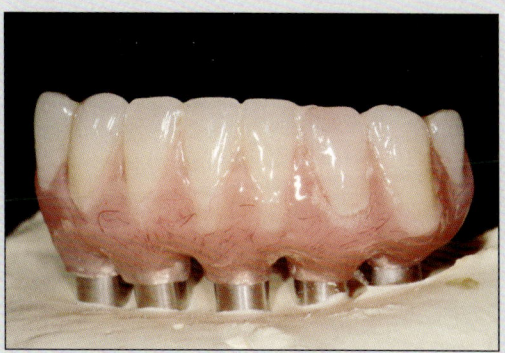

Fig 3b Fixed prothesis ready for delivery after removing flange and cantilever.

serted and torqued to 32 Ncm, and temporary titanium copings were attached to the abutments using 20-mm guide pins. Rubber dam was placed to isolate and expose the coping surfaces, and the denture was placed in the mouth and checked for proper occlusion and clearance. Once the fit was verified, a syringe filled with a soupy mixture of Jet acrylic resin (Lang Dental, Wheeling, IL) was injected into the recess, and the patient was closed to maximum intercuspation (centric occlusion) for 10 minutes.[22] Centric occlusion was used to position the mandibular prosthesis because the patient had been placed under general anesthesia. After the resin had polymerized, the prosthesis was removed, multiunit abutment replicas were attached to it, and the assembly was placed in a patty of low-expansion dental stone (Resin Rock, Whip Mix, Louisville, KY) (Figs 2a to 2e).

The posterior maxilla was isolated and prepared for placement of 40-mm zygoma implants, which were then placed in submerged fashion via closure of the mucoperiosteal flap. Immediate loading of the implants in the mandible and the use of zygoma implants in the maxilla eliminated the need for 2-stage surgery and bone grafting to the posterior maxilla, thus reducing the overall treatment time by 6 to 8 months.

The denture was carefully removed from the mouth to ensure that acrylic resin surrounded each coping. The abutments were covered with healing caps and the tissues were approximated with double-layered closure.

Laboratory and Clinical Techniques

After the dental stone was completely set, the assembly was removed, and the underside of the coping area was augmented via incremental applications of autopolymerizing acrylic resin. Care was taken to avoid the attachment surface of each coping. The assembly was then placed in a pressure pot of warm water at 25 psi for a complete dense cure. The flanges were subsequently removed, as were the posterior occlusal extensions to the second premolars. The prosthesis was designed with a scalloped underside and a convex shape to permit cleaning, particularly between the abutments (Figs 3a and 3b).

The prosthesis was delivered the next day. As it was being inserted in the patient's mouth, care was taken not to trap tissue between the coping and the abutment. All coping screws were then torqued to 15 Ncm. Complete seating was verified by direct visualization and radiographic techniques (Fig 4a). The access openings were covered with cotton and closed with Cavit (3M ESPE, St Paul, MN), although resin composite also could be used. The patient was advised to maintain a soft diet while wearing the prosthesis. The stone cast was retained for later use as a verification index during the second phase of treatment. The prosthesis was removed after 90 days. At that time each implant was percussed to confirm integration, and the soft tissue around the implant abutments was deemed superior (Fig 4b).

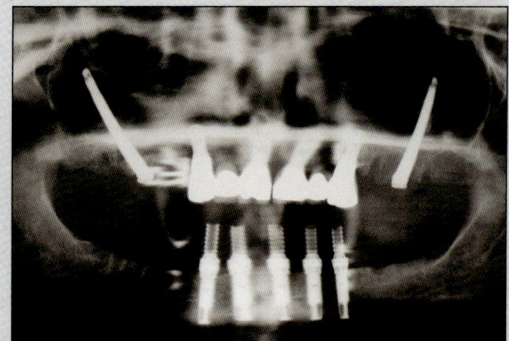

Fig 4a Panoramic radiograph depicting placement of five interforaminal implants with titanium copings using immediate restoration and two zygoma implants.

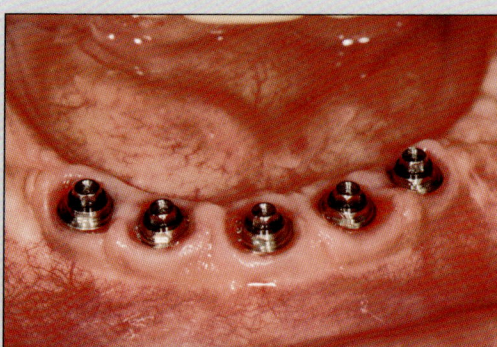

Fig 4b Abutment/soft tissue condition after removal of immediate load prosthesis.

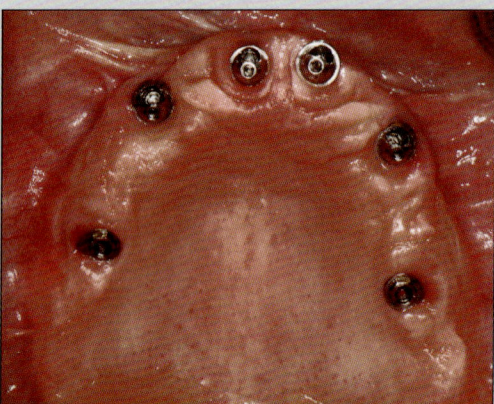

Fig 5a Maxillary view of the four standard implants with angulated abutment that had been in place for 10 years and the recently added zygoma implants.

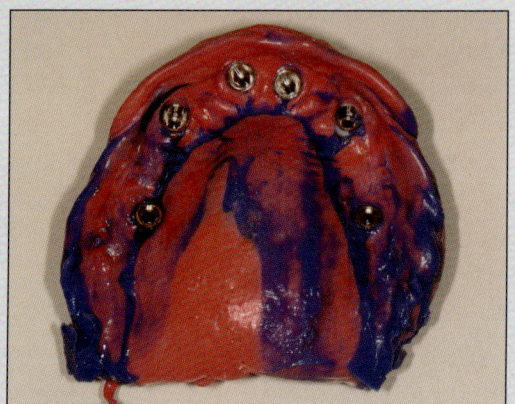

Fig 5b Open tray transfer of six implants in the maxilla.

The position of the implants in both arches was transferred to the laboratory by means of standard and custom impression trays using the open tray (ie, pick-up) technique (Figs 5a and 5b). In the laboratory, a verification pattern of the maxillary denture was made with acrylic resin (Fix 6a), sectioned, and then reassembled in the mouth with autopolymerizing acrylic resin (GC America, Alsip, IL). When the pattern was removed from the mouth, abutment replicas were attached to it, and the entire assembly was placed in low-expansion dental stone (Resin Rock) to prepare laboratory verification indices (Figs 6b and 6c) to use for reference in framework scanning and fabrication.

The acrylic resin verification pattern was used to fabricate a wax try-in of the prosthetic framework with set denture teeth (Figs 7a to 7c). Esthetics and phonetics were verified, and the linguoalveolar seal was evaluated. Occlusion was verified intraorally via comparison with the articulator registration (Figs 7d to 7f).

The waxup and verification indices were returned to the laboratory, and the entire screw-retained tooth setup was duplicated with low-shrinkage autopolymerizing acrylic pattern resin (GC America). A silicone-based material (Sil-Tech, Ivoclar-Vivadent, Amherst, NY) for the matrix was then used as a reference for cutback (Figs 8a and 8b). After cut-

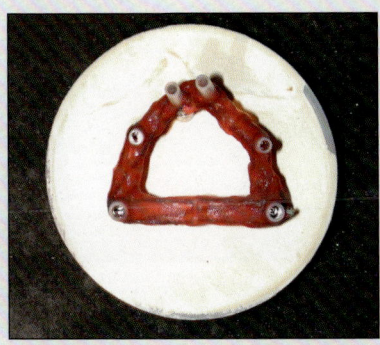

Fig 6a Implant verification assembly created after joining the copings in mouth and attaching implant/abutment replicas immersed in low-expansion dental stone.

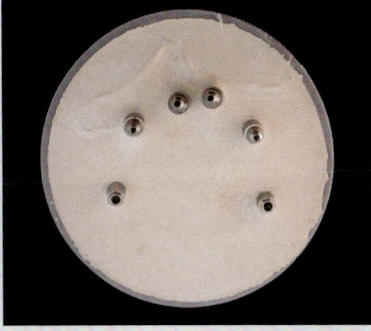

Fig 6b Maxillary implant verification index.

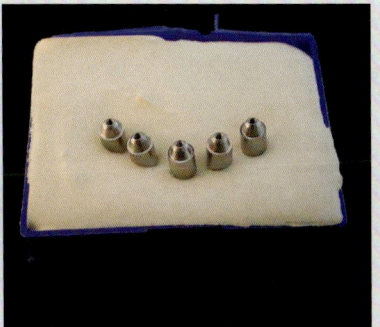

Fig 6c Mandibular implant verification index.

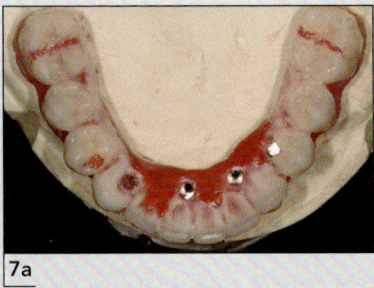

7a

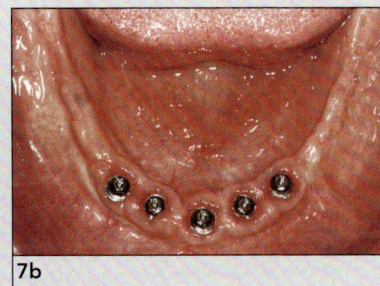

7b

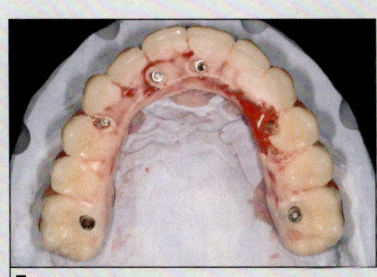

7c

Fig 7a Waxup of mandibular prosthesis supported on acrylic resin structure ready for try-in.

Fig 7b Occlusal view of five anterior mandibular implants.

Fig 7c Waxup occlusal view of maxillary implant distribution and location.

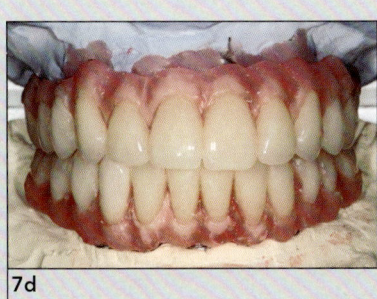

7d

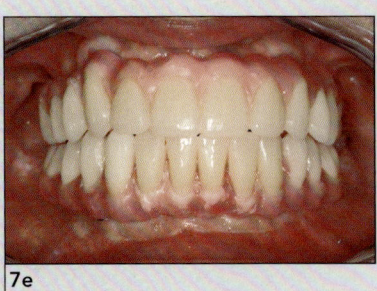

7e

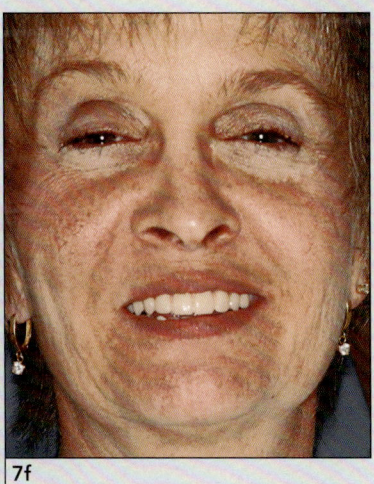

7f

Fig 7d Frontal view of waxup on articulator.

Fig 7e Esthetic try-in verified intraorally for registering centric relation.

Fig 7f Try-in of wax model for esthetic verification of facial and lip support.

back was completed to ensure adequate space for the prosthetic tooth opaquing and lamination/securing material, the screw-retained resin framework was prepared for scanning by rechecking it for passive fit with the verification index.

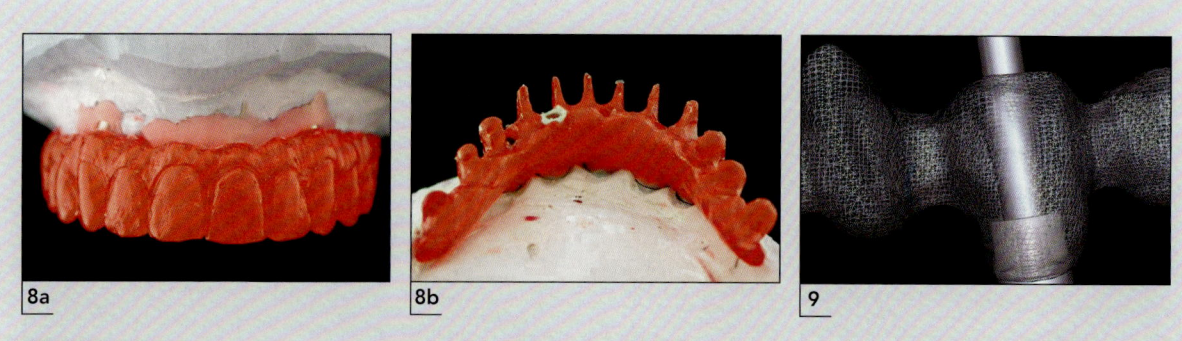

Fig 8a Full contoured acrylic resin duplicate of waxup.

Fig 8b Occlusal view of maxillary waxup indicating excellent placement of implants. Cutback of full contoured acrylic resin duplicate to make framework for scanning.

Fig 9 Point cloud dataset obtained after scanning to determine external and internal contours.

The two scanning options for CAM-milled frameworks are to send the resin pattern with the verification indices to the production lab, or have them both scanned onsite using the Forte scanner (Nobel Biocare); in either case, the framework would be returned as with other Procera products.

For the present case, outsourcing was used: the resin frameworks and the verification indices were sent to the manufacturer, where two separate types of scanning were performed for each abutment platform interface.

The first scanning captured the data for each spatial coordinate of the centroids—x = lateral, y = sagittal, and z = vertical—by means of an extremely accurate tracing method. Either the abutment or implant platform may be used for fabrication of these restorations.

In the second scanning, a laser scanner captured the external shape of the resin framework, generating a point cloud dataset reflecting external framework contours (Fig 9). To avoid surface reflection and enhance light absorption, the resin pattern was coated with a white contrast media. This improved the overall quality of data output gathered by the laser beam. Had the Forte scanner been used, the second scanning would have been unnecessary. These two data subsets were oriented and combined in a virtual setting that resulted in a complete three-dimensional internal-external dataset of the structure.

At present, there are two material alternatives for producing screw-retained framework superstructures: commercially pure titanium grade 2 or yttrium-stabilized tetragonal zirconia polycrystals (Y-TZP zirconia) ready to be CAM-milled. The manufacturer recommends that Y-TZP zirconia frameworks be veneered with zirconia porcelain (Nobel Rondo, Nobel Biocare). Cantilevered extension the size of one molar is acceptable assuming that conventional anteroposterior spread, vertical height, bone quality, and implant stability are achieved.

The new scanning alternatives can be obtained directly from the manufacturer by capturing both resin framework contour as well as measuring the spatial implant/abutment position with an advanced scanner capable of surveying and compiling multiple datasets. As mentioned above, the Procera software calculates correct data compilation, finally generating a three-dimensional virtual image of the screw-retained implant framework (Figs 10a and 10b). The three-dimensional file is sent for CAM manufacturing, obtaining a completely homogeneous, stress-free milled framework in commercially pure titanium.

Incorrect fit between the prosthesis and the implant/abutment generates a dynamic preload on the bone, contributing to an overload situation with potential loss of the implants. Extrapolation of extremely accurate x-, y-, and z-dimension im-

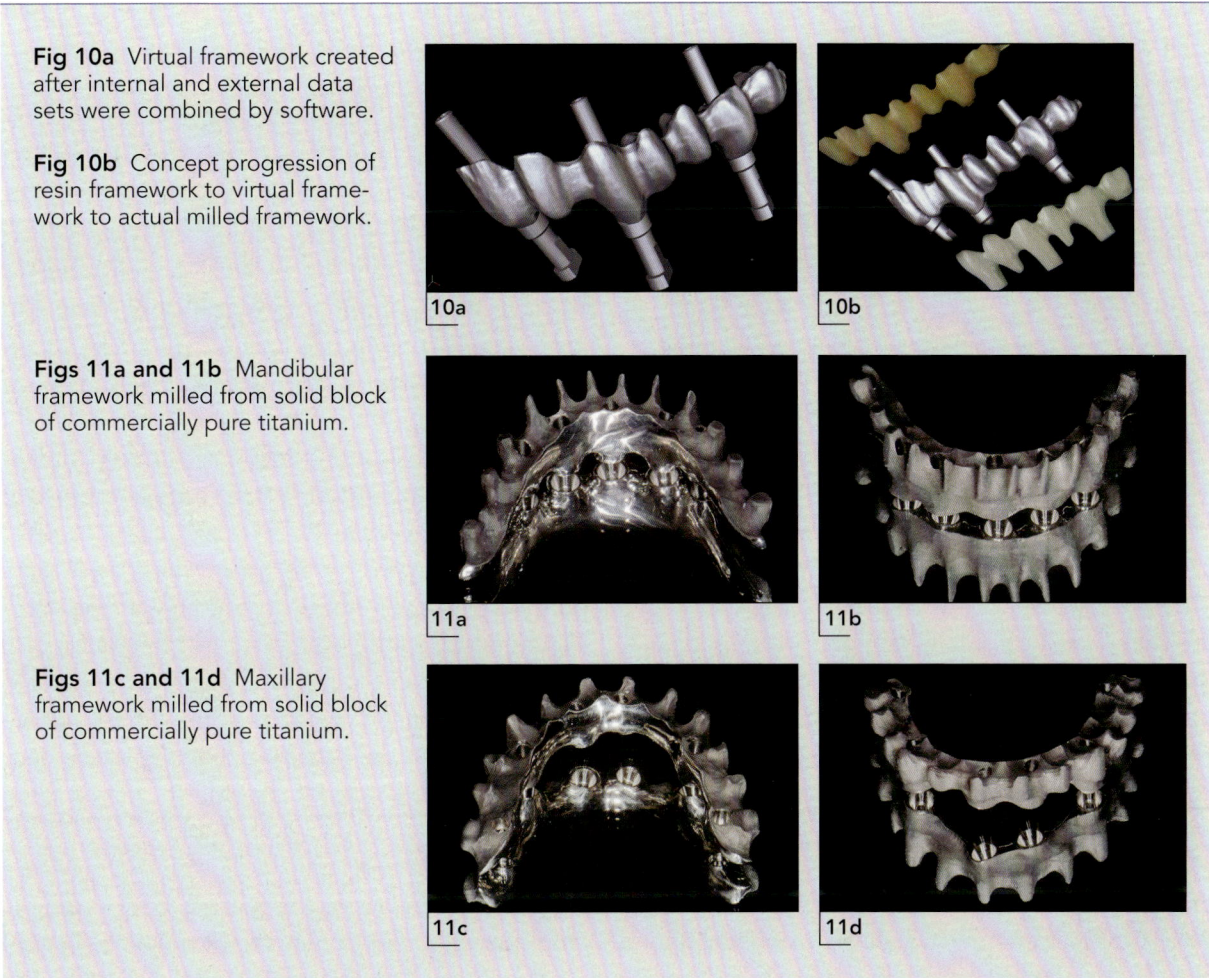

Fig 10a Virtual framework created after internal and external data sets were combined by software.

Fig 10b Concept progression of resin framework to virtual framework to actual milled framework.

Figs 11a and 11b Mandibular framework milled from solid block of commercially pure titanium.

Figs 11c and 11d Maxillary framework milled from solid block of commercially pure titanium.

plant/abutment position measurements results in an extraordinarily well-fitting framework within 15 μm, resulting in minimal or no strain transferred to the bone.

Appropriate considerations for any cross-sectional framework design within the confines of the total intraoral space and predetermined tooth setup are of imperative concern. Cross-sectional design has been tested, and metal undersides with either an L- or U-shaped configuration are most resistant to deformation.[23] Therefore, in order to achieve esthetic results and provide sufficient space for veneering material while maximizing the cross-sectional framework volume and avoiding buccolingual prosthesis bulkiness, the hybrid design of a metal underside may prevail over so-called wrap-around bar designs (Figs 11a to 11d).

Both lingual and intaglio prosthetic surfaces were finished with polished titanium, although 2 to 3 mm of acrylic resin could have been substituted. Titanium or bisphenol A-glycidylmethacryate (BIS-GMA) intaglio surfaces also provide superior hygiene maintenance since acrylic resin is prone to aging and water absorption, creating potential plaque-retentive conditions.

Most important, increased cross-sectional volume, especially in overall height, is achieved by creating retention posts that are a homogeneous part of the titanium framework. This maximizes the overall mechanical strength of the framework, supporting veneering material and allowing a retentive and resistant form. Designs of reinforced acrylic pontics have been successful in many patients over long periods of observation.[24]

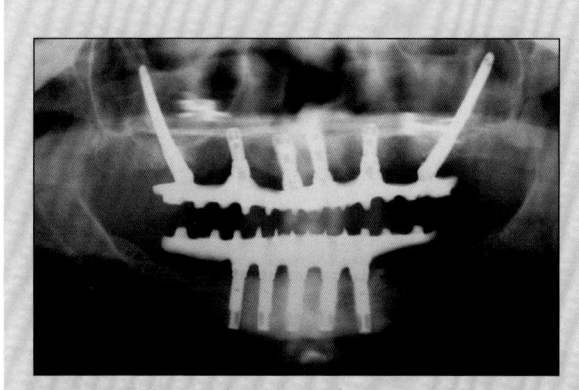

Fig 12 Radiograph taken at framework try-in to verify seating.

The frameworks for both arches were tried in to determine fit, which was verified via a panoramic radiograph for complete seating. Soft tissues in the area of the zygoma implants slightly impeded framework placement as direct-to-implant connections were used in this area (Fig 12).

The frameworks were returned to the laboratory for lamination with resin composite and attachment of the prosthetic teeth. Use of polymethyl methacrylate was debated due to the inherent acrylic-resin–metal microgap, water absorption, and general esthetic deterioration. To address these negative aspects, the prostheses were processed in accordance with a technique that has been used by one of this article's authors for most CAD/CAM titanium frameworks since 1992. It has been well documented that in combination with air abrasion, the silica-coated metal surface increases surface wettability and consistently enhances bond strength, especially in the case of titanium.[25–27]

In this case, the Rocatec technique (3M ESPE) was used to develop thermal energy by accelerating the 110-μm alumina particles against the metal surface. The energy created is sufficient to melt the quartz, smearing each silica particle onto the metal surface. Next, traditional polymethyl methacrylate acrylic (PMMA) resin-based pink and dentin opaque was applied onto the titanium surface (Ivocron SR, I7 customized shades of pink, Crown and Bridge; Ivoclar-Vivadent), eliminating the metal-resin gap. The prosthesis was veneered using several shades of pink and dentin material in a reverse porcelain buildup technique, followed by autopolymerization processes conducted under controlled temperatures that were increased to minimize undesirable behaviors of the PMMA resin.

The connector material between the PMMA resin and the final resin composite layer is then used to cover only the gingival, lingual, and intaglio surfaces of the prosthesis. Application of an acrylic resin primer (Dentacolor Connector, Heraeus Kulzer, Armonk, NY) provides transitional activation layers between the PMMA resin and BIS-GMA resin composite that have a very similar pattern of activation since the reactive methacrylate groups are similar.[28]

The restorations were finished in the usual fashion with fastened polishing protectors, and were disinfected prior to insertion (Figs 13a to 13g).

A trial placement of both restorations was first verified radiographically, and the clinical refinements included occlusal correction and attainment of cleansable areas with floss (Figs 14a to 14c). After attainment of desired occlusion and verification of the cleansable areas, closure of the access openings was accomplished with cotton pellets and flowable resin composite (Revolution, Sybron Dental Specialties, Newport Beach, CA) (Figs 15a and 15b).

CONCLUSION

This technique is a compilation of the latest methods of computerized manufacturing of titanium frameworks that may improve the accuracy of multiple-implant screw-retained restorations. The ease of obtaining a properly fitting framework makes this technique easier than conventional cast frameworks or those made passively by resin luting techniques. It may serve as the best means to achieve optimal fit and maximum anchorage for restorations using multiple dental implants. The use of immediate loading in the anterior mandible has become an important treatment, greatly reducing the time and difficulty associated with traditional

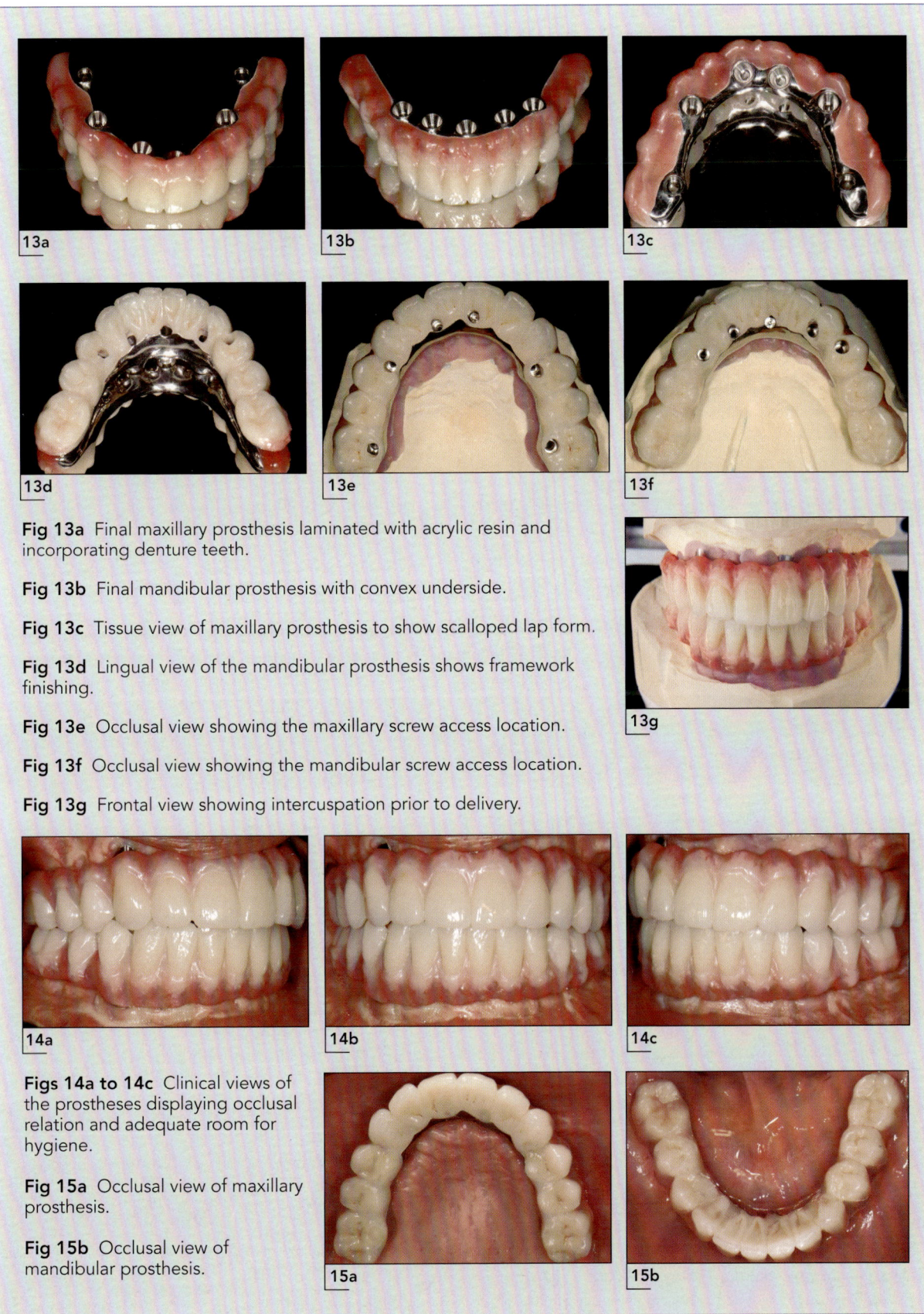

Fig 13a Final maxillary prosthesis laminated with acrylic resin and incorporating denture teeth.

Fig 13b Final mandibular prosthesis with convex underside.

Fig 13c Tissue view of maxillary prosthesis to show scalloped lap form.

Fig 13d Lingual view of the mandibular prosthesis shows framework finishing.

Fig 13e Occlusal view showing the maxillary screw access location.

Fig 13f Occlusal view showing the mandibular screw access location.

Fig 13g Frontal view showing intercuspation prior to delivery.

Figs 14a to 14c Clinical views of the prostheses displaying occlusal relation and adequate room for hygiene.

Fig 15a Occlusal view of maxillary prosthesis.

Fig 15b Occlusal view of mandibular prosthesis.

2-stage techniques. The additional use of zygoma implants has become a reasonable alternative to sinus augmentation of the posterior maxilla, allowing a shorter treatment period and reducing the donor site morbidity often associated with bone grafts. Combinations of these technologies will propel traditional implant treatment forward, enhancing patient satisfaction by reducing treatment time and increasing the level of precision.

ACKNOWLEDGMENTS

The authors wish to acknowledge Nobel Biocare USA for its support in the fabrication of the prostheses.

REFERENCES

1. Assif D, Nissan J, Varsano I, Singer A. Accuracy of implant impression splinted techniques: Effect of splinting material. Int J Oral Maxillofac Implants 1999;14:885–888.

2. Naconecy MM, Teixeira ER, Shinkai RS, Frasca LC, Cervieri A. Evaluation of the accuracy of 3 transfer techniques for implant-supported prostheses with multiple abutments. Int J Oral Maxillofac Implants 2004;19:192–198.

3. Ortorp A, Jemt T, Back T. Photogrammetry and conventional impressions for recording implant positions: A comparative laboratory study. Clin Implant Dent Relat Res 2005;7:43–50.

4. Carr AB, Stewart RB. Full-arch implant framework casting accuracy: Preliminary in vitro observation for in vivo testing. J Prosthodont 1993;2:2–8.

5. Chang TL, Maruyama C, White SN, Son S, Caputo AA. Dimensional accuracy analysis of implant framework castings from 2 casting systems. Int J Oral Maxillofac Implants 2005;20:720–725.

6. Hellden LB, Derand T, Johansson S, Lindberg A. The CrescoTi Precision method: Description of a simplified method to fabricate titanium superstructures with passive fit to osseointegrated implants. J Prosthet Dent 1999;82:487–491.

7. Stumpel LJ 3rd, Quon SJ. Adhesive abutment cylinder luting. J Prosthet Dent 1993;69:398–400.

8. Riedy SJ, Lang BR, Lang BE. Fit of implant frameworks fabricated by different techniques. J Prosthet Dent 1997;78:596–604.

9. Hellden LB, Derand T. Description and evaluation of a simplified method to achieve passive fit between cast titanium frameworks and implants. Int J Oral Maxillofac Implants 1998;13:190–196.

10. Stumpel LJ 3rd. The adhesive-corrected implant framework. J Calif Dent Assoc 1994;22:47–50, 52–53.

11. Carr AB, Gerard DA, Larsen PE. The response of bone in primates around unloaded dental implants supporting prostheses with different levels of fit. J Prosthet Dent 1996;76:500–509.

12. Clelland NL, Papazoglou E, Carr AB, Gilat A. Comparison of strains transferred to a bone simulant among implant overdenture bars with various levels of misfit. J Prosthodont 1995;4:243–250.

13. Rasmussen EJ. Alternative prosthodontic technique for tissue-integrated prostheses. J Prosthet Dent 1987;57:198–204.

14. Tames R, McGlumphy E, El-Gendy T, Wilson R. The OSU frame: A novel approach to fabricating immediate load fixed-detachable prostheses. J Oral Maxillofac Surg 2004;62(9 Suppl 2):17–21.

15. Rocci A, Martignoni M, Gottlow J. Immediate loading in the maxilla using flapless surgery, implants placed in predetermined positions, and prefabricated provisional restorations: A retrospective 3-year clinical study. Clin Implant Dent Relat Res 2003;5 Suppl 1:29–36.

16. Salama H, Rose LF, Salama M, Betts NJ. Immediate loading of bilaterally splinted titanium root-form implants in fixed prosthodontics—A technique reexamined: Two case reports. Int J Periodontics Restorative Dent 1995;15:344–361.

17. Takahashi T, Gunne J. Fit of implant frameworks: An in vitro comparison between two fabrication techniques. J Prosthet Dent 2003;89:256–260.

18. Jemt T, Henry P, Linden B, Naert I, Weber H, Wendelhag I. Implant-supported laser-welded titanium and conventional cast frameworks in the partially edentulous jaw: A 5-year prospective multicenter study. Int J Prosthodont 2003;16:415–421.

19. Ortorp A, Jemt T, Back T, Jalevik T. Comparisons of precision of fit between cast and CNC-milled titanium implant frameworks for the edentulous mandible. Int J Prosthodont 2003;16:194–200.

20. Jemt T, Back T, Petersson A. Precision of CNC-milled titanium frameworks for implant treatment in the edentulous jaw. Int J Prosthodont 1999;12:209–215.

21. Parel SM. The single-piece milled titanium implant bridge. Dent Today 2003;22:96–99.

22. Balshi TJ, Wolfinger GJ. Teeth in a day. Implant Dent 2001;10:231–233.

23. Stewart RB, Staab GH. Cross-sectional design and fatigue durability of cantilevered sections of fixed implant-supported prostheses. J Prosthodont 1995;4:188–194.

24. Brånemark P. The Osseointegration Book: From Calvarium to Calcaneus. Chicago: Quintessence, 2005.

25. Sharp B, Morton D, Clark AE. Effectiveness of metal surface treatments in controlling microleakage of the acrylic resin-metal framework interface. J Prosthet Dent 2000;84:617–622.

26. Zitzmann NU, Marinello CP. A review of clinical and technical considerations for fixed and removable implant prostheses in the edentulous mandible. Int J Prosthodont 2002;15:65–72.

27. Watanabe I, Kurtz KS, Kabcenell JL, Okabe T. Effect of sandblasting and silicoating on bond strength of polymer-glass composite to cast titanium. J Prosthet Dent 1999;82:462–467.

28. Papazoglou E, Vasilas AI. Shear bond strengths for composite and autopolymerized acrylic resins bonded to acrylic resin denture teeth. J Prosthet Dent 1999;82:573–578.